Tai Chi Dreaming

A Scientific Study of Tai Chi for Health as Mind-Body Exercise for Health, Fitness & Wellbeing

Elva Arthy and Dr Denis Arthy

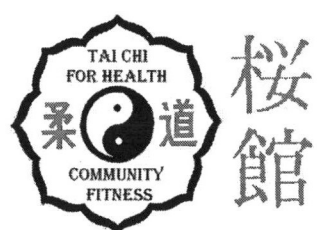

National Library of Australia

National Library of Australia
Cataloguing-in-Publication Data

Arthy, Elva, and Arthy, Denis
Tai Chi Dreaming: a scientific study of tai chi for health as mind-body exercise for health, fitness & wellbeing

Bibliography
Includes index
ISBN 978 0 646 53323 0

1. Tai Chi – Study and Teaching   2. Health I. Title.

613.7148

Published in Australia in 2010
Tai Chi for Health & Community Fitness
ABN: 73482976952
260 Bloomfield St, Cleveland QLD, 4163, Australia
Ph +61 7 3286 2779   Fax +61 7 3286 2110
Email: elvamar@bigpond.net.au
Website: www.taichiforhealth.multiply.com

First edition of this book was published in Australia in 2009 by Tai Chi for Health & Community Fitness
Under the title of Australia Dreaming: tai chi for health advanced instructor training course
ISBN 978 0 646 51095 8

Front Cover & Art Work by Gail Higgins
Gail Higgins website - www.gailhiggins.com.au
Photos and Design by Denis Arthy

Printed in Australia by Love of Books
Website: www.loveofbooks.com.au

CONTENTS

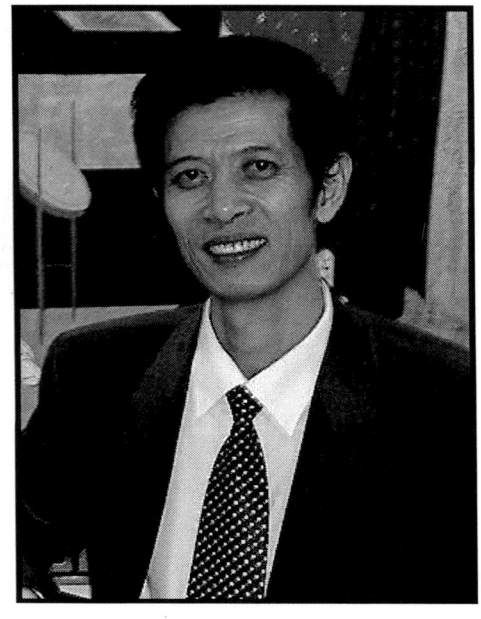

Foreword by Dr Henry Zheng

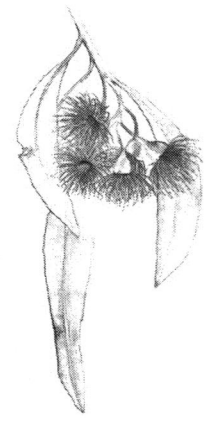

According to the World Health Organization, "physical inactivity" is identified as one of the major health risks in the modern age and is estimated to annually cause 1.9 million deaths and the estimated loss of a staggering 19 million "healthy life years". The optimistic factor here is that this particular risk can be within the control of the individual and is also considered to have reversible effects on the health and wellbeing of those who choose to become active. The policy implications and responsibilities for government are thus profound for addressing this reversibility factor. While modern technology has fundamentally changed our lifestyles, it has come at a huge cost for so many with compelling scientific evidence linking the modern epidemics such as obesity, diabetes and cardiovascular disease directly to the lack of physical activity. There are more than one billion adults worldwide who are overweight and at least 300 million who are clinically obese. Among these, about half a million people in North America and Western Europe combined will die each year from obesity-related diseases, and this is increasing. Research evidence has been mounting for the past 50 years on the efficacy of physical activity in reducing the risk of and preventing sedentary lifestyle-induced diseases. However, translating research evidence into safe, effective and sustainable practice remains a daunting task far from being achieved.

Tai Chi represents a form of exercise that has yet to be embraced and properly understood in the West for its immense healing and therapeutic value and the enormous potential for reversing the fortunes of those afflicted with the modern disease of chronic "physical inactivity". In this regard, two distinguished Australian Tai Chi experts, Elva Arthy and Dr Denis Arthy, through their publication - *Tai Chi Dreaming – A Scientific Study of Mind-Body Exercise for Health, Fitness & Wellbeing* - have made a timely and invaluable contribution to the search for and promotion of evidence-based "best practice" at the general population level to address this modern malaise of "physical inactivity". Their publication confronts the myths and misinformation which hamper the public health efforts to promote Tai Chi as an ideal exercise intervention strategy. But it is much more than this. Despite well-documented health benefits of Tai Chi, there is still considerable lack of proper understanding of the scientific value Tai Chi for health and an even puzzling disregard for the urgent need to engage with a modern "duty-of-care" approach to the teaching Tai Chi for health where "one-size" clearly does not, and should not fit all.

Drawing on their considerable knowledge and expertise in teaching Tai Chi for community health over many years, with their *Tai Chi Dreaming* Elva and Denis offer a scientific approach to the learning, practicing and teaching of Tai Chi for Health. From modern teaching knowledge & skills, to the essential knowledge of the human body, to a comprehensive knowledge of tai Chi, to a modern duty of care and other legal and ethical responsibilities, to an in-depth study of 73 Sun style tai chi, to the beautiful 15 form Qigong set *Australia Dreaming* and to advanced levels of instructor training, *Tai Chi Dreaming* fills a knowledge gap in the quest for effective learning and teaching of Tai Chi for health. It is an excellent textbook for all students and tai chi teachers to acquire an essential Tai Chi knowledge and an invaluable training manual for advanced level Tai Chi Instructors to enhance their career development. To maintain good health and fitness is a "Dreaming" we all have irrespective of age, gender or race. *Tai Chi Dreaming* symbolises our common aspiration for health and fitness and offers an ideal and modern way for realising our dream for a better, happier, and healthier life for us all.

Henry Zheng PhD
Exercise Science Researcher
National Accreditation Course Presenter
Exercise Medicine Australia, Castlereagh St, Sydney, Australia

Foreword by
Dr Bob McBrien

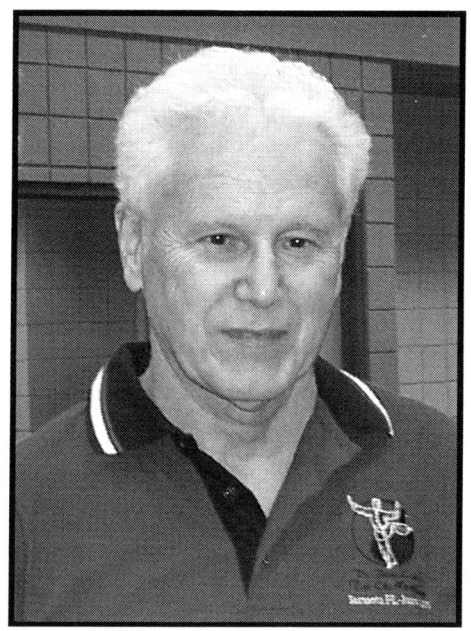

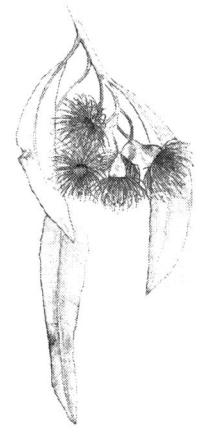

During the summer of 2007, at a Tai Chi for Health Workshop on a beautiful college campus in Massachusetts, I first learned about *Australia Dreaming* by the Arthys. With a unique combination of scholarly research, an extensive understanding of Tai Chi as a health-promoting exercise based on personal study, training with masters of tai chi chuan and martial arts and years of teaching martial arts and tai chi, the authors offer a comprehensive textbook for instructors seeking to advance their understanding of modern Tai Chi for Health programs.

In presenting their advanced training course for instructors of Tai Chi for Health classes, the authors provide six units of study which offer knowledge and skills to prepare teachers who will make a difference in the lives of students from all walks of life. A key goal is that *Australia Dreaming* will especially benefit the least advantaged in society. They are to be applauded for their concern for the disadvantaged.

Studying the units on: teaching principles and methods; the human body and exercise safety concerns; a modern framework for understanding how tai chi promotes health; important information about duty of care and risk management; a study of the Sun 73 Form; and the requirements for achieving accreditation as an advanced instructor, many readers will recognize that here is a curriculum that resembles a university course of study. A scan of the bibliography will confirm the level of scholarly effort here.

Beyond the "academic" qualities of this text, the creative and sensitive fusion of Australian images and Tai Chi movements" found in Elva Arthy's Australia Dreaming Qigong places the text in its own category. With a goal for honoring the indigenous people of Australia, the special set of Sun style forms seek to evoke images of the Australian environment. The beautiful art of Gail Higgins ensures us that the images will be easily recognized by indigenous and non-indigenous Australians, just as it will be admired by students of tai chi for health around the world. Not only does this special program honor Australia's first people and celebrate the global nature of tai chi for health programs, it offers readers a gift of experiencing Australia's natural beauty. It brought me strong feelings of peace within.

The ancient saying, "When the student is ready, the teacher will appear," is appropriate here. As a student and instructor of Tai Chi for Health, trained in Dr. Paul Lam's system of special programs, I am a ready student. With the Australia Dreaming text I realize that two fine teachers have appeared. I am delighted to have this resource to guide me as I grow in my new "healing profession." I believe this work will benefit all those who wish to make a difference.

Bob McBrien PhD
Licensed Clinical Professional Counselor
Diplomate in Adlerian Psychology
Fellow of the American Institute of Stress
Authorized Master Trainer: Tai Chi for Arthritis
Salisbury, Maryland, USA

Elva Arthy - Author

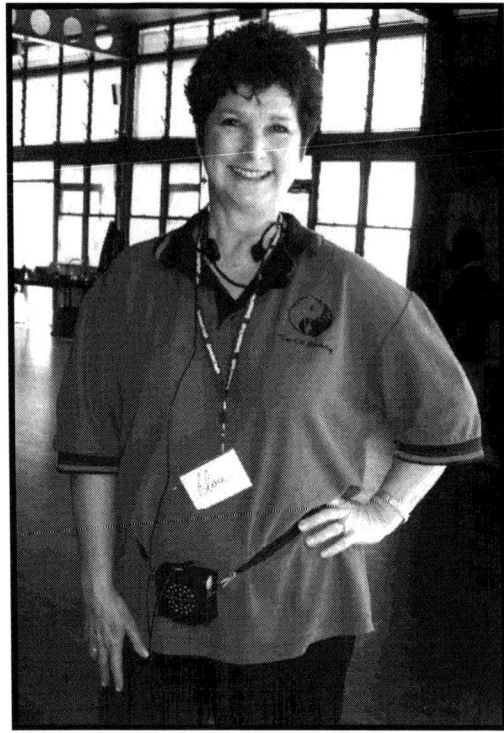

Elva has been a teacher of movement, dance and exercise for forty nine years. At aged 15, she won a scholarship to the Queensland Opera Company performing in *Carmen* and *The Magic Flute* while studying singing, movement, Laban-Carpenter and the Alexander Technique. She achieved her Advanced certificate with the Royal Academy of Dancing (London) – classical ballet - while studying various forms of Folk dance – Ukraine, Scottish, Irish, Italian, Hungarian – as well as contemporary, modern, jazz and tap. She began her teaching apprenticeship aged 13 with Jill Cadden in Brisbane. She choreographed dances for and performed in various charity performances including the Lord Mayor's "Christmas in Storyland" at the Brisbane City Hall for many years.

She was later a professional dancer with JC Williamsons performing in *Half a Sixpence* which toured Australia with Mark McManus. Upon returning to Brisbane, she worked as a dance teacher, choreographer and performance coach for examination students. Since 1982, she has been a community based Fitness Instructor pioneering the specialised field of Gentle Exercise for older adults as an accredited Fitness Trainer with Fitness Australia. She now runs her own training and consulting school – *Tai Chi for Health & Community Fitness,* which is geared towards the health and fitness industries as well as the community and corporate areas.

As a Master Trainer for Dr Paul Lam's Tai Chi for Health programs, she has organised over 50 Tai Chi for Health (TCH) workshops in Queensland and trained over 650 Tai Chi for Health Instructors/Leaders since 2002. She has assisted Dr Paul Lam in the training of new Master Trainers of the Tai Chi for Arthritis (TCA) Instructor/ Leader Training program in Sydney and Korea. As Master Trainer, she has conducted and taught in numerous TCA Instructor Training Courses in Australia, New Zealand, USA and Korea. In addition, she has taught Sun Style Tai Chi at an advanced level in Australia and the USA.

Elva holds a Bachelor of Arts University of Qld with specialist studies in Human Movement, Anthropology & Psychology. At the First International Tai Chi for Health Conference held in Seoul, Korea in 2006, Elva presented a paper co-authored with her husband Denis, on "How to Teach Tai Chi for Health Effectively". She is the Tai Chi Instructor and presenter on the DVD titled *INSPIRE - Tai Chi and Yoga for Adults with Bleeding Disorders* produced by Haemophilia Foundation Australia and distributed in Australia and overseas including Europe, India, USA, UK and Canada released in April 2005. Since 1999, she has attended numerous workshops in Australia, China and the USA where her Tai Chi and Qigong studies include – Yang 42, Yang 24, Chen 36, Sun 73 and Mulan Qigong. She is accredited with Alice Liping Yuan's Exercise Medicine's Tai Chi for Health and Falls Injury and Prevention Program and Mulan Qiong and is a registered Tai Chi Instructor with Sakurakan-QUBBA with her school *Tai Chi for Health & Community Fitness.*

Through her school, Elva has pioneered with Denis the Tai Chi for Health Advanced Instructor Training course to provide an extension for teaching expertise and alternative pathway for TCA Leaders and others at an advanced level who do not wish to pursue the traditional Kung Fu martial arts instructor training. She is the author of *Raging Ageing Gentle Exercise Manual for Design and Delivery,* a manual used as a resource for health and fitness professionals and carers of older adults. The manual is also a suitable and effective program for other persons in the community who have some health limitations or who may simply wish to exercise more gently. This is a set text in the training of community-based carers. In recognition of Elva's significant contribution over twenty five years in the Redlands to providing community based gentle exercise activities and supporting numerous charity activities and community events, Elva was awarded the *Most Outstanding Woman Making a Difference 2007* at the "Women Making a Difference Awards" hosted by the Redlands Women Information Network (RWIN) in Queensland, Australia: "*As a teacher, Elva's personal qualities are always inspirational. She creates a friendly and happy atmosphere in her classes, using fun music and leading by example. She gives individual attention to all participants and encourages her students to get the technique correct rather than leaving them to continue to make the same mistakes*". Elva's life interests include teaching, travel, piano, cooking and orchids.

Dr Denis Arthy - Author

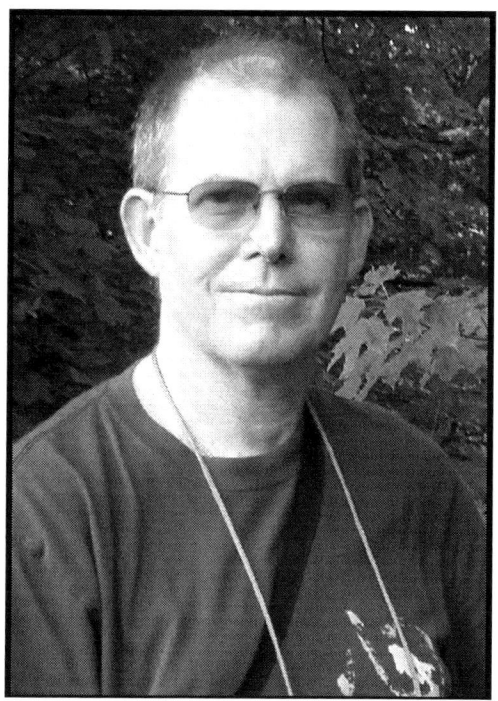

Denis has been involved with the "gentle" or "yielding" martial arts since the early 1960s, firstly in Judo and Jujitsu with Geoff Geurts (the founder of Sakurakan-QUBBA) as his first teacher, and in later years in a traditional "hard-soft" style of Okinawan Karate-do. When Denis was 48 years of age, his health was such that he had to give up playing tennis due to a combination of chronic neck and shoulder injuries and the ill effects of a sedentary lifestyle, having spent the previous fifteen years researching and studying as a part-time student while working full time as a Student Counsellor at the Queensland University of Technology (QUT). He had formed the idea, like so many men, that it was time to retire from challenging forms of exercise and was looking to take up lawn bowls. Then he met Shihan John Dalmedo and Goju Ryu Karate-do.

After eight years of solid mental and physical training in the martial arts, eight hours formal class instruction a week, Denis completed a grading in Sydney held by Grandmaster (10th Dan) Kazuo Saito and was awarded his 3rd Dan and his Instructor's certificate in Karate-Do registered in Japan. During this time, Denis obtained his 1st Dan black belt in Judo and 1st Kyu in Jujitsu with Shihan Bill Cadoo and trained with Sifu Keith McGregor in traditional Yang style of Kung Fu Tai Chi Chuan through Sakurakan-QUBBA. Denis is a registered Martial Arts Instructor and Tai Chi Instructor with that organisation.

Seven years ago, Denis began to explore the commonalities of "internal" or "yielding" Asian martial arts styles and formed his own part-time school called *Gentle Arts of Self Defence*. He now teaches Martial Arts for Health, Tai Chi for Relaxation and Karate-Do for self defence incorporating techniques and principles from Judo, Jujitsu and Kung Fu Tai Chi Chuan into a practical self-defence curriculum.

Since the year 2000, Denis attended numerous Tai Chi for Health workshops in Australia, China and the USA where his Tai Chi for Health and Qigong studies include – 24 Form Mulan Quan Bare Hands, 8 Form Mulan Qigong, Chen 36, Yang 42, Sun 73 and Yang 24. He is also an accredited and certified Tai Chi Instructor with Alice Liping Yuan's Tai Chi for Health & Falls and Injury Prevention program (Exercise Medicine Australia) and Dr Paul Lam's Tai Chi for Arthritis program (Tai Chi Productions). Over the years, Denis has assisted his wife Elva in her Tai Chi for Health activities and they both worked together in researching, writing and creating the Tai Chi for Health Advanced Instructor Training course. Denis also began to research the origins of a modern and scientific approach to health, exercise and movement in the Asian martial arts through the genius of Professor Jigoro Kano as the founder of Judo and the genius of Master Sun Lutang the creator of Sun Style Tai Chi Chuan. At *The First International Conference for Tai Chi for Health* held in Seoul, Korea in December 2006, Denis presented a paper titled *The Genius of Sun Lutang: Concepts and Principles of Tai Chi for Health* and co-authored another paper titled *Text and Context of How to Teach Tai Chi for Health Effectively* with his wife Elva which she presented. Also at that conference, he was involved in teaching in the advanced workshop *Explore the Depth of Tai Chi for Arthritis* for Dr Lam's Master Trainers and for other advanced Tai Chi for Health students.

Denis worked for over twenty years at QUT as a Student Counsellor during which time he assisted thousands of Australian, overseas and migrant students with their careers, study, English language skills, financial and personal problems and issues. At the same time as a part time student himself he completed an Honours Bachelor of Arts degree (BA Hons) in the Faculties of Humanities, a Masters of Science degree (MSc) in the Faculty of Science and a Doctor of Philosophy (PhD) in the Faculty of Arts at Griffith University and published numerous articles in national and international professional journals. During this time Denis was actively involved as an executive member of the Queensland Ethnic Broadcasting Association Inc contributing to the successful application for a community based radio licence in Brisbane (now 4EB) in the early years of multiculturalism in Australia. Prior to working at QUT, he qualified with Honours as an accountant with CPA Australia and is now working full time for the Australian government in the Department of the Treasury. His life interests include meeting people from different cultures, studying languages, global politics, anthropological and historical studies in the fields of education, government and the Asian martial arts.

Gail Higgins – Wild Life Artist

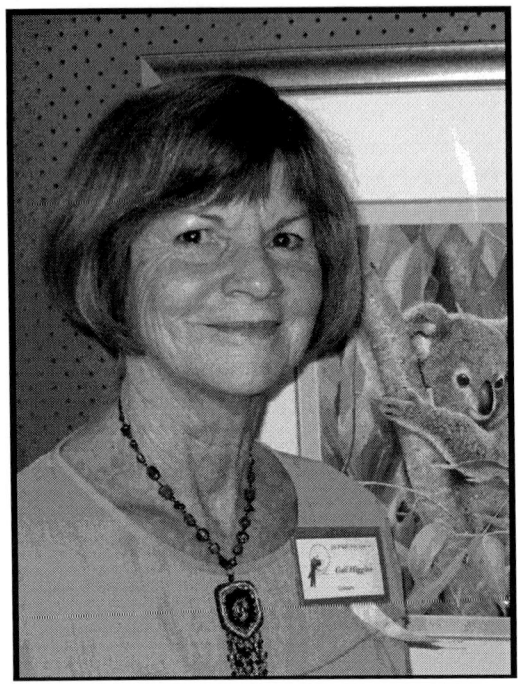

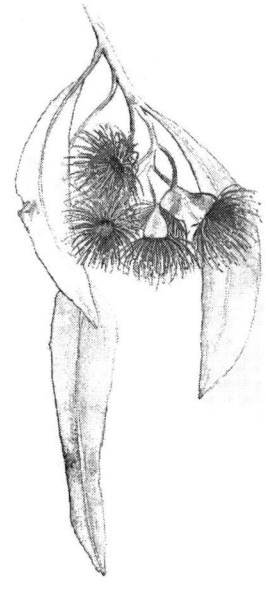

After commencing art lessons in 1995 Gail became increasingly interested in painting Australia's beautiful native flora and fauna and now devotes more and more of her time to painting birds and the research that involves.

A winner of many major awards, including Silver Medallist at the International Wildlife Art Society 2004 exhibition in Bristol, UK , The Pastel Acquisitive Award at Pine Rivers Art Awards 2006, major award winner at Courier Mail Art Show 2005, Gail has also won many major awards at QWASI exhibitions. She was invited to by Australia Zoo to create awareness of native flora and fauna found in the Steve Irwin Wildlife Reserve, Cape York with a solo exhibition on Steve Irwin Day, November 2008

She has had several articles published in *Australian Artist* and *Australian Birdkeeper* magazines. In 2005, with Sandra Temple, she produced *Aussie Friends in our own backyard*, an art and education book for children, based on images of their wildlife paintings.

After completing a Cert IV in Assessment and Workplace Training, in 2003 Gail commenced her own art classes and in 2007 moved into her teaching studio in Wynnum.   She is now sought after to conduct workshops in pastel - her favourite medium because of the vibrancy and the tactile nature of pastels. This year her workshops will be held at Pine Rivers, Boonah, Kenilworth and Kingfisher Bay Resort during Birdweek.

In 2006 she was awarded Master Pastellist status with the Pastel Society of Australia.   She was accepted as an exhibiting member of the Queensland Wildlife Artists Society in 1997 and is currently Secretary, a position she has held for many years. She is a member of the *Nature in the Raw* group of wildlife artists and the Old Schoolhouse Gallery in Cleveland where her work can be found.

She is motivated by the belief that wildlife art is not only about the art, but also about the environment in which we live -- wildlife artists can do much to call attention to the plight of our beautiful and disappearing wildlife through artistic endeavour.

When Gail is asked why she paints wildlife particularly, she says that she finds it difficult to explain except to say that she cannot help herself – She is never as happy as when she is painting birds.   There is a type of compulsion in her, she says, to hold a pastel or brush to try to capture on paper the beauty and unique characteristics of birds.

She has the hope that her paintings will encourage others to give thought to wildlife and to the environment, and to believe that the natural world is precious and worth preserving.

**Graduates of 2007-09
Tai Chi for Health Advanced
Instructor Training Course**

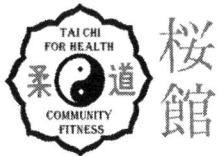 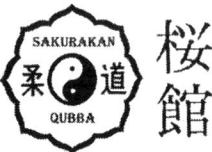

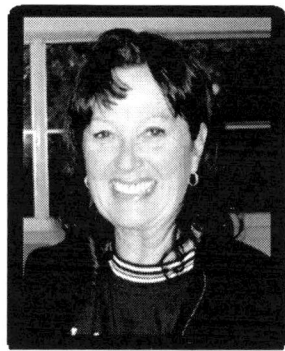
Cheryl Shirvington

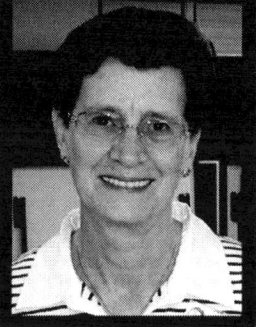
Jan Davis

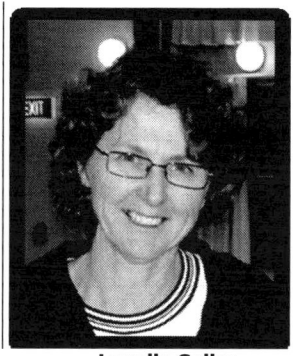
Lynelle Seiler

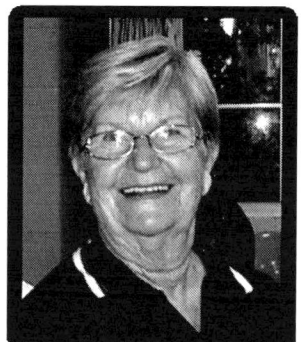
Maureen Lee

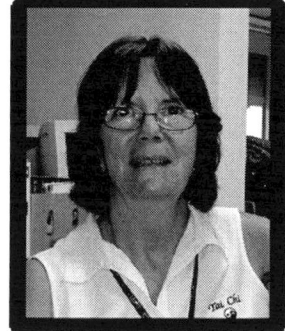
Ann Davis

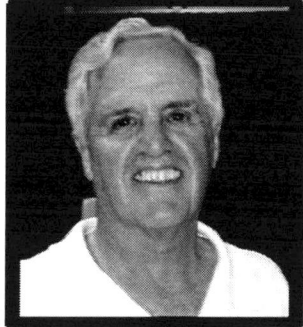
Leon Davis

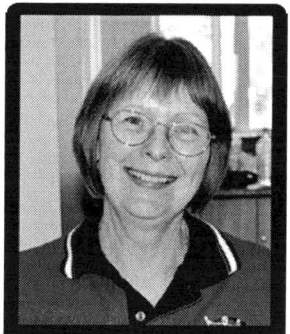
Kathryn Baker

Workshops Participants 1st Workshop July 2007

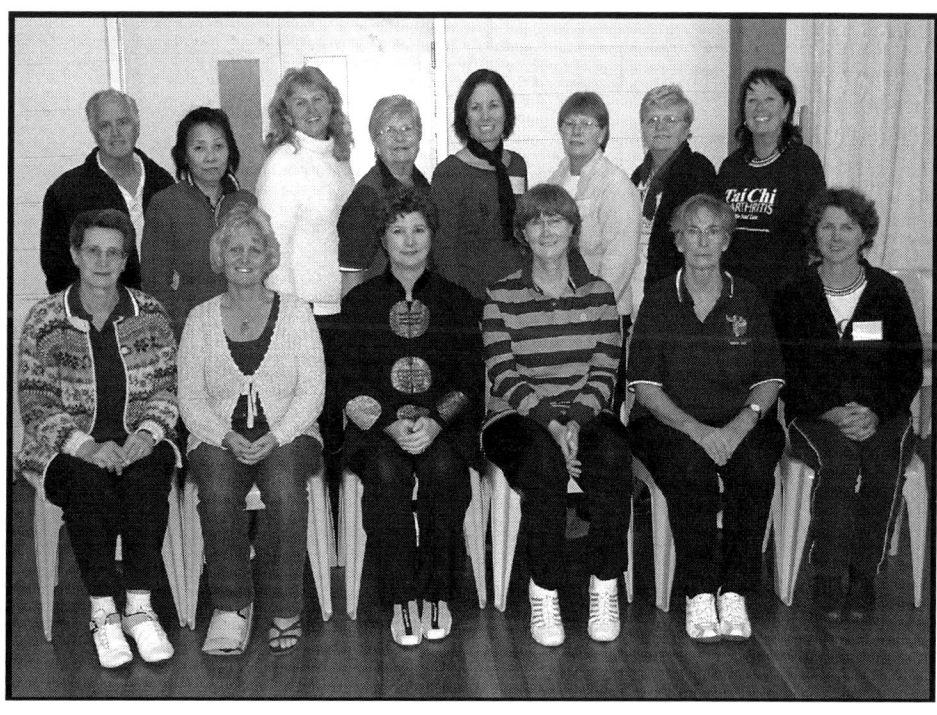

Graduates of 2007-09
Tai Chi for Health Advanced Instructor Training Course

When I first started teaching *Tai Chi [TCA program], it became very clear to me very quickly that I didn't know enough. I needed to know more about everything concerned about teaching, but I couldn't find any course that suited my needs. Then I heard that Elva and Denis were offering a new Advanced Instructor Training course over a 12 month period. Lucky me, being isolated in rural New South Wales, I jumped at the opportunity. Best thing I ever did! This course is brimming with information, teaching methods, history of Tai Chi, seminars, discussion groups, teaching practice, legal obligations, practicals, assignments and lots of Duty of Care and safety. All of this is covered in detail in the workshop manuals and at the workshops. I could not have wished for anything better in all areas. ... This is an exciting course, I recommend it to everyone who is already teaching or wishes to teach Tai Chi for Health. Your class will be interesting, informative and above all – Safe.* **Cheryl Shirvington**

I am excited *about your Tai Chi for Health Advanced Instructor Training book and I am very happy to support you. As a fifth Dan in Judo, as a Level 2 Coach and Judo Instructor accredited with the Australian Sports Commission and as having been awarded the Order of Australia medal and the Australian Sports Medal, I retired from active participation in Judo in early 2000 and began as a student with traditional Yang Style Tai Chi. Judo had been my life for forty three years, in one sport, with a lot of great memories, it was my life. Within a few years, I attended my first Tai Chi for Health Leader course in 2003 and began teaching the Tai Chi for Arthritis program. I now enjoy my Tai Chi, I love teaching and I am very particular that I teach Tai Chi in a traditional and Safe way. The Tai Chi for Health Advanced Instructor Training Course has helped me to obtain this goal. I believe there is a real need for this course in the Tai Chi community for the serious teachers wanting to teach competently and safely.* **Janice Davis**

From the very first Advanced Instructors' Workshop, *taken over twelve months, it was evident there was a high standard and the more I learned the more I realised there was so much more to learn. The twelve months Course was exciting as I enjoyed the learning, feeling my ability to teach and my confidence growing in leaps and bounds. In this Course there was not a subject uncovered in the workshops and assignments, with discussions, lots of teaching and performance practice. The quality of Tai Chi for both my students and my own has vastly improved which I believe is a huge benefit to my students' wellbeing and quality of life. As a result, since completing the Advanced Instructor Training course, the classes have taken on a new dimension with numbers continuing to grow, enhancing their interest in Tai Chi as a health art.* **Maureen Lee**

I am a Fitness Instructor *who initially discovered Tai Chi for Arthritis (TCA) program and loved it and its benefits. I teach in rural Queensland and hence I don't have opportunities to go to a variety classes to broaden my skills and base of knowledge of healthy activity options. The Tai Chi for Health (TCH) Advanced Instructor Training course was a great chance for me to do that. TCH firstly was a lot of fun and secondly gave me a depth of knowledge and skills to strengthen my teaching, while giving me a chance as well to learn something for my own satisfaction. I have copious valuable notes in the manuals to refer to as the need arises and I feel well placed in the "safety of clients" as a result of the course. I know I am a better teacher of TCA/TCH having completed the course.* **Lynelle Seiler**

After completing the Advanced Instructor training course, *my level of teaching students has greatly improved. I feel my communication with my students has developed considerably and I am more able to help students to move their body gently to increase strength, flexibility and co-ordinate breathing with movement in a safe and positive manner. I now have a clear understanding about legal matters and ethics and I am continually aware of safety issues with my students. I have always enjoyed teaching Tai Chi but now I am more considerate and understand that each person is different. I am much more open to how they do their Tai Chi, how they can modify and feel happy about themselves.* **Leon Davis**

Before the Advanced Instructor Training course, *I used to only teach the movements without any understanding of so many things. But now the course has given me much more confidence in teaching and communicating with my students. I have increased my knowledge of the concept of co-ordination of mind and body and actually how to teach that. Also I am more aware of posture and alignment of joints and now have a much better understanding about breathing and energy flow. I have tuned into the physical barriers some of my students have and I can now see the pain signals. Teaching has become more meaningful for me and I feel much satisfaction in guiding them to find their own Tai Chi.* **Ann Davis**

Attending the workshops with Elva and Denis *gives me the lift I need to continue with my Tai Chi. Learning, practicing and catching up with the other students and both Elva and Denis is a rewarding experience. All I learn I pass onto my students and between us we find a deeper and enriching understanding of our Tai Chi.* **Kathryn Baker**

Preface - Tai Chi Dreaming

The first edition of our book was overwhelming in the support generously given by so many in the appreciation and value of our publication. In looking to a second edition, we examined the impact of the previous title - *Australia Dreaming* - in the international arena and the inherent cultural and geographic limits which such a title might constrain the general reader in wanting to explore the central feature of our *Tai Chi Dreaming*. And this, we believe, is that the "magic" and "miracle" of a Tai Chi for Health can be readily understood scientifically as a powerful mind-body exercise capable of making a significant difference to wide range of people in regard to their health, fitness and wellbeing.

By changing the title of our book, we effectively created a more accurate reflection of the content and the intention of *Tai Chi Dreaming* as being about MAKING A DIFFERENCE. In this second edition, we have included a new Foreword written by Dr Henry Zheng from *Exercise Medicine Australia*, an organisation with the Tai Chi Master Alice Liping Yuan as the Principal Instructor dedicated to teaching, and promoting the "magic" and "beauty" of Tai Chi for Health through a modern scientific framework of evidence based research and reasoning. The friendship, enthusiasm and support of our book from Alice and Henry is indeed most valued as is also from Dr Bob McBrien who has written the Foreword to the first edition.

Tai Chi Dreaming is a valuable resource for all involved in teaching and learning Tai Chi for Health. As the language of Tai Chi for the beginning student can be daunting, the book aims to de-mystify and empower the student to understand the generative power of yin-yang theory in relation to a "safe, secular and scientific" and modern approach to exercise, health and well-being. As a teaching resource, the focus is on learning to teach Tai Chi for Health as a safe and effective form of exercise using modern teaching techniques in accordance with evidence based, secular and scientific reasoning and a curriculum graded from beginners to advanced levels of expertise. The idea of a curriculum is not about grading the Tai Chi student who may never have any interest in teaching, but about developing levels of expertise and competence for teaching beyond a basic level for those who have no interest in pursuing the instructor training of the traditional Kung Fu Tai Chi Chuan martial artist.

The concept of advanced levels of instructor training is also offered as a template for other Tai Chi for Health organisations and practitioners to develop similar courses. Access to higher levels of Instructor training, we believe, should be made available to all those who qualify and be consistent with modern pedagogic principles which demand open and transparent access to education and training outcomes on the basis of graded levels of academic standards, achievement and merit.

The book includes an in-depth study of the Sun 73 Tai Chi Form with the focus on teaching and on how to be able to modify each form and movement using strategies which are safe and effective for a wide range of people. The book also provides a detailed description of the *Australia Dreaming: Tribute to Our Ancestors* Qigong set derived from Sun style Tai Chi first performed by Elva in the USA in 2003. Included in the book are drawings depicting the Australian landscape as a background to the Qigong set. These drawings have been specially created by Elva's sister, the internationally recognised Australian Wildlife Artist, Gail Higgins.

In the delivery of Tai Chi for Health exercise programs, we strongly believe that teaching expertise should be valued as an equal player with and parallel the development of practical skills and the focus on scientific research. In *Tai Chi Dreaming*, the emphasis is on learning to teach Tai Chi for Health as a safe and effective form of exercise in accordance with modern ethical and legal duty-of-care requirements which affirm evidence based and secular reasoning and a scientific understanding of health and wellness issues. Our approach is conceptually represented in the teaching dynamics of our *Matrix of Performance* where the focus is not on a "One Size Fits All" but on the modernisation processes of the Asian martial arts pioneered by Professor Jigoro Kano and Master Sun Lutang, processes which promote safety factors, ethical, scientific and modern pedagogic principles in the transmission of knowledge about physical education.

Our principal motivation for producing *Tai Chi Dreaming* was to highlight and address the central role of the teacher properly trained and prepared to be able to make a difference for a wide range of people – the teacher who can motivate and encourage all participants regardless of age, gender, race, health, mobility, fitness and cultural factors. The following personal story encapsulates the essence of what we believe is a good tai chi teacher who understands that one-size does not fit all and has the capacity, skills and training to modify and adapt the tai chi program to suit the particular needs of the participant:

> *I have been doing Tai Chi for about eight years. My interest in Tai Chi started after a trip to China in 2001, where I observed different types of Tai Chi in the parks all over China. They encouraged all visitors to join in and I found it to be a fantastic experience. Upon my return to Australia, I found a Tai Chi class here and joined the group.*

> *Unfortunately in October of 2004, I suffered a stroke which took me out of action for a while. After being out for about six months, I tried to rejoin my class, but it became apparent that it did not accommodate someone, who was recovering from a stroke like me. I thought that Tai Chi was no longer something I could do and I left the class very upset and disheartened as I always enjoyed my Tai Chi and it was a big part of my life.*

Luckily, I stumbled on another Tai Chi Class nearby which practised and taught the Tai Chi for Health programs by a teacher who was trained through your advanced level instructor training course. I have been doing this class now with this Tai Chi teacher now for four years and thoroughly enjoy it. For me the reason of now wanting to become a tai chi teacher comes from the joy and help Tai Chi has given me before and after my stroke.

I believe if I can be half as good a teacher as my teacher is, I can make a difference to people's lives especially if they do suffer health problems. Tai Chi gives a lot and more people should have the opportunity to learn it.

We believe that our *Tai Chi Dreaming* is about making a difference to the quality of teaching and enhancing the capacity to learn. It is a valuable resource readily accessible to not only the tai Chi teacher in search of better ways of teaching Tai Chi for Health exercise programs, but to anyone who is looking to make a difference to their own personal health, fitness and wellbeing through the "magic" and "miracle of a modern Tai Chi for Health as being understood in terms of evidence based reasoning and practiced within a modern duty-of-care.

We offer our *Tai Chi Dreaming* to all those who seek a modern approach to significantly improving teaching expertise and to find creative and safe ways to MAKING A DIFFERENCE to the health and wellbeing of anyone who shares the magic, modern journey of a Tai Chi for Health accessible to all people, old and young, regardless of race, creed or colour and which must include those least advantaged in society.

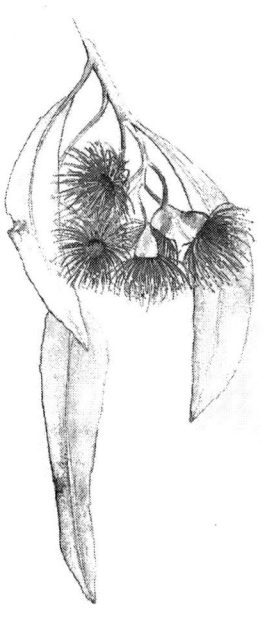

Preface - Australia Dreaming

OUR ACKNOWLEDGEMENTS for the existence of this book *Australia Dreaming: Tai Chi for Health Advanced Instructor Training Course* begin by paying tribute to our ancestral mothers, women over the millennia who gave birth to nurture our very existence. We acknowledge Aboriginal Australians as the First Australians who through their *Dreamtime Stories* culture of over 40,000 years lived in harmony with the Australian landscape. The reference in this book to an *Australia Dreaming* pays special tribute to the history of this ancient land, offering a pathway for reconciliation between ancient and modern cultures, between East and West.

By so doing, we offer *Australia Dreaming* as our tribute to ancestors of all Australians regardless of their ethnic, tribal and cultural origins and also to a global community of people striving for a more peaceful, happy, healthy and harmonious co-existence. In the latter part of the twentieth century, modern Australia had been struggling to emerge as a multi-cultural society that attempted to embrace diversity within a democratic and ethical framework of a *Fair Go for All*. This has in large measure been achieved by lifting the seductive veil of the British colonial myth of white superiority from the Australian landscape and its common humanity. (see Reynolds, 2000)

Over two centuries ago, Aboriginal Australians, were invaded by Britain, their lands taken and "peacefully settled" by white man's technologies of martial power adopting the British legal doctrine of *Terra Nullius* [1] as the system of government. Their traditional culture was radically challenged by the British establishment newly armed with the pseudo sciences of eugenics and phrenology (Reynolds, 2005) aiming to "Civilise and Christianise" [2] the native population. Aboriginal Australians had to wait nearly two centuries before they could begin to be recognised as Australian citizens. (Atwood and Marcus, 2009; see also Australian Government 2009a) The "white-fellas" history and myth of "peaceful settlement" in colonising an empty continent (*Terra Nullius*) was challenged in 1992 by the controversial Mabo decision in the Australian High Court. (CLR, 1992)

It was not until February 2008 that Prime Minister Kevin Rudd on behalf of the Australian government in a televised speech to the parliament also challenged the pervasive myths of a British colonial past which had survived virtually intact into the 1970s, referring to compelling historical evidence, including the tens of thousands of stories of forced separation offering the long overdue "Apology" to Indigenous Australians for the "Stolen Generation". (Rudd, 2008)

Australia has been significantly transformed from its British colonial past to becoming a modern nation through post Second World War mass migration of "New Australians" arriving from Europe dreaming of a new life in the antipodes. It was not until after 1973, however, with the legal demise of the "White Australia policy" [3] that migration began to include people from different parts of Asia. This brought to Australia many people whose traditions and culture have greatly enriched the fabric of modern Australian society and assisted in the further transformation from the mono-cultural white Australia as part of the British Empire to a modern and multi-cultural Australia. This post War mass migration included people who brought with them traditional forms of knowledge of the Asian Martial Arts from Japan, China and Korea thus breaking down traditional cultural divisions and gender barriers facilitating participation for all, men and women, Asians and non-Asians. This included access to traditional forms of secret knowledge of Chinese "Kung-fu" and later to modern "Wushu" martial arts, both of which featured Tai Chi Chuan practised by many as an effective form of gentle exercise, health enhancement, moving meditation, and for some as a spiritual and healing journey.

The beginnings of the modernisation of the Asian Martial Arts, however, can historically be attributed to the genius of Professor Jigoro Kano who literally paved the way in bridging the gulf between Eastern and Western cultures in the late nineteenth century, and in promoting safety factors, ethical and modern pedagogic principles in the transmission of knowledge about physical education. From the late nineteenth century, he spent his life as an educator pioneering the transformation of the Japanese martial arts into a modern physical education program by combining the elements of ethics, health, safety, physical development and significantly for our purposes within a system of graded levels of achievement to be included in schools. He employed the latest European and American pedagogical methods especially John Dewey in teaching students to reject the "win at all costs" mentality, affirming instead the ethical and intellectual principles of "Maximum Efficiency with Minimum Effort" and "Mutual Welfare and Benefit" promoting the focus of physical education as being for the "benefit of humanity". He tirelessly promoted these ideas and ideals internationally by travelling to China, America and Europe influencing such people as Moshe Feldenkrais and Mikonosuke Kawaishi. He is also responsible for an

---

[1] The British treated Australia as *Terra Nullius,* as unowned land. Under British colonial law, Aboriginal Australians had no property rights in the land, and colonization accordingly vested ownership of the entire continent in the British government. The doctrine of *Terra Nullius* remained the law in Australia throughout the colonial period, and indeed right up to the Mabo High Court decision in 1992. (Banner, 2005)

[2] This was the terminology used in colonising native populations throughout the British Empire in the nineteenth century, reflected in the broader government strategy of "Shaping the Good Citizen" as a pedagogic technology based on a Christian philanthropic practice committed to the ethical formation of the "good citizen". (Arthy 1996, 1996a and 1997)

[3] White Australia policy is the term used to describe a collection of government policies from 1901 to 1973 that intentionally restricted non-white migration to Australia.

Asian Martial Art (Judo) to gain widespread international recognition and the first to become an official Olympic sport, having represented Japan from 1909 on the International Olympic Committee and at subsequent Olympic Games. (see Kano, 1994 & 2005; and Wikpedia, 2009)

The beginnings of the modernisation of Tai Chi Chuan being transformed from a combative and dangerous "martial art" into a modern and effective form of exercise accessible to all, can be traced to the genius of Sun Lutang in China in the early twentieth century. He was responsible for having laid the intellectual and ethical framework for the liberation of a martial Tai Chi from the secret knowledge of the "brotherhood of the boxers" and the emergence of a cross-cultural and modern approach to health, well-being and exercise. We pay special tribute to these two Asian ancestors, Professor Jigoro Kano and Sun Lutang, both of whom who were responsible for the modernisation of the Asian Martial Arts, paving the way for future developments in physical education and exercise programs accessible to all.

In the latter part of the twentieth century in Australia, and following in the pioneering footsteps of Sun Lutang, Dr Paul Lam, a Sydney Medical Doctor and an internationally recognized Tai Chi Master, broke with the martial traditions of Tai Chi in developing Tai Chi as a Safe, Secular and Scientific program specifically aimed at the health management of arthritis. Dr Lam was part of a new wave of Asian migration that effectively began with the demise of the "White Australia policy" in the early 1970s formalised by the new Whitlam Labor government which soon introduced multiculturalism into Australia. In the late 1990s, in consultation with a number of health professionals, Dr Lam introduced a Safe, Secular and Scientific form of physical activity and exercise which has been successfully promoted internationally.

In the 1990s Alice Liping Yuan and Henry Zheng migrated to Australia from the People's Republic of China bringing with them modern Chinese forms of Wushu including Tai Chi and Qigong both practised as health enhancement exercises. They migrated to Australia with their own "Dreaming" as "New Australians" to transform a Tai Chi traditionally practiced as a martial art into a modern Tai Chi for Health accessible to all Australians through the formation of *Exercise Medicine Australia* within a modern Duty of Care based on science and an evidence based approach to health and wellness. We thus pay tribute to all "New Australians" who brought with them the secret, the traditional and modern forms of knowledge we understand collectively as the Asian Martial Arts not only from Asia but also from Europe.

Part of this post-war migration included the "New Australian" Geoff Geurts who brought with him from Holland in the late 1950s the modernised, highly effective and accessible form of martial knowledge [4] including Mikonosuke Kawaishi's European approach to Judo, the "Gentle Way", a martial art which has a great deal in common with the "energy efficient" principle of the martial art Kung Fu Tai Chi Chuan. Geoff Geurts was responsible for the formation of a grading and accreditation authority, Sakurakan-QUBBA. [5] We also pay tribute to another "New Australian", Bill Cadoo who migrated from Scotland in the 1950s, to be graded by Geoff Geurt's as his first Black Belt in Australia. He became the Chief Instructor and Technical Advisor of Sakurakan-QUBBA since the untimely death of Geoff Geurts in 1969.

One of the first graduates of our Tai Chi for Health Advanced Instructor Training course in 2008 was Jan Davis. In 1966, Jan was one of the first women in Australia to be graded to Black Belt level in an Asian martial art, and she was the first woman to be graded to Shodan Black Belt in Judo by Geoff Geurts though Sakurakan-QUBBA. This was nearly a decade before equal opportunity legislation was enacted in Australia to remove discrimination against women in the workplace and society. Jan later earned her fifth Dan in Judo through the Judo Federation of Australia and she was accredited as a level 2 Coach and Judo Instructor through the Australian Sports Commission. For her outstanding achievements and meritorious services to Judo, she was awarded the Order of Australia medal in 1985 and later the Australian Sports medal in 2000 in recognition of her 41 years involvement in judo and positive influence on young people. After having retired from active participation in Judo, Jan began as a student with traditional Yang Style Tai Chi. Within a few years, she attended her first Tai Chi for Health Instructor training course in 2003.

Our *Australia Dreaming* has thus emerged as part of a new age of harmony between peoples from different cultures, aiming to transform past cultural and martial practices into modern forms of health improvement and physical exercise through a modern Duty of Care to "Do No Harm" affirming evidence based reasoning, and a scientific understanding of health and wellness issues. Our contribution to a New *Australia Dreaming* is to provide a "training the trainer" course that is significantly different from the Kung Fu Tai Chi for Martial arts training regime, thus contributing to the knowledge of teaching Tai Chi for Health at an advanced level using modern teaching techniques and principles which are Safe, Secular and Scientific.

---

[4] "The Power of the Great Master doesn't consist of his muscular strength, but in the superiority of his great mind "Geoff Geurts 1960.

[5] This is the non-profit organisation which now includes Chinese forms of the martial arts as well as Martial Arts for Health and Tai Chi for Health activities supporting the Tai Chi for Health Advanced Instructor Training course.

THE ORIGIN of the name of this book *Australia Dreaming* has its beginnings in a Qigong set first published and presented by Elva when she taught the Sun 73 Tai Chi form in 2003 at a week long workshop held by Dr Lam in Connecticut in the United States of America. The response by the Tai Chi community was powerfully emotional offering a challenge and invitation for people wanting to know and understand more about Australia, the First Australians and their creation myths and stories. That was six years ago and with further performances of this Qigong set, similar responses have been made by Tai Chi people who felt refreshed by the revelation that traditional Tai Chi imagery of harmony manifested in the Dao, in the Way of Nature was not a cultural and historical concept that belonged exclusively to the traditional and original Chinese owners and the lineage of a secret knowledge transmitted by the "brotherhood of the boxers", the Kung Fu Tai Chi Chuan martial artists.

They understood that an *Australia Dreaming* was a Qigong set devised for the health enhancement and participation by all people. This *Australia Dreaming* offered imagery of the natural beauty of the Australian landscape that very quietly and respectfully affirmed the existence of Aboriginal Australians, of an another ancient culture other than the ancient Chinese culture and its creation myths of Daoism and the harmonious Way of Nature.

To these Tai Chi people, the *Australia Dreaming* Qigong set was something that bridged cultural divisions not only of East and West, but between two ancient cultures highlighting the universal spirit of humanity. For some Tai Chi people, there was the intellectual connection between the Chinese Dao, the Way of Nature with the Dreamtime imagery of the First Australians found in the landscape of Nature both expressed as creation myths and stories. Tai Chi and Qigong could thus be perceived of as art forms and as vibrant health giving exercises which have the power to transcend these apparently radically different cultures as well as having the power to personalise the way of learning to be in harmony with oneself, other people and the environment. In the original *Australia Dreaming* created by Elva in 2003, reference was made in the opening movement to a "Piccaninny Dawn", as a cultural and historical reference to Aboriginal Australians, to evoke the imagery of a baby crying just before dawn and that the baby was black, not white, as a recognition and affirmation of the life force of a small Aboriginal child.

At that time, Elva had created the *Australia Dreaming* Qigong set in good faith after having consulted with Aboriginal Australians who reported that they did had not have any issue with the use of this term nor with other terms or concepts such as the Rainbow Serpent in the way in which they were being used. We have now formed the view, however, that, the term "Piccaninny" can be viewed by some as at best patronising and at worst offensive. As this term is also not unique to Australia and has international usage apparently being of Irish origins, we have removed this particular historical reference to describe an Aboriginal baby term from the Qigong set.

In examining the ethical question of cultural sensitivities for indigenous Australians, our dilemma was, do we remove all references to indigenous Australians in our book and thus avoid the possible claim of "cultural appropriation". This would have been a very easy option, but we decided that by removing all references to or acknowledgement of the ancient culture of the First Australians in the imagery of the Australian landscape, this would lead us into an intellectual form of cultural apartheid whereby the ancient Australian landscape has expunged the presence of the First Australians.

In arriving at this conclusion, we were mindful of related cultural issues as outlined in the special report commissioned by ATSIC in 1999 *Our Culture: Our Future -- Report on Australian Indigenous Cultural and Intellectual Property Rights*. (ATSIC, 1999) We understand and accept that other references such as Rainbow Serpent, Guardian Spirit have special significance to many Aboriginal Australians, but we also understand that these concepts represent cultural and archetypal expression of creation myths and totemic forms of spirituality that exist in other cultures.[6]

We therefore have rejected the idea that we should switch the indigenous Australian human factor in the imagery of the Qigong set to non-indigenous Australians being part of this magical and beautiful Australian landscape, with white European squatters, farmers, miners, backpackers exercising in an open field who see nothing else but the landscape empty of other humans. The imagery of a "White Australian" within the Qigong set enjoying the beauty of a day in the bush or outback would thus not present any problem. It would have been nice and safe and easy to find appropriate words and imagery with some oblique reference to Jolly Jumbucks and Swagmen whistling Waltzing Matilda, ironically testing copyright boundary claims by overseas owners in the USA of this powerful "White Australian" icon of national sentiment.

Or alternatively, we could have juxtaposed with the Australian landscape a Chinese Kung-fu martial arts character (someone perhaps like David Carradine) facing the sunrise, experiencing the day unfolding, seeing

---

[6] For the mythological representation of the Rainbow Serpent existing in other cultures (see Reptilian Agenda, 2009; Reinman, 2009; Tunneshende, 2001; see Stookey, 2004 for Rainbow Serpent myths from Australia, Africa, India, Asia, Eastern Europe and North and South America, where the rainbow is associated with the great serpent symbol of both water and the earth's fertility; see also Australian Government 2009b

nothing else other than the Australian landscape, empty of other people - but to this persona transported from an Asian ancient culture this would not be simply a form of exercise and training for combat, but it would represent another face of the Dao, the Way of Nature, where emptiness within Nature itself is a prized spiritual virtue and of immense existential value. This may even have pleased some in the Tai Chi world, but we felt it would have seemed strangely romantic and out of place in the Ozzie bush especially with a Chips Rafferty (or a John Wayne) character waiting in the wings to engage in cross-cultural combat, Hollywood style.

Whichever way, had we removed all references to the First Australians we believe this would have resulted in a *Terra Nullius* Qigong set using an empty Australian landscape. We would have been safe and secure in publishing the absence of any reference to an *Australia Dreaming* which we believe affirms the ecological and cultural connections between the ancient and the modern, between East and West, between the First and New Australians and the rest of humanity.

In 2003 when Elva first presented her *Australia Dreaming* in Connecticut, she had the "audacity to hope" that it would make it more accessible and acceptable to Aboriginal communities by including references to indigenous Australians as part of the imagery of the Australian landscape. She also had the hope that one day that *Australia Dreaming* might become part of a range of exercise and educational programs at the community and school classroom levels for indigenous and non-indigenous Australians, thus bridging the enormous chasm of knowledge between East and West as well as contributing to improve the appalling health which exists within many indigenous communities throughout Australia.

For those who feel that an *Australia Dreaming: Tai Chi for Health* can only belong to the descendants of the traditional owners of the secret knowledge of the Kung-fu Tai Chi Chuan martial arts, the Chinese "brotherhood of the boxers" and to the descendants of the First Australians, we offer as the inspiration to find a better world in Barack Obama 's own *Dreaming,* in his own *Audacity of Hope* (Obama, 2006) and the prophetic words of Martin Luther King's *Dreaming*:

> I have a DREAM that my four little children
> Will one day live in a nation
> Where they will not be judged
> By the color of their skin
> But by the content of their character

We offer our *Australia Dreaming* to all those who seek to find a modern approach to significantly improving teaching expertise and to find creative and safe ways to MAKING A DIFFERENCE to the health and wellbeing of not only all Australians, but to anyone who shares the magic, modern journey of a Tai Chi for Health accessible to all people, old and young, regardless of race, creed or colour and which must include those least advantaged in society.

We dedicate this book to our children Ben, Tara, Zoe, to our grandchildren Jarron, Tiahana and Riley and to the children of the world as they are all our future.

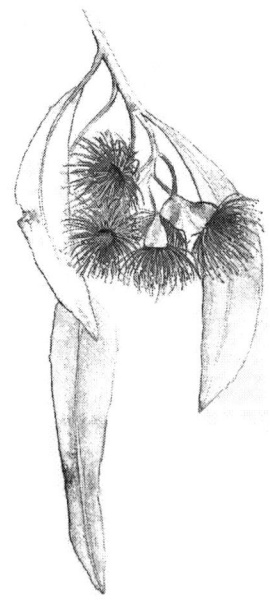

Introduction

Tai Chi for Health - Making a Difference

The overall aims of developing the Advanced Instructor Training Course for Tai Chi for Health are to provide:

- Teaching expertise at a high level of competency for the Tai Chi for Health Instructor who is capable and confident in the delivery of a range of safe exercise programs in the local community

- A basic understanding of necessary legal and ethical responsibilities of the Tai Chi for Health Instructor where the primary aim in a modern Duty of Care is - to do no harm

- An in-depth knowledge of and performance training in Sun Style Tai Chi, a style of Tai Chi highly suitable for an extensive range of people who are interested in modern, Safe, Secular and Scientific exercise programs aimed at enhancing health, fitness and well-being

In the last few years, there has been a growing need in Australia for an advanced level of Instructor training in Tai Chi for Health, which offers a different and viable pathway from that of the traditional Tai Chi for Martial Arts Instructor training that exists at present.

Current Tai Chi for Health Leader and Instructor training programs do not offer graded levels of progression to become a Tai Chi for Health Instructor other than through the traditional Martial Arts approach of Kung Fu Tai Chi Chuan, which specifies in Australia that you must complete the Level 1 Coaching course through the Australian Kung Fu & Wushu Federation (AKWF) before you can be called a Tai Chi Instructor.

Legally, however, anyone can call themselves an "Instructor" without any proper formal training and some people do just that leaving themselves, their students and others exposed and vulnerable to Duty of Care issues, and for some, the legal fine print of liability insurance and to other related legal and ethical matters.

We are unaware of any other similar course available within Australia or within the world as this training is specifically aimed at teaching how to teach TAI CHI FOR HEALTH, as a modern and effective form of exercise at an advanced level, and not teaching the martial art, Kung Fu Tai Chi Chuan.

In Australia, this journey of discovery into Tai Chi for Health has already begun for those who have completed basic level of the Tai Chi for Arthritis Leader course and other similar courses offered by Dr Paul Lam (see Tai Chi Productions, 2009) and of the Tai Chi for Health & Falls Injury Prevention Instructor training program and other similar Tai Chi and Qigong courses offered by Alice Liping Yuan (see Exercise Medicine Australia, 2009). What is new with the Tai Chi for Health Advanced Instructor Training program is the extension of a teacher training focus from a basic level to advanced levels necessary for an independent, responsible and proficient Tai Chi for Health Instructor.

We believe it is an exciting and pioneering development in the world of Tai Chi for Health. Our view is that Tai Chi for Health should be about MAKING A DIFFERENCE through a holistic approach to a Safe, Secular and Scientific exercise program, and with this initiative we both feel we can make some small contribution to this end.

This book will also be a valuable resource for all Tai Chi students, not only those who are involved in teaching Tai Chi for Health, but also those who wish to better understand the historical, cultural and philosophical origins of a modern Tai Chi for Health. In addition, we hope that the ideas contained in this book will encourage others better positioned to develop Instructor Training courses and exercise programs based not only on other Tai Chi forms and styles but also on other Asian martial styles and forms.

Our approach is conceptually represented in the teaching dynamics of our *Matrix of Performance* where the emphasis throughout the course is not on "One Size Fits All" but in the modernisation processes of the Asian martial arts pioneered by Jigoro Kano and Sun Lutang, processes which promote safety factors, ethical, scientific and modern pedagogic principles in the transmission of knowledge about physical education

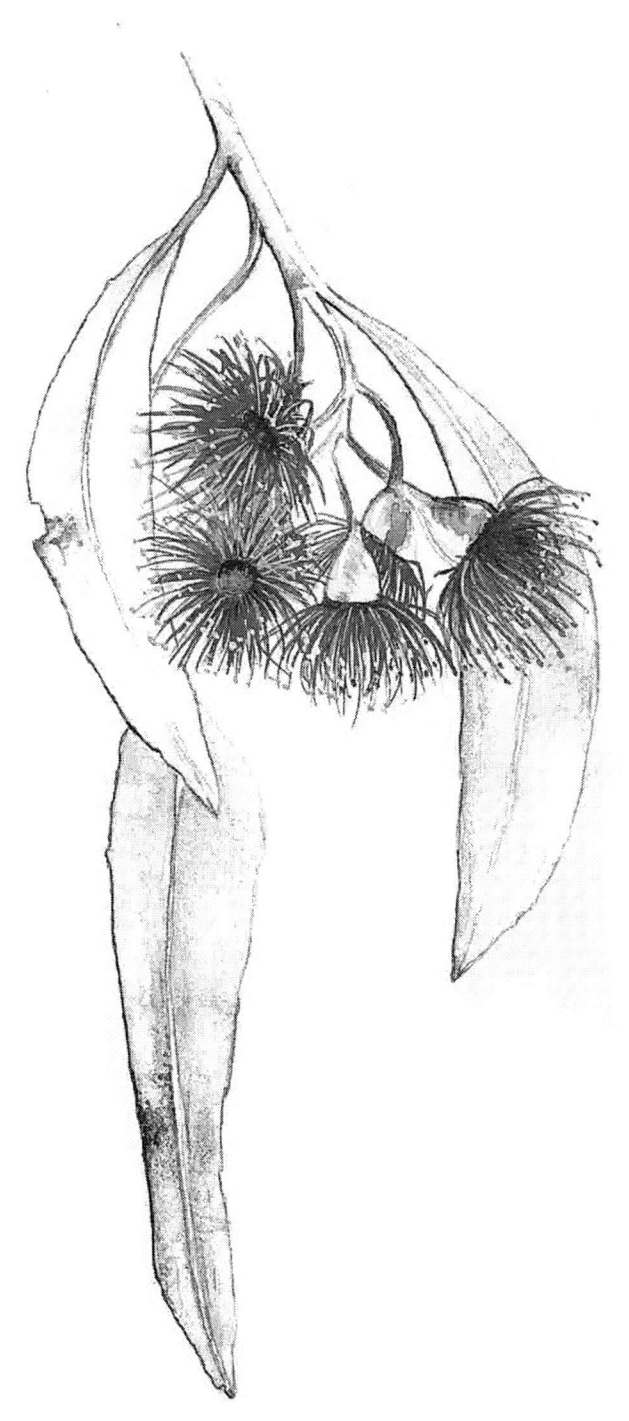

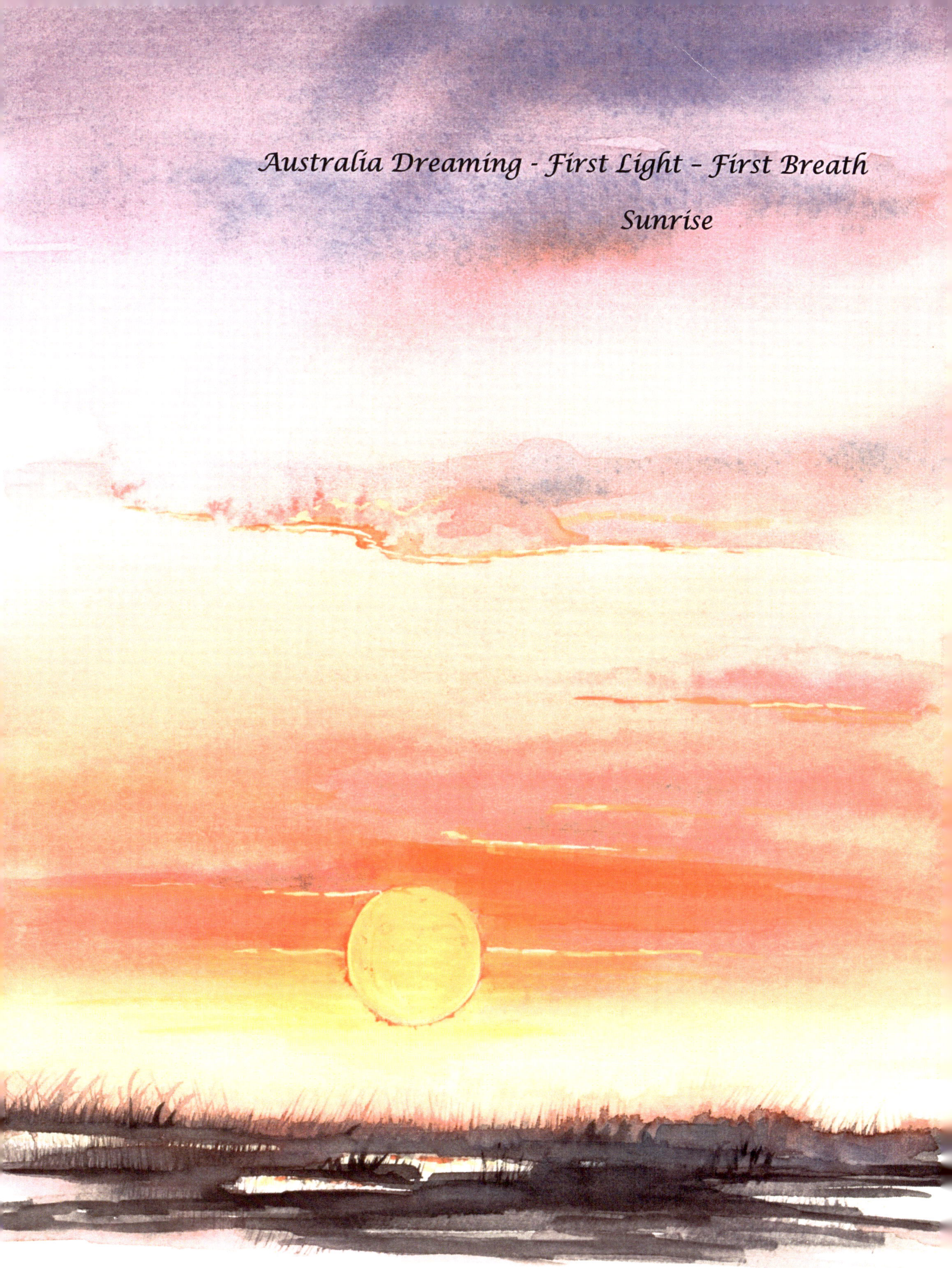

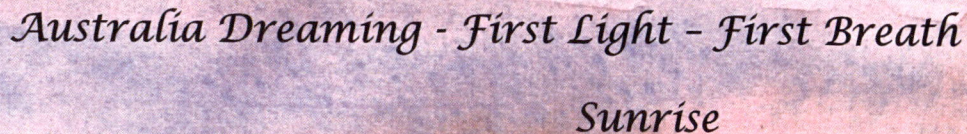

Australia Dreaming - First Light - First Breath

Sunrise

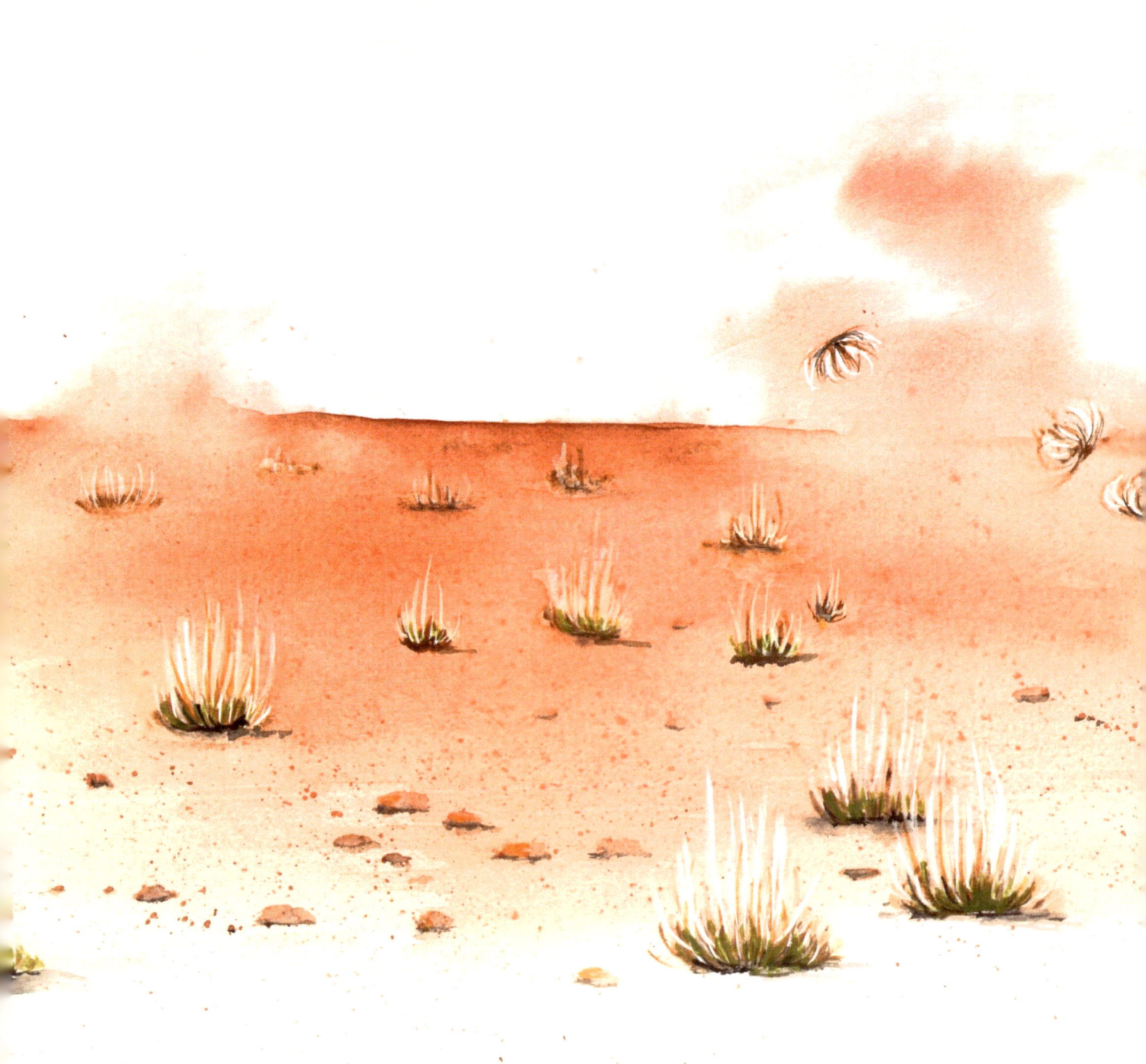

Australia Dreaming - Desert Wind Sweeps the Nullarbor

Australia Dreaming – Blue Sky, White Clouds

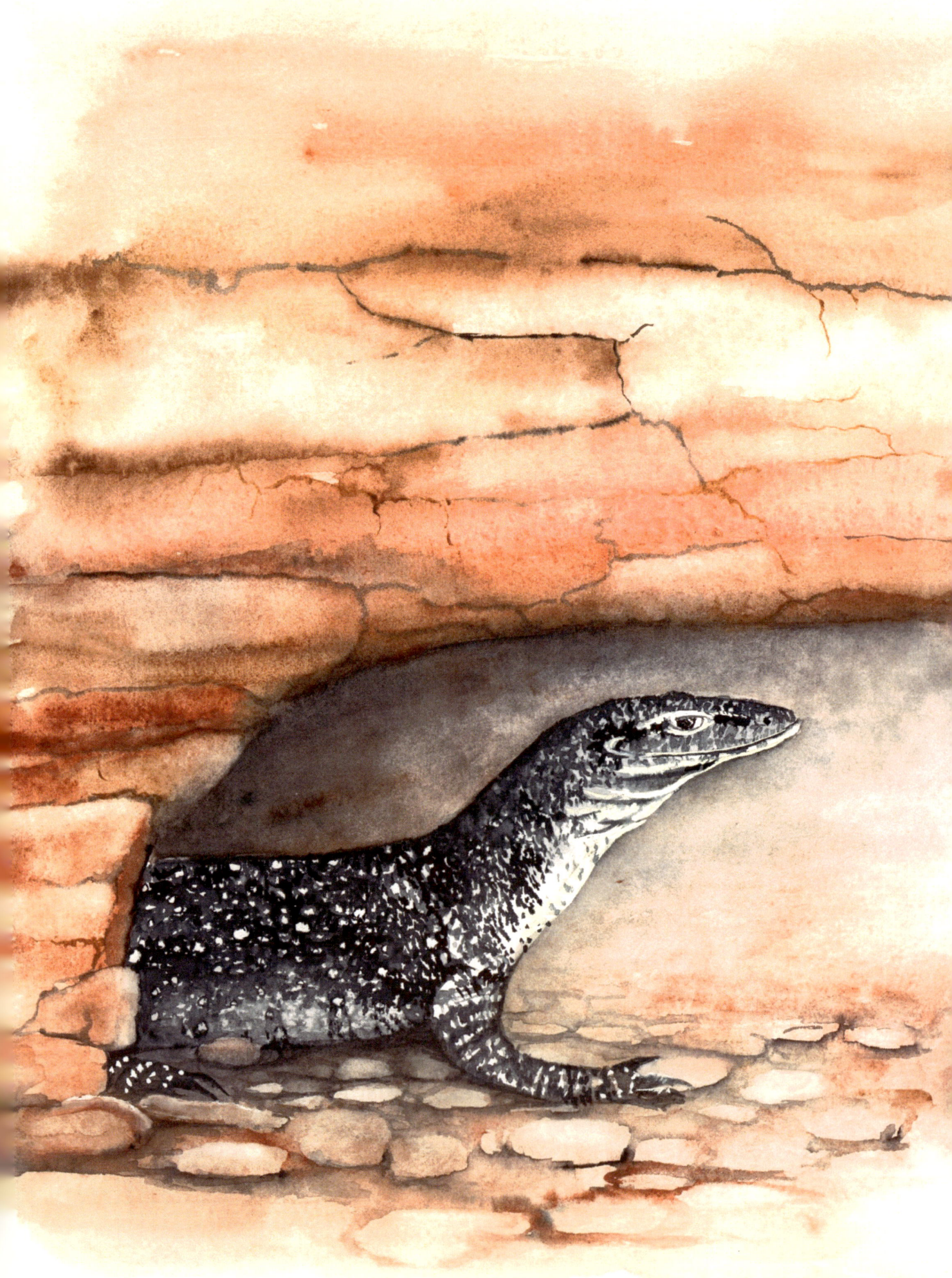

Australia Dreaming - Goanna Hides from the Sun

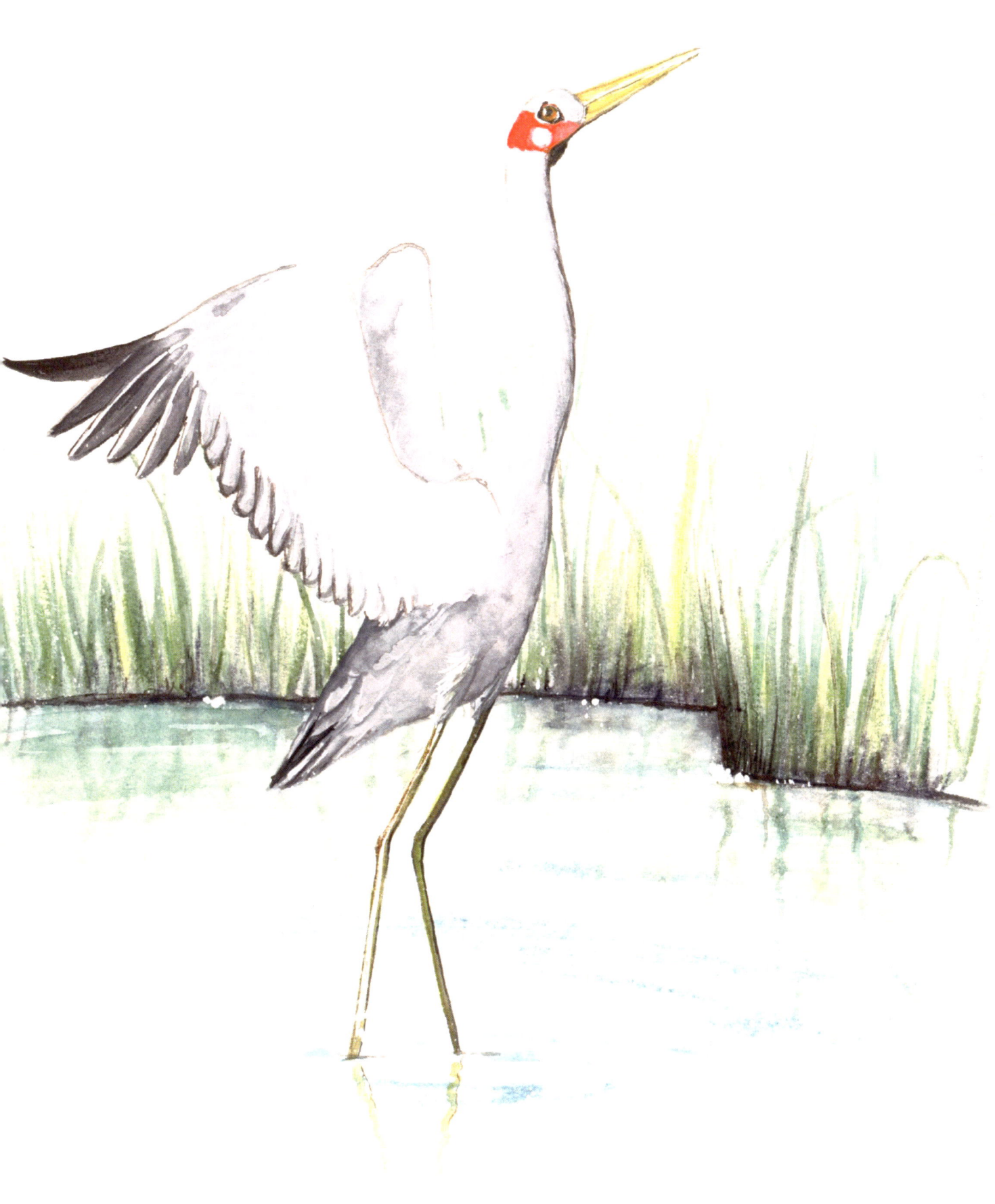

Australia Dreaming - Perentie Waits

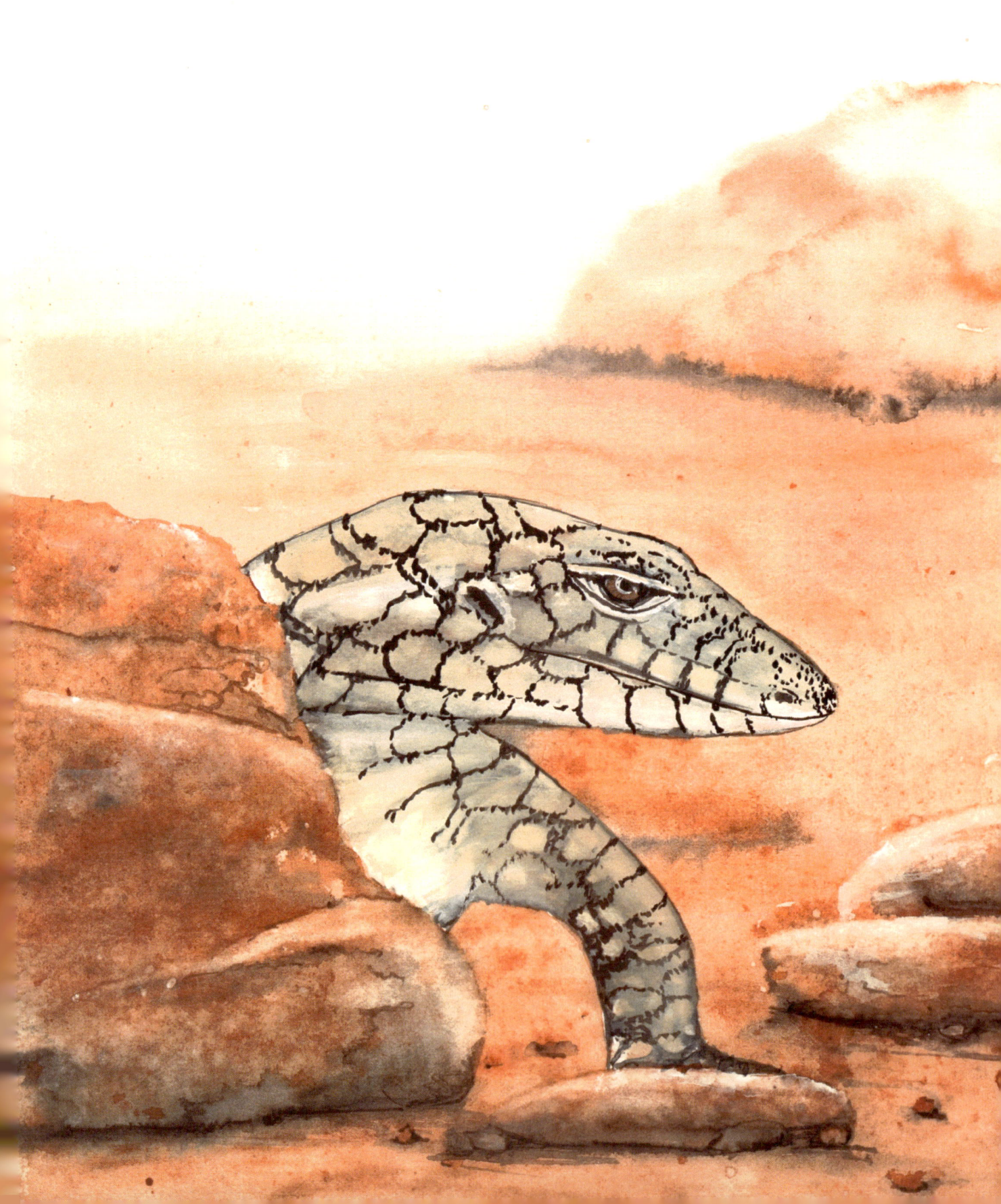

Australia Dreaming - Jabiru Takes Flight

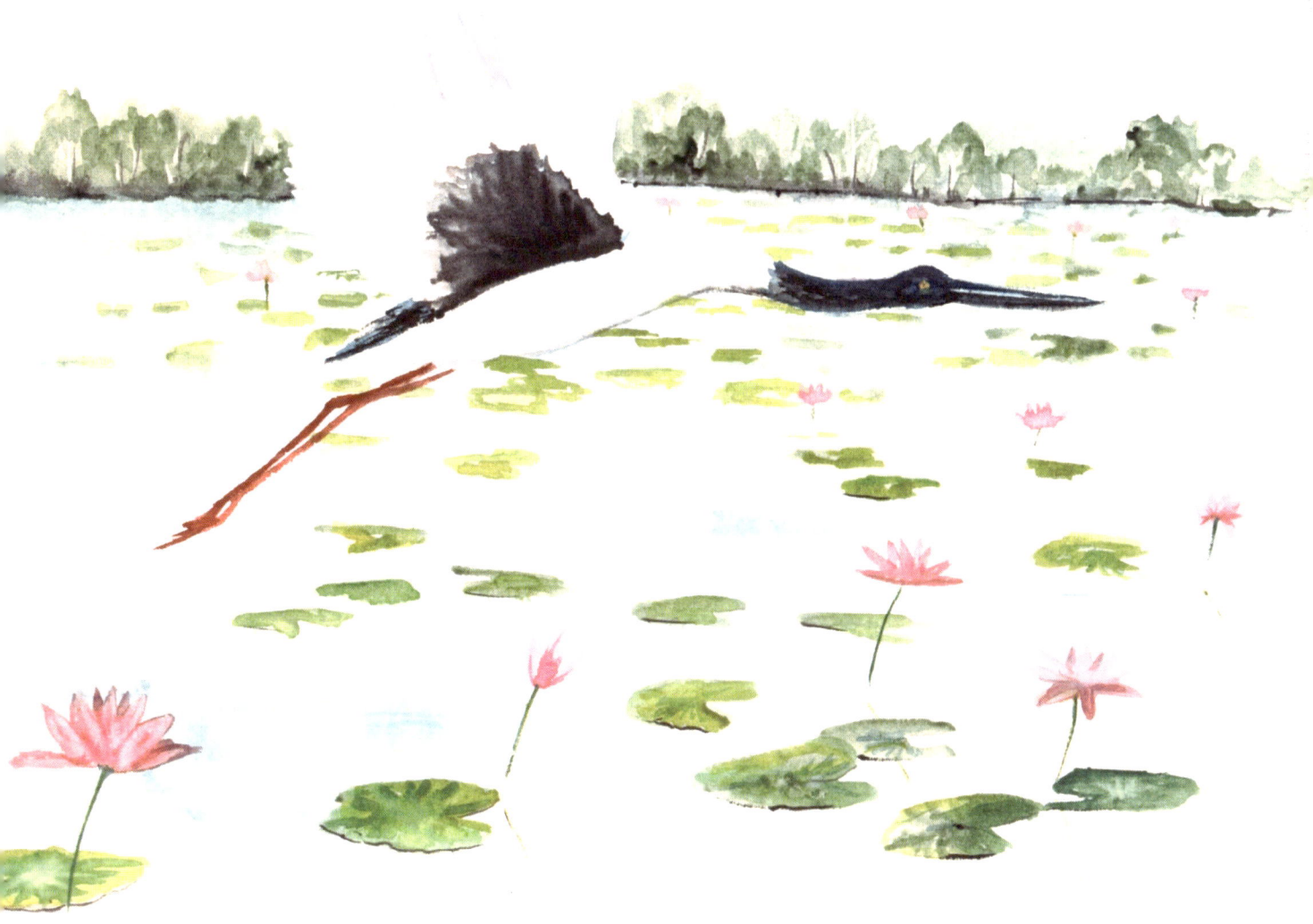

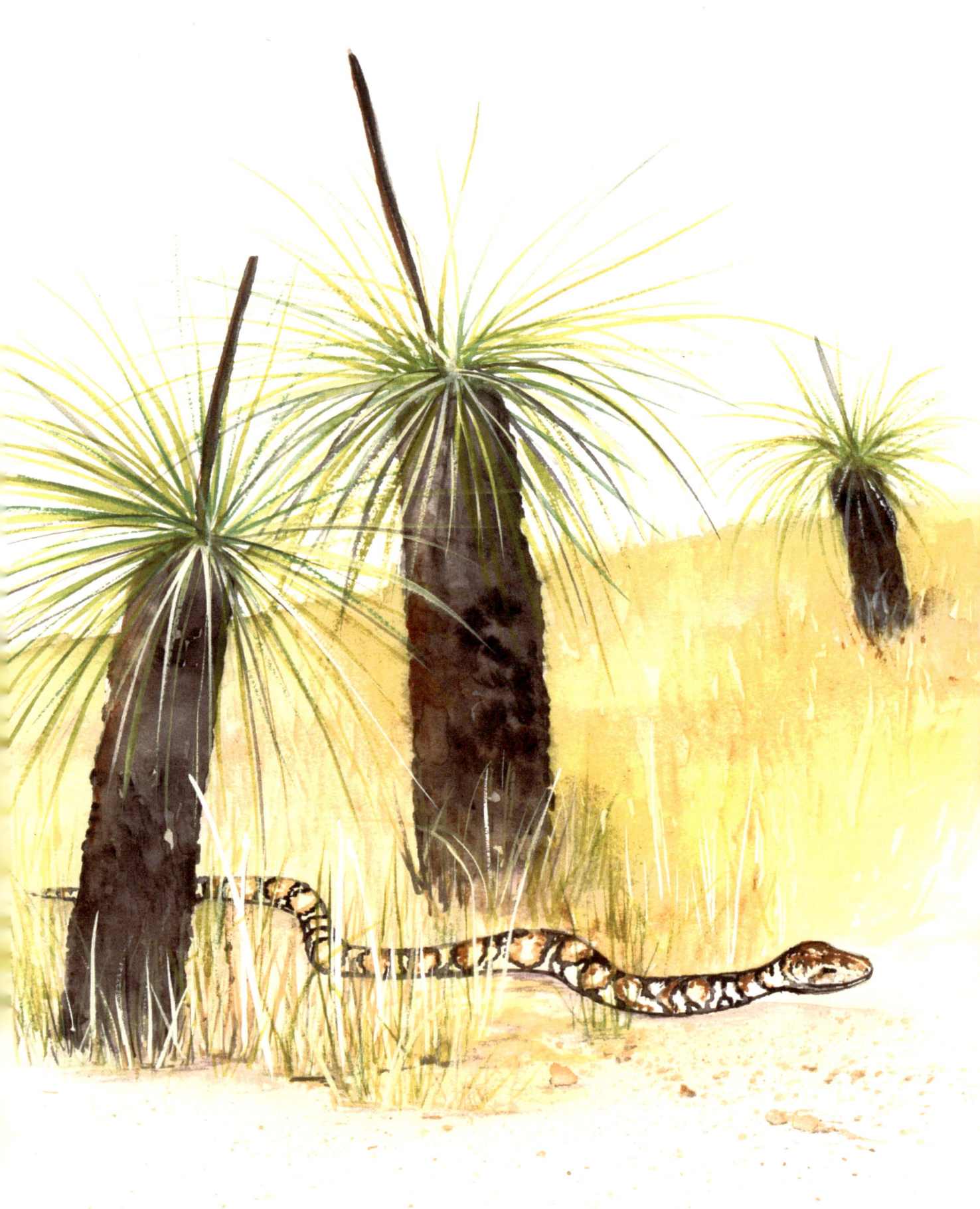

Australia Dreaming - Rainbow Serpent Guardian Spirit

Australia Dreaming – Sunset -End of Day

Australia Dreaming – Southern Cross – Dreamtime

UNIT 100
TEACHING KNOWLEDGE & SKILLS

Unit Overview	1.10	Teaching Principles
	1.20	Communication
	1.30	Preparation
	1.40	Techniques of Teaching
	1.50	Imagery & Concepts
	1.60	Music
	1.70	Modification for Tai Chi [1] for Health
	1.80	Working with Special People

1.10   TEACHING PRINCIPLES OVERVIEW

1.11   Objectives
1.12   Classification of Participants
1.13   Barriers to Participation
1.14   Participants Are Discouraged
1.15   An Instructor Needs
1.16   Duties And Responsibilities Of The Instructor
1.17   Setting the Standards
1.18   Duty of Care & Contraindications

1.11   Objectives - To learn to plan and deliver Tai Chi for Health classes which foster the following:

- Enjoyment, fun, distraction from concerns
- Continuing regular participation and activity
- Education and support
- Social interaction and co-operation
- Improvement of overall health and function
- Development and maintenance of musculo-skeletal strength and endurance
- Development and maintenance of flexibility, mobility, balance and co-ordination
- Learning of relaxation skills
- All of the above, to encourage and maintain quality of life and independent living

1.12   Classification of Participants for Instruction - Tai Chi for Health encompasses a full range of fitness levels. Age is not a reliable guide to group classification. There are 80 year olds who run marathons and 80 year olds who are bed-ridden or chair-bound. There are 50 year olds with biological ages a decade lower than their chronological age and 50 year olds or younger who are sedentary, unfit and already in serious chronic disease situations and disability.

Just as a classification by age is not reliable, neither are the broad groups of "young aged", "active aged" or "frail aged". People in their fifties usually don't want to be classified as "aged" anything and many who may be classed as "frail" very often are not. They may have a disability, which precludes their participation in more active classes.

A more user-friendly classification is to design classes aimed at different levels of participation (see also page 62):

Level A - Fit and active, absence of serious health disorders
Level B - Active, controlled health conditions
Level C - Restricted ability, limited capacity

With Tai Chi it is therefore possible to combine Levels A and B in the one class very successfully. Level C would rarely be combined because of the broader issues of safety. However, many people begin Tai Chi with chair work and if they are being incorporated into an already established class, this is an ideal way to introduce them to the brain/body work of Tai Chi. On the other hand, if there are several people who are confined to a chair, the progress is better if they have a session of their own for some time as there are other issues than physical limitations to consider. Private tuition is indeed an option, which can have very good therapeutic results. Refer Matrix of Performance Levels for Duty of Care for a more detailed analysis of different categories of participants in relation to levels of performance within Tai Chi for Health (see Unit 3.40).

This broad categorisation for physical activity can be a useful guide for the types of people who come to Tai Chi. Unlike "Fitness classes" where students are expected to and are told to "work at the their own level and pace", and where they generally seem to follow the Instructor's example to the letter, the Tai Chi for Health affords the

---

[1] The spelling system used here is Wades-Giles which is still used for familiar Chinese words such at Tai Chi, Tai Chi Chuan, and Kung Fu rather than the Pinying spelling of Tai Ji, Taijquan and Gong Fu. The Pinying spelling system will be used for all other Chinese words.

opportunity for all people to be safely included in any class. That is, at least all those people who can walk unaided should be able to successfully and happily blend into the one class. In so doing it is therefore the professional responsibility of the Instructor to teach the participant to (1) realise and accept their limitations and (2) understand and accept that change takes time – and is not an instant fix. In saying that, it is also important to teach that change will occur and the value of visualisation so that the participant has the opportunity to improve more quickly.

To safely and happily accommodate the different levels of capabilities into a regular Tai Chi class takes the persistence of Instructors to educate and encourage their students to discover what it means to think and feel for themselves, to relax and accept a level of comfort that is commensurable for training and "not working to please the Instructor" with their progress but working to discover how to feel more well with the guidance of someone who can lead them in their discovery. The role of the teacher is one of guiding and coaching and encouraging- as well as teaching.

1.13   Barriers to Participation
- Self concept "physical inability" to exercise
- Stereotype of older/working individual sitting back and taking a well deserved rest
- Attitudes of expected behaviour of significant others in their lives
- Fears concerning the harmful effects of exercise
- Belief that they have/do work hard all their lives and don't need exercise
- Lack of opportunity to attend lessons
- Unwillingness to attend not knowing anyone in the class
- Lack of transportation
- Misinformation concerning Tai Chi
- Inappropriate self image - poor body shape, too fat, too thin, slow
- Clumsy, uncoordinated, unmusical.
- Chronic pain
- Financial
- Mental processing deterioration – cognitive decline
- Fatigue
- Religious bias
- Anything foreign in concept
- The main barrier – perceived lack of time

1.14   Participants are Discouraged by
- The instructor with her/his hand on the light switch at the end of the class - the tight schedule – too busy to listen
- The soloist performer
- Sloppy or unprepared work
- Lack of confidentiality
- Music too loud, too modern, too old, too fast, too slow, too "foreign", too much
- Being expected to absorb complex moves too quickly
- Instructor not knowing their name
- Attention being drawn to them in class
- Patronising behaviour
- Unpunctuality
- Going overtime
- Ageism in all its forms
- Favouritism
- Disinterest in their social activities
- Social isolation in the class
- Not being aware of improvements
- Lack of encouragement
- A misplaced word or look

1.15   An Instructor Needs
- To like her/his participants – to be a people person
- To look fit and healthy and enthusiastic on most days
- To lead by example – don't teach when ill
- To enjoy her/his work and have fun
- To care
- To have good posture, alignment, technique.
- To have the capacity to be creative, to develop and expose participants to new ideas.
- To have clear enunciation, good and consistent cueing and effective voice projection (or use of a microphone)
- To be encouraging to treat participants equally

- To be versatile, flexible
- To be updated via workshops and personal research
- To make mistakes sometimes
- To BE THERE

1.16   Duties and Responsibilities of the Tai Chi for Health Instructor - Help others to achieve a better quality of life in their daily activities and to encourage them to improve the range of activities in which they are able to participate to enrich their enjoyment and well being by:
- Care and assistance
- Public Relations
- Education
- Quality Programming
- Encouraging, Motivating, Participating
- Assessing and Evaluating
- Referring to Health Professionals

The importance of your role as their point of contact will make a positive impact on their
- Physical Needs
- Mental Needs
- Emotional Needs
- Social Needs

Need for Networking Resources at your disposal through sharing of information, records, filing, contacts
- Medical/Health personnel
- Senior Citizens
- Outpatients workshops
- Veterans Affairs
- Arthritis Foundation
- Scrapbooks on relevant health issues
- Diabetes Australia
- Guest speakers
- Returned Services League
- Publications
- National Heart Foundation
- Fitness Industry workshops
- Local Government resources
- Health and Community Care

1.17   Setting the Standards
What resources do I need to provide really good quality care for my class?
What and who is my support network?
What are my goals?
What do I expect to achieve?
What criteria in class structure do I need to consider?
Resources:
- Screening
- Safety
- Safe and effective class delivery
- Continuing education for me and my students
Networking
- Set up your own participant filing system
- List health professional contacts
- Compile topical issues and information from professional sources which may interest participants
- Contact participants' medical advisers when appropriate
- Participate in community health & fitness related functions
- Market your class particulars
Goals and Achievements
- Expect that your participants will improve their quality of life
- Expect that you will feel satisfaction in the quality of your classes
- Expect respect and gratitude from your participants
- Expect a gentler physical working load on your body
- Expect a great health program for yourself
- Expect your working life to be a pleasure
- Expect as good if not better financial reward for your output
- Expect to enjoy your participants and your work

Class Structure
- Warm-up
- Qigong
- Training Exercises
- Revision
- Something New
- Cool-down
- (Happiness)

Program Planning

1. Your Tai Chi class should include consideration of:
   (a) Physical/Mental
   - Strength, Conditioning, Co-ordination, Flexibility, Balance, Relaxation – and all of the other benefits of Tai Chi will be taken care of in each class
   - Alignment and Posture
   - Safe physical activity
   - Maintenance of health to Improvements to health
   - Improved Breathing
   - Intention to do no harm
   (b) Social/Emotional.
   - Belonging - to a group with similar goals in mind
   - Self worth - sense of well being, seeing others coping with difficulties
   - Awareness of improvement in performance
   - Accomplishment - sense of achievement
   - Appreciation - of one's own body and movement capabilities
   - Feeling of control
   - Loss of powerlessness
   - Something to strive towards
   - Something to look forward to
   - Enjoyment in participation
   - Development of social interaction and cooperation

2. Limiting Factors for people participating in Tai Chi may include:
   - Kyphosis - Lordosis - Scoliosis - Sacro-iliac instability
   - Osteo and Rheumatoid Arthritis and sub groups
   - Shortened muscles - stiffer ligaments - weaker cartilage
   - Systolic and Diastolic increases and decreases
   - Joint Replacements - Cardiac and other organ surgery – Minimal coordination capabilities
   - Poor balance - Poor circulation - Pain - Cancer - Some brain dysfunction
   - Depression - Extremes of body weight and composition - Accident disabilities - Hearing impairment
   - Breathing difficulties - Reduced thermo-regulation - Vision impairment
   - Slow reaction times - Sensory deprivation – Osteoporosis - Dementia
   - Stroke - Medication - In-elasticity and fragility of skin - Cardio-vascular insufficiency

The very many conditions for ill health should alert Tai Chi instructors to be very much aware that students should not be expected to learn at the same pace or in the same way. Begin work on the lowest common denominator and teach them how to work at a comfortable level – not what they think you expect. Working at a comfortable level with a focussed mind is the best way to improve strength, flexibility and conditioning. The most important Duty of Care is to teach students how to connect with themselves and work at a comfortable level. Many students do not know how to feel parts of the body, and do not understand why they should work at a comfortable level. Many simply want to work hard both for their teacher and because their mental conditioning expects that they should. – otherwise they feel some self imposed guilt. This attitude change takes perseverance to overcome. When this is achieved exercise (Tai Chi) becomes a joy.

3. Creative Ideas
   - Use a variety of techniques to explain and demonstrate form and principles
   - Use a repertoire of music that is not invasive and does not interfere with focus and concentration
   - Be resourceful and adaptable
   - Watch your students for how they modify to suit their bodies
   - Be accepting of what they offer. It is their Tai Chi – not yours. Many teachers make the mistake of being too rigid and too demanding – this is the main reason that students stop coming to class

1.18   Duty of Care & Contraindications - The main focus on the legal and ethical responsibilities of the modern Tai Chi for Health Instructor is addressed in Unit 400.

The consideration of a Tai Chi for Health Instructor (or any one teaching physical activity) is the intention to do no harm. This means that nothing in your teaching, what you say, your expectations, how you handle your students, how long you keep them working, how many repetitions, your failure to explain about the pain rule and so forth – nothing – that you do or say or fail to do should harm your student. This means that your student should not be worse off for attending classes with you.

Your concern is to make everything safe yet still be effective – even if it takes some time to achieve. This is where learning how to modify has its greatest strength. Knowledge of the body, the bones and how they are aligned, how the muscles work, the role of the nervous system, what the principles and concepts mean, how they work, how Tai Chi works all helps to understand the need for modification and the rationale for it. In Tai Chi practice there are many interesting and effective stretches and strengthening methods. In the modern approach of Tai Chi for Health, there is a real danger of teachers going beyond their understanding and trying to do exercises and stretches that are really only suitable for the trained athlete/martial artist or experienced Tai Chi practitioner. The over-riding consideration for the Tai Chi for Health Instructor is to do no harm.

Secondary to this is to understand that many students have not had years of training and conditioning and may have many health problems and restrictions (see Unit 1.17). They are not training for competition or for self defence but have come to class for a better quality of life through their own self management. Teaching the student how to understand their bodies and working within a comfort level that is about 70% of what they perceive to be their maximum in the beginning will help to achieve this aim. Trying interesting and risky moves "to try something new" or "to be like the teacher" does not meet this aim. This is one reason why the behaviour of the Instructor could compromise the understanding of the student. If the instructor, for example, does ballistic stretches, ham string stretches or deep squats before a TCA class this might give the impression that it is all right to do this sort of practice at home. The physical conditioning and training of someone who has been working with Tai Chi for many years will be harder and should be more advanced than the beginner or person with health problems. Being aware of who is in the class and who is watching should always be a consideration for what is being presented.

Many participants at a Tai Chi class may experience these effects of a de-conditioned lifestyle
- Decreased aerobic capacity, anaerobic power and capacity
- Decreased muscular strength and power
- Decreased flexibility
- Decreased ability to balance
- Decreased maximum heart rate
- Decreased oxygen uptake
- Decreased bone density
- Decreased cognitive ability
- Decreased sensitivity to visual and aural acuity
- Slower reaction and movement times
- Increased body weight
- Decreased pulmonary and cardiovascular efficiency

Attending such a class as Tai Chi for Health having it available and accessible with a competent and caring instructor can eliminate, reduce or slow down many of he affects of ageing and inactivity and will certainly improve the health and well being and quality of life for most if not all who participate.

1.20   COMMUNICATIONS OVERVIEW
   1.21   Motivation
   1.22   Communication
   1.23   Communicating Effectively
   1.24   Making a Connection
   1.25   Pitfalls to Avoid
   1.26   General Class Information
   1.27   Making a Connection (Extract from Arthy and Arthy, 2006)

1.21   Motivation - Everyone who has decided to be more physically active as part of their lifestyle knows how movement can clear the cobwebs, fight off fatigue and send the "blues" packing. Getting motivated is all that is needed. How is it achieved for the student of Tai Chi?

M	Movement (for better quality of life)
O	Organise (better time management to fit gentle calming activity into your life)
T	Time (find some time every day – give it the importance your health deserves)
I	Inspiration (to do the things you want to do)
V	Valuable (and meaningful improvement to your health)
A	Activities (feeling better so more things to do)
T	Tenacity (don't give up – every day some improvement - persevere!)
I	Investigate (ways to feel more comfortable when doing Tai Ch – don't push)
O	Optimistic (be positive about everything- look on the bright side)
N	Never Alone (with your Tai Chi practice and Tai Chi friends)

How does the instructor motivate the students?

The Instructor:
- Bright & pleasant personality
- Ability to provide leadership
- Good, clear instruction
- Encouraging manner
- Comment on progress
- Positive attitude to performance in participants
- Provide non-competitive atmosphere
- Ensure successful participation for all participants at their own level
- Awareness for music preferences
- Encourage improvisation of movement patterns
- Not drawing attention to correction of an individual participant
- Should be seen and heard easily
- Start on time, finish on time
- Take genuine interest in participants
- Encourage exercise commitment by participants
- Do not show off
- Look well, fit and groomed
- Relax and enjoy your class
- Remember how you were as a beginner

The Program:
- Will be well designed from a scientific basis
- Will be free from exercises with potential musculo-skeletal risks
- Will be designed with consideration of the students attending
- Will use a variety of teaching and learning techniques and skills
- Will be geared to class capabilities
- Will be enjoyable and safe

Report Progress:
- Point out to participants that you can see their efforts and accept them
- Point out when they can work for longer periods
- Point out when they have learned something new
- Point out when improvements to form and ability are achieved

Additional Activities:
- Workshops
- Competitions
- Social functions (for pleasure or fund raising for the community)
- Availability before and/or after class for consultation
- Rewards for improvements
- Rewards for bringing a friend

Identification:
- Wearing of a T-shirt with logo or a track suit, bag, badge etc
- Special costume days - Easter (bunny ears and tail), St. Patrick's Day (wear green) Mad Hatters Day (funny hat) for a laugh or two
- Participating in parades or displays as a group
- Being involved in or organising some of their social activities
- Becoming involved in community activities such at Breast Cancer Awareness etc
- Seniors Week, Clean-Up Australia

Education:
- Instruction and reinforcement of the need to be physically active

- Modification of segments to individual needs
- Explanation of program structure
- Cautioning against unsafe or contraindicated exercise practices
- Working within personal limits, estimating perceived exertion
- Teaching muscle groups, posture, alignment, functional fitness when appropriate
- Using correct footwear and clothing
- Learning how to increase use of water during exercise (and after)
- Writing newsletter to suit needs and progress of the class
- Participating in public talks and meetings to increase awareness of Tai Chi

Be Yourself: Using vocal and manual dynamics sometimes:
- That's The Best You've Ever Done
- Where's My Camera
- I Wish I Had That On Film
- It Can't Be Done Better Than That
- I'm Going To Retire - You're Amazing

Often just a great smile will say 100 words. Remember that "beautiful" "good" etc have no meaning in themselves for people to build on. Better to say something like "the posture was perfect – you looked so calm. I really enjoyed watching you". They might think –"I felt calm, too. I enjoyed that."

If the Instructor is prepared, enthusiastic and motivating, and takes special care not to be demanding: if the participants feel comfortable and enjoy what they are doing - whether their work is "good" or not, then the class will be successful in its objectives. They will want to come again, and again. Many will enjoy a greater feeling of independence and wellbeing and they will be better equipped to enjoy their preferred activities and the normal events of daily living.

1.22   Communication

Clarity of Teaching

Good reciprocal visibility

Communication:
- Instructor's voice should be audible – if not use a mic
- Music must not be over-riding or too soft
- Be consistent & generous with cueing
- Use descriptive words consistently
- Avoid repetitive use of fill-in words - "OK"
- Maintain eye-contact
- Talk to the whole class - avoid favouritism, cliques
- Motivate with personality, manner & attitude
- Dress appropriately
- Give feedback
- Get feedback
- Educate about pain

Poor Communication Skills will lead to
- Class frustration
- Reduced motivation
- Poor attention span
- Poor alignment
- Reduced performance
- Reduced fitness benefits
- Reduced attendance
- Potential for harm

Things to say that make people feel great

"MAY I" Asking permission implies that it is up to the other person to make the decision and that they have the authority to grant or deny permission

"I'D LIKE YOUR ADVICE   or   I'D LIKE YOUR OPINION" Suggests that the other person has a knowledge or wisdom that you could benefit from

"YOU'RE RIGHT" A verbal pat on the back and an acknowledgment of their input

"CAN YOU SPARE A FEW MINUTES?" Implies that you respect the other person's busy schedule and that you think their time is valuable

"PLEASE" The one word that makes relationships much smoother. "Please" implies respect.

Demonstration of Student Performance - The performance of the students may not reach the expectation of the Instructor. This may result from:
- Beginner has learning difficulties due to
  - Lack of fitness
  - Not understanding cueing
  - Unfamiliarity with movements
  - Poor movement memory (untrained)
  - Anxiety - feeling awkward, lack of confidence
- Lack of focused practice, repetition and consolidation which eliminates many of the problems of remembering
- The teacher not willing to allow the student to perform the movements with the teacher watching

Correction:
- As a group
- As individual (be subtle)
- By contrasting and correcting

1.23   Communicating Effectively – Be very clear about the difference between Teaching and Demonstrating. Demonstrating is where the teacher (or student) shows some Tai Chi for others to see. As far as communications goes, it is a one way process. They could be demonstration to a wishing well. There is no connection. Teaching however, should be a two way process. It involves information output from the teacher and reception of input from the participant who has the correct information that can be understood and processed.

Sometimes during a demonstration it is necessary for the instructor to tell the student what to look for – otherwise they have only a visual input – and less than effective processing.

A   Effective Output requires of the teacher:
- Visibility
- Audibility
- Clarity and precision of instruction
- Selection of the correct knowledge appropriate at the time

B   Effective Input for the student requires from the teacher:
- Eye contact
- Constant monitoring of responses, body alignment, facial expression, loss of concentration, confusion, signs of physical stress, boredom, lack of control
- Selection of the correct information for the student to understand in a language they comprehend and are able to process

"A" must be modified according to "B" for Effective Teaching

In addition to offering a balanced, well-designed Tai Chi class for improved health, providing a structured activity for people to look forward to, an outlet for physical expression and creativity and an opportunity for social contact are all, in themselves, very important aspects of the embodiment of a modern Tai Chi class.

Make sure you know the reasons why your participants are becoming involved (for enjoyment, socialising opportunities, hopes of increased fitness, relief from pain etc). This will help you to be mindful of why people come to class – and not get lost on what you want to teach them. In any real class situation, the reasons why people attend are as varied as are the health and fitness levels of the participants. Simply being aware of their reason for attending will enable you to offer them some feedback from time to time. Just by reading your records will refresh your memory about why people want to do Tai Chi or try out Tai Chi. You can mark it off (in a notebook) so that no one is forgotten.

1.24   Making A Connection - What does "making a connection" mean? Most teachers are interested in communicating better and value the connection with their students. Communication is a two way process. If something is transmitted and it is not received it is only a one way process. Information is going out but nothing is coming back. Here there is no communication, there is no connection between the two. Information needs to be sent to the student, the student needs to hear it and or see it, absorb it, understand it, come up with an output and send the message back to the teacher either my doing an action or expressing in some way their inability to do it. Then there is a communication between the two.

Here the student is the pivotal factor. The teacher has many possibilities for transmitting information and has a large repertoire to choose from. The skill here is knowing what or how much information to select and what to pass on to the student. The student needs to be able to receive cues, be able to process, then either perform or express in some way they have that information so that the teacher receives some feedback from the student. For communication to be efficient, there has to be some interaction between the student and the teacher.

The better the interaction, the better the outcome:
- The teacher sends information to the student
- The student sends information to the teacher

The communication from the teacher to the student should have:
- Accurate technique with clear, clean movements
- Language both verbal and non-verbal should be clear simple, consistent and reassuring
- Skills for observing and receiving information and messages from the student
- Quality personal behaviour, calm, interested and happy

The communication between the student and the teacher is shown via:
- Technique – everything offered by the student is acceptable as long as it is safe
- Behaviour in class as outlined by teacher at commencement
- Language encouraged without fear – natural verbal and non-verbal expression

To really connect with your students avoid standing in the centre at the front at all times "in the teacher position" (see Unit 1.44). While they are practising, walk around and make some contact. Your keen interest in their efforts will result in you being able to comment positively on some aspect of their presentation and you have the opportunity to offer something really helpful for their progress.

1.25   Pitfalls to Avoid
- Don't be a clockwork listener going through the motions - saying the same things to Betty as you say to Flora
- Don't use unrealistic reassurance
- Don't talk to others nearby as if the person is not there
- Don't hurry important conversations or start them when you know or strongly suspect you'll run out of time. If you're short of time, say so, in a pleasant manner. Don't let your body language say it for you
- Don't give medical advice - EVER. Don't even be tempted to give hasty advice regarding significant issues to your students. Reserve general health information for your educational component and give a mini-workshop. Remember - you are trained in EXERCISE not MEDICINE
- Don't assume they know what you mean
- Don't assume you know what they mean
- Don't get too personal

1.26   General Class Information Education/Information Component - Timing of educational input for your participants is important. If before the class, it should be brief e.g. teaching or reminding them of "Rate of Perceived Exertion" or "How to know what is comfortable" or "The importance of water for exercisers". Or" when should I rest in class" – so many topics.

When the educational component comes into the class is a matter for the instructor to decide. If the class is long and you have a tea break – this is a good time. Also if the weather is very hot this is another opportunity to allow them to sit for a while but still be learning about Tai Chi or how Tai Chi works. As participants do not have to concentrate on balance and co-ordination etc., you are more likely to have their attention.

By waiting until after the class, you lose your captive audience. Many will leave immediately following the class. Be aware of the Calendar of Events e.g. Heart Week, Arthritis Week or Back Care and so forth. A few comments can be appropriate, informative and helpful. If you feel inclined, you may choose to become involved in a more practical way at a community level. This also gives people a feeling of belonging and having a connection with the outside world.

Keep a file of topical health and fitness issues that you feel may be of interest to your participants. Store articles in clear sheets in a folder and take to class. Keep a file of topics (at home), pamphlets and references for your own information to improve your networking in the local area such as clinics, courses offered through the health department or hospital, lists of classes in other fields such as swimming, sporting activities, yoga, relaxation courses and further education through your local community or education facility.

Hold a morning tea or "bring-a-plate" after class on a regular basis (say once a month or once a term) and suggest a topic for casual discussion. You act as facilitator. Sometimes it is just fun to have a jokes day.

Where an instructor holds a pivotal position in a town or district, it is sometimes possible for them to engage an expert in their field to address the class (perhaps once or twice a year).   Often a representative from the Heart

Foundation can educate on the value of exercise, a physiotherapist (eg from the Home Nursing Services) will speak on Incontinence, a rep from the dairy industry can speak on the value of calcium in the diet. There are many Government bodies who are only too pleased to have the opportunity to impart their information to a waiting and interested audience. Most visitors bring leaflets, and demonstrating materials to make their presentation and some bring free samples, which will delight your class members. Participants are usually happy to donate a gold coin (if required), which will usually cover expenses of professionals or make a donation. If you publicise your presentation and open it up to the public, you are not only performing a service to the community but you may get a few new participants as well.

1.27 Extract from Paper – Teaching Effectively (Arthy and Arthy, 2006)

Connections between Teacher and Student
The relationship between the teacher and the student has a huge bearing on the effectiveness of teaching. There are some Tai Chi teachers whose connections to the student is about "showing knowledge" and not "sharing knowledge". These teachers show their knowledge through demonstrating their Tai Chi skills while using a style of language that fails to communicate, in particular to the beginning Tai Chi student. Little or no effort is made to find a common language with the student, instead choosing a syntax and vocabulary that is difficult, metaphysical, mysterious and sometimes incomprehensible. The expected student's role here is to accept these new forms of knowledge as an act of faith, thus bypassing the intellect being encouraged to feel positive energy and emotions, to get in touch with their inner feelings and chi by copying and following in the faceless shadow of the Tai Chi teacher. This style of teaching makes certain assumptions about how knowledge is integrated and internalised, the effect of which is to significantly delay the acquisition of knowledge and skills about Tai Chi by the individual student. This approach by a Tai Chi teacher who may well be very knowledgeable about Tai Chi in "showing" this knowledge, unfortunately inhibits the student to begin to take personal responsibility for their own health and development of skills and knowledge and fails to generate "mind-body" awareness, a prerequisite for independent learning and development.

There may be some TCH Instructors who may have limited knowledge of Kung Fu Tai Chi Chuan, or who may have a considerable amount of prior teaching experience, and may have many students who are highly motivated and enthusiastic. In the short term, students might flock to them, and lessons will have a palpable vibe and happiness. In the longer term, these teachers will only continue to be effective with an ongoing commitment to acquiring more forms of knowledge about Tai Chi and how Tai Chi works in relation to various levels of health, age and fitness. As they renew their knowledge and skills, such teachers continue to be motivating and nurturing by refreshing, learning, enhancing, exploring the many layers of knowledge about Tai Chi, health and fitness to invigorate and inspire their students.

Initially, it is the TCH Instructor's responsibility to find out why the student wishes to attend the TCH class. It may seem an impossible task to seek out these answers that on the surface seem unimportant. The students have enrolled, paid their fee and they are there to learn. Everyone can see how a student seems to be, but very few take the time to see who they are. This is not the same as knowing intimate details as the TCH Instructor always needs to maintain a professional teacher-student relationship. It is about knowing why they are at the class, knowing what their expectations are. Making a connection! Giving them the opportunity to tell you about themselves! They know that you are the teacher and through reputation or written material or through recommendation, they will have certain expectations about you both as a teacher and about what they will be learning.

One of the most difficult aspects of teaching is holding on to beginners. The teacher will want to hold on to them long enough for them to not only make a connection with you the teacher but with themselves, particularly in relation to "mind-body" awareness. When students come to you and leave, the teacher may feel a strong sense of loss. This is a loss of opportunity to learn about Tai Chi, to make a connection with them, for them to make a connection with themselves, with their body, to discover or re-discover the power of the mind and receive knowledge to enhance their health. This sort of knowledge takes quite a bit longer – as teachers we know that but if we can't make the right connection with them in those early days our chances of holding them will be minimal. If you are expecting your students to stay with you – you need to find out why they are coming and more specifically what they their needs are.

It is therefore essential for the teacher to find this out very early in the relationship. You can rely on your memory if you have people skills, or you can keep a little card system where the student actually states their reasons for attending. Creating an early knowledge and understanding of the student's needs and goals is a great advantage for the teacher and has excellent beneficial outcomes for all students. Reviewing needs and goals is also very worthwhile in the medium to longer term.

For many of us teaching TCH, our lessons take the same format – greetings, warm-up, revision, learn something new, cool-down, be positive, be encouraging, have fun. But it is often the subtleties that make people feel comfortable or uncomfortable. If you are able to create a teaching environment that is not only welcoming and friendly, but also accepting, if you can teach in a generalised manner that treats everyone equally and with respect, and if you can develop of sense of humour and optimism, people will want to be there. Tai Chi should be pleasant, friendly, and non-threatening at a personal level. You need to create an environment that is a pleasant experience where people feel happy and want to be there. It follows that if they want to be there, they will get to know other people in a socially non-threatening, uplifting and positive environment. You will then have the opportunity to share what you have to offer.

We need students to periodically recognise that they have learned something new, to have made a change, through a review process of reflecting back. We need to confirm with the student that they must continue to take personal responsibility in maintaining or improving their health. They have a part to play, as we have a part to play in teaching, not only the form, principles but about the "mind-body" connections and how that relates to personal development and health improvement. We have to constantly maintain that relationship of connection.

From the first lesson you can give them the personal responsibility to practise. You may need to have written guidelines in the beginning to help them learn more effectively – but that will soon pass as they begin to focus and begin to train to memorise as they train the body. If you notice that improvement, even without being obvious, this is very encouraging for a new student. Eye to eye contact with an accepting attitude is all that is often required for the student to feel encouraged.

The teaching skill of the TCH Instructor will be most evident in the efforts made by the students. When being tough was part of accepting criticism and correction, it was a necessary condition for effective martial conduct. In TCH, it is accepted and expected that simulated and real forms of assault for learning self defence purposes is not part of the curriculum. In a few Tai Chi schools, self-defence is the reason why students are learning. It is understandable in a violent world that some might be attracted to learning self defence through the intrinsic intelligence of Kung Fu Tai Chi Chuan as a martial art, than with some of the more physical, full contact forms of the Martial Arts where exceptional physicality is often a necessary prerequisite for success. It is important for any prospective student to understand, however, that many Tai Chi schools simply do not teach self-defence in any practical form. Some Kung Fu Martial Arts Instructors would claim that very few Tai Chi schools teach any form of martial arts or any form of self-defence. (see Zorya, 2006; and Montaigue, 2004)

A vital part of teaching TCH is for the TCH Instructor, however, is to understand that many students do not want to put themselves into confrontational situations of learning or even understanding the self-defence applications of Kung Fu Tai Chi Chuan. Feelings of making strikes and warding off blows are not conducive to happy and relaxed thoughts, especially for the beginner. For some students, however, it may be a revelation that Kung Fu Tai Chi Chuan, is a martial art and a few may express some interest in understanding the martial application or context. Understanding the "forces" involved" can make a huge difference to how a movement is co-ordinated and to how the form "feels", that is whether awkward or flowing. Some may find that the knowledge of the biomechanics of "forces" is very helpful to the quality of their teaching. The extent to how this should be managed by the TCH Instructor is dependent on the objectives of the TCH group itself and the teacher's understanding of forces and biomechanics of movement.

The central point for our purposes is that the TCH Instructor needs to ensure that all students are able to participate in a comfortable and relaxed environment. Minimising correction is an important part of effective teaching. Except for matters of safety and issues related to mutual respect within the class, there is not a place for "this is wrong" or "this is a better way" – which implies the first way was not acceptable. A teacher can always be positive about their students' efforts and gradually work towards improvement by teaching and demonstrating principles and encouraging practice. The TCH Instructor will find that the teaching will be truly effective if students understand that their Tai Chi is not something that should be compared with other students' levels of performance. What is important to develop is an understanding about the "mind-body" connections, a conscious reflection on what the body is doing at any point in time and to generate an enthusiasm for the continuing Tai Chi journey itself, and not the finish lines in the struggles and races of competitive egos.

We need to learn to focus not at an end result, but on the process or journey interrupted at periodic intervals where we are able to consciously reflect on a set of characteristics, principles, strategies that allow us to know we are on the right track, so that we might be more effective in our teaching role. Our students should have a degree of happiness, not necessarily happy-delirious, but happy and satisfied enough with their progress, happy in their relationship with you as their teacher, happy in the social environment you have created. They should achieve some skills with respect to the expectations of fitness and their improvement should be, but not necessarily always be visible. In other words they should exhibit some of the outcomes of good TCH teaching. The TCH Instructor will be able to see a difference or improvement and they will be able to know that it feels better. Knowing that "it feels better" is perhaps the single most important motivator for students continuing with their Tai Chi.

The success or otherwise of "mind-body" connections are most evident through the "show me" phase of the "1,2,3" method (Stepwise Progressive Method) in the teaching cycle of the TCH Instructor. The idea is to work towards achieving a level of independence from the teacher that will allow students to practise safely with a clear understanding of what they are doing, and allow them to strengthen and realign their Tai Chi form independent from the class environment. The TCH Instructor should teach in such a way that the student will be seeking more knowledge and more guidance from you as the TCH Instructor and finding that mental quietness and inner strength is at their fingertips. It might even come as a surprise!

It is the nature of human beings to yearn for freedom, equality and dignity. If we accept that others have a right to peace and happiness equal to our own, do we not have a responsibility to help those in need? ... When we do not know someone or do not feel connected to an individual or group, we tend to overlook their needs. Yet the development of human society requires that people help each other. (Dalai Lama, 2000)

1.30   PREPARATION OVERVIEW
    1.31   Class Structure
    1.32   Measuring Exercise Effort
    1.33   Movement That Matters

1.31   Class Structure

General - This section outlines three components to a Tai Chi Class
Warm-up, Conditioning and Cool Down

Warm-Up - The warm-up component is probably the most important part of any exercise class including Tai Chi. In fact, all exercise activities should have an adequate warm-up suitable for the exercise program involved in order to prepare the heart and the muscles for work. If the warm-up is inadequate the body will not be prepared for the activity and the risk of injury is increased. Use slow controlled breathing, visualisation and body awareness teaching techniques. Use phrases that will help the class to focus on the task, and away from problems they may be encountering in their daily lives. Cue participants to become more self-aware by using such phrases as: "Focus on lifting up through the top of the head and lengthen the spine" or "Allow your arms to float up". so that their focus can be directed to the task in a meaningful way. Once the participants have been trained, there may be no need for many words at all during this phase.

To begin, an opening section of smooth co-ordinated, controlled gentle movements will warm the body, calm and deepen the breathing and focus the mind. A walk around the room by everyone including the instructor perhaps enhanced with bright music is a greeting activity that promotes friendship and co-operation and is also a great way to start a class. Remember to walk in the opposite direction to your participants and make eye contact with everyone. This is the safest because it allows the instructor to check for signs that may suggest the student is unwell. It also gives the teacher the opportunity to greet every participant and is an excellent way to build confidence and trust. The walking around for a few minutes begins the preparation for the heart and circulatory systems to prepare for the work ahead.

Research highlights the importance of longer warm-up phase in an older adults class suggesting a Warm-up phase of 30% of a 60 minute class - about 18 minutes (Cisar & Kravitz, 1989) or 20 minutes (Myers & Gonda, 1986). Also keep in mind that 60% of adults have some type of visual dysfunction at age 55 (alone) which should affect how you design your program, how you cue and how you technically perform your work. If you add into this the statistics for Arthritis and other chronic diseases and longer warm-up period can easily be justified. Unfortunately, many people practising Tai Chi often do an inadequate warm-up for the condition of their bodies. If a long warm-up seems excessive, remember there are many excellent moves you can perform in the warm-up phase that can be of real value to participants. Movements from the form can be broken up into legs or arms with repetitions to help prepare the body and quieten the mind (see Training Exercises Unit 3.20). Learning to breathe gently with these exercises also helps to calm and focus.

The warm-ups for the various Tai Chi for Health programs including - Tai Chi for Arthritis, Back Pain, Diabetes, and Osteoporosis by Dr Paul Lam (see Tai Chi Productions 2009) and Tai Chi for Health & Falls Injury Prevention, Tai Chi for Health Heart and Qigong for Health & Fitness – 8 Form and 24 Bare Hand Mulan by Alice Liping Yuan (Exercise Medicine Australia, 2009) contain complete sets of gentle stretches for the major segments of the body – neck, shoulders, spine, hips, knees, ankles and hands. These sets (including Warm-ups see Unit 3.20) represent an ideal segment of the lesson to slowly introduce Tai Chi principles and concepts, and developing an awareness of "mind-body" connections. Specifically, the warm-ups allow time to focus the mind on body parts without the complication of moving away from the base of support where the focus is on balancing and controlling these movements. It also is an opportunity to discover what is a comfortable and safe level within which to work and move. Some students who no longer have to simply copy can be encouraged to develop the segment as a Qigong exercise, to concentrate on breathing as a stand-alone exercise.

One of the main outcomes of the Warm-up phase in Tai Chi is that it sets the focus and quietens down the thinking processes of many students who find it difficult to stop thinking about daily matters. This does not mean that the mind becomes dull – in fact the complete opposite. "Clear the Mind" does not really mean think about nothing but it sets the focus by "listening" to the body breath. It can be is a real bonus for the beginning student discovering the bliss of the warm-ups. Many advanced students can instantly go into this quiet place and begin the process of preparing the body for meaningful work.

When students are developing their strengths and have already gained good techniques, balance and control, these warm-ups can be lengthened to include other exercises and drills to extend the warm-up phase of the lesson and better prepare the student for their work (see Unit 3.20).

Conditioning - Beginners will always need an aerobic phase of at least 20 to 30 minutes – ideally every day. These people need to build their aerobic fitness and will do so with encouragement and guidance. With consistent attendance and practice they will be increasing the time they are able to move continuously and thereby increase their endurance. A review of 31 controlled experimental studies and clinical trials (Li et al, 2001) shows that people who attend Tai Chi regularly can expect and aerobic uptake of around 55%. This level of endurance equates to a brisk walk. In addition these studies also show Tai Chi is beneficial to immune capacity, mental control, flexibility, balance control, improves muscle strength and reduces the risk of falls in the elderly.

People who are practising Tai Chi with chronic pain may need to rest every 10 or 15 minutes or even more frequently when they first start class. A recent study (Song et al, 2003), shows that within a relatively short period of time people with chronic pain will be able to participate for longer and longer periods with less pain of up to 30%. The focus helps to distract from the pain, but more importantly over a period of time, they will build up strength and conditioning and improve functional fitness and quality of life.

The conditioning phase of a Tai Chi class is the main section of the lesson. Tai Chi gives an aerobic conditioning that is better obtained through evenly paced work. To maximise the aerobic conditioning it is better to choose a level (of knee bend) to work within and try to keep that level throughout. Finding the comfortable level, which is just under "the edge" is in itself a challenge. By keeping the arm and leg movements smooth and flowing and even with regard to the amount of muscle recruitment used, the heart will beat at an even pace and will of course be more than when the student is standing around or moving spasmodically. This is why it is proper technique to lower and close slowly after a complete set and to either walk around gently and continuously before starting again or begin a repeat immediately. This extends the aerobic outcome and helps to build stamina. Improving aerobic conditioning or" endurance" or" fitness" can be achieved readily and easily by repeating the forms in succession.

Seniors can obtain cardio-respiratory benefits from as low as 30% Maximum Heart Rate. Thirty minutes per day spread over 3, ten minute periods, has been shown to have benefits including improved insulin and lipid levels. Feeling better also lifts mood and confidence and quality of life. When the physical activity has to be broken down in such a way the warm-ups alone using the techniques outlined in the principles and concepts of Tai Chi would have a beneficial effect of health. Considering this type of exercise is gentle, flowing and relatively easy to do, it can be done to music, and it can be thought of something pleasant to do and enjoyable rather than something that HAS to be done to stay well. Moving regularly and consistently should not only enhance mood but should also have a positive effect on appetite and sleep.

Cool Down - This section deals with bringing the body back to homeostasis and is achieved by gentle stretches, letting go of tension and deep abdominal breathing. The cool-down will facilitate a safer change from active work to the completion of the class and signal a return to normal activities. Normally this section takes about 5 to 6 minutes and when it is performed in a circle is a pleasant and unifying "close" to the class followed by the "Tai Chi for Health Salute" (see Unit 3.21).

1.32   Measuring Exercise Effort - In exercise prescription, the classical method of prescribing intensity has been heart rate. To improve fitness, an exercise heart rate for older persons of, say, 50 - 60% of maximum (usually determined as 220 minus the age of the participant) is used. But despite its usefulness in the past, using heart rate as a measure of exercise effort may be problematic and is now outdated and unnecessary. One reason cited for this is the complication of medications. In fact, even in the fitness industry most trainers no longer use this method as it is not as effective as participants setting their own comfortable levels and progressing with guidance from the trainer. Practising Tai Chi is an excellent training for the student to learn how to recognise and read the body and to take personal responsibility on how to work safely.

Using the classic Heart Rate formula has run into difficulty because:
- Maximum heart Rate (M.H.R.) decreases with age
- Heart rates are affected by medications
- There is often inaccuracy in reporting
- Heart rates can vary between different types of exercise

For these reasons and others, the Rate of Perceived Exertion (RPE) scale was developed by Swedish Exercise Physiologist, Gunner Borg (1982). RPE involves asking a person to rate how intense an activity is on a scale of 1 to 20 and structuring an exercise program around that intensity.

RPE can be used to assess a person's perception of effort, or to enable him or her to produce a level of effort for a desired result. In other words, the scale (1-20) can be used to find out the individual reaction to an exercise load. For someone who is unfit, walking up stairs may rate a 13; for a fit person this may only be a 7. It can also be used to get different individuals to work at the appropriate intensity for their level of fitness, to increase or decrease their working load for benefit and safety.

However it can be far more accurate to teach the person how to relate to the body, how to feel when work is too hard, how to pull back to a level which causes no distress, how to adjust to the level of exertion on a day to day basis, and how to work just under the "edge" and gradually increase their capacity when they are stronger or when they feel like it.   In Tai Chi RPE can be used to give a beginning student an idea of working at a comfortable level. Any method that helps a person new to exercise or someone who is trying a new type of exercise needs to understand and know where they should work and not work where they think they should be working.

In a Tai Chi for Health class it is expected that all participants work at a level in which they feel comfortable on that day and learn to read the body, pull back and make adjustments when needed.

1.33   Movement that matters - This concept encourages moves, which are specific to real-life situations and is particularly relevant to students with some loss of function or people who are de-conditioned through illness or inactivity. These types of exercises are known as "movement that matters" or functional fitness and can certainly be discussed before the beginning of a term and at the end of a block of lessons. Pointing out to students their improvements with normal, necessary every day tasks can improve their confidence and sense of achievement. Instead of watching themselves decline, it is a very pleasant realisation to see actual improvements – some of which can be significant.

Listed below are some of the daily activities that Tai Chi could improve:
- Reaching for the seat belt
- Backing out of the garage
- Rising from a chair
- Combing hair
- Reaching to back of collar
- Fixing a twisted belt
- Doing up a zip or bra
- Being able to reach for groceries from the shelf
- Putting on stockings or socks
- Walking backwards
- Being able to change direction
- Toe clearance
- Stepping backwards or sideways
- Looking over the shoulder
- Turning a tap
- Getting in or out of a car
- Looking behind
- Reaching up
- Shaking a tablecloth
- Lifting a bucket
- {A punch or a kick that will count}
- Balancing
- Reaction time or readiness.................and many more

1.40   TECHNIQUES OF TEACHING OVERVIEW
      1.41   Introduction
      1.42   Teaching Methods
      1.43   Teaching Image
      1.44   Teaching Positions
      1.45   Constructive Caring
      1.46   Cueing

1.41   Introduction - Techniques are the "Tools of Trade" for teachers of movement. Teaching Tai Chi is at the very basic level the delivery of physical exercise but is of course much more. Recent developments of pioneers of Tai Chi for Health such as Dr Paul Lam (see Tai Chi Productions, 2009) and Alice Liping Yuan & Henry Zheng (see Exercise Medicine Australia, 2009) in Australia have revolutionised the exchange of information from teacher to student in the Tai Chi for Health world. This willingness to open up knowledge by simplifying information with a very solid foundation enables the non-traditional teacher to deliver Tai Chi safely and effectively to a much wider audience than at any time in the history of Tai Chi.

Techniques are short-cuts. In a modern teaching setting these snippets of teaching techniques considerably diminish the time it usually takes to learn the complex art of Tai Chi using the more traditional methods of slow conceptualisation and understanding through contemplation and introspection.   Some of the more complex techniques do take a long time for some people to grasp (such as acquiring a quiet mind), but if practising Tai Chi is seen as a "work in progress ', a changing evolving body with many facets of input, having time to absorb and reflect and connect is something that is often difficult for the beginner. Having short-cuts to the learning process is not only ideal for many people but some would say necessary in modern society. Many people have said Tai Chi is a journey and so it is. Being able to learn the pattern, understand the basic principles of movement and balance, and having an awareness of the mind working with the body means that more and more people (many of whom may have serious health concerns can receive some if not most of the health benefits attributed to Tai Chi. Making Tai Chi accessible means that many people can have a more healthful life – as well as those who practise Tai Chi for other purposes (such as a martial art, self defence, competition, longevity and an art form).

Having techniques for teaching aims to provide a resource for easy and considered learning for the student. A modern approach to how people learn has been to discover that people learn in very different ways. Learning Theory teaches that there are many different ways that people learn. For example, some students learn quickly and others are painfully slow. A quick learner usually means a good brain but a slow learner does not always mean poor brain function. Experienced teachers understand that some people respond to visual cues efficiently. They can copy not only movements but the nuances of movement such as weight change, rhythm, alignment, balance and connectedness in a highly co-ordinated and accurate manner. Others respond to aural cueing in particular. Some people respond better by studying the written work and committing it to memory, (because they are used to learning that way) mapping out all the directions and co-ordinations mentally before putting the body into action. Even once people have learned the basic shape of the movements, being able to understand the principles of movement is not the same for everyone. Being versatile in how concepts can be explained is one of those tools, which is a valuable asset to teaching. Here the emphasis is being able to put the principles and concepts of Tai Chi for Health into a language that is clear and meaningful.

Often people who are "slow learners" are great analysers. They recognise a lot of detail and are overwhelmed by the volume of information they are seeing and try to process it accurately and exactly and immediately. They are unable to filter off cues and are absolutely aware of a lot of information at the same time. Others have a very high standard they expect to attain (sometimes immediately also). They are disappointed and annoyed that they cannot replicate the movements and skill of the teacher. This is one of the lessons of Tai Chi – we have to crawl before we can walk. Above all, we learn patience. Not expecting perfection is a great asset not only for the student but also for a teacher. Many teachers do realise that their role in the class with Tai Chi is all about the journey of the student. How they learn, and how they do their Tai Chi (as long as it is safe) is surely the right of the student. The skill of the instructor will draw out the very best from the student and it is the role of the Instructor to find an easy way for each student to learn and have a happy experience when they are learning and discovering Tai Chi. It should not be a painful, frustrating or embarrassing experience for anyone.

Only allowing the "normal" way to learn, that is by memorising and copying, is taking a somewhat rigid view as to "how people learn". Many modern Tai Chi teachers make it a practice not to give hand outs of written material for beginning students. The rationale is that they have to learn to commit to memory and not rely on the teacher. This is certainly true for students who have already learned the shape of the set and applied some of the principles. They should be able to use their mind to control their movement and energy levels. But what does it matter how students learn in the beginning – as long as they learn and you can pass on information to help them (in their journey). Sometimes people have no awareness of feeling body parts. They cannot even begin to connect the cognitive brain to parts of their body like where their hand is placed, let alone being able to memorise movement patterns for balance, stability and alignment. However, if they can take some written word home it is often enough to start the thinking and analysing processes. After a few years (or less) generally people settle down and become not only competent but strong and confident and do not require such coaxing and encouragement. Improvements in their health is encouragement enough.

1.42 Teaching Methods - One of the most useful methods of teaching Tai Chi efficiently and safely is Dr Lam's Stepwise Progressive Method (see Lam, 2006a). He uses a method used in many disciplines for teaching movement, but he has tailored it especially for teaching Tai Chi. This method involves three phases: Watch Me, Follow Me and Show Me. The "Show Me" phase is a valuable asset in teaching because it allows the student the opportunity to practice independently from the teacher and to be able practise alone much sooner.

Other advantages of the Stepwise Progressive Method are:
• The student has the opportunity to learn and consolidate by repetition, which is the most successful method of keeping information. In schools it is called Rote Learning.
• It enables the teacher to pace the introduction of new work suitable to the students' ability and memory.
• It gives the students confidence and a sense of achievement
• It allows the teacher to adequately observe and correct for safety
• It is efficient in the long term

The Stepwise Progressive Method incorporates sectional or separate practice for hands and legs as an important tool for teaching difficult moves. To illustrate the importance of this tool, a student who learns piano will use "sectional practice" when learning a new or difficult section. This involves learning the hands separately and thoroughly, then putting them together. This method for Tai Chi usually means fewer "mistakes" and is more efficient than learning upper and lower body together. In teaching Tai Chi, this can be a useful method for teaching difficult forms. Waving Hands in the Cloud for example and Deflect Downwards to Parry, Parry and Punch can be easier to teach in this way because the movements are highly co-ordinated. Focussing on either the legs or the arms means that all the attention is directed to one segment of the body. There is less distraction trying to control other parts of the body and the student is able to focus better, build better neural pathways and consolidate quicker. With sectional practice students usually feel less frustrated and more capable.

The traditional way of teaching Tai Chi is the Follow and Copy Method where the form is practised with the teacher leading the students with his/her back to the students who are simply copying every movement without any form of direct instruction from the teacher. This method has no place in a modern Tai Chi for Health class without some form of supervision as it does not address a modern Duty of Care and relies on the rationale of a Discovery Learning Method. Turning the back to the students is not in the best interests of safety unless the teacher is able to delegate this role while watching the performance which is being modelled by competent students or assistant teachers. This scenario thus combines the Follow Me and Watch Me phases into an effective strategy to facilitate direct instruction for safety and corrections of the form.

Many teachers of Tai Chi are resistant to modern methods of teaching, such as cueing, mirror image teaching, which requires the teacher to face the students and maintain a visual connection. Some Tai Chi teachers might claim that the Follow and Copy Method with the teacher facing away from the class has been the long honoured way as part of the traditional approach to teaching. However, we now live in a modern society where people are much better informed about their legal rights to have no harm done to them by a service provider and will be more likely to litigate for negligence. With the teacher not keeping an eye on the students there is a significantly increased element of risk of injury. Considering that a complete set may take some minutes, and considering that many of our health and fitness professionals are taking on people in ill health and chronic conditions as students, physical changes can occur in a few seconds.

In addition, the traditional Follow and Copy Method relies on the rationale of the Discovery Learning Method which allows the student to feel and to discover for themselves what is happening to their body and this happens without direct instruction or correction. As students practise over lengthy periods of time, sometimes over months and years, there may eventually be some form of awakening and discovery. Here students are left to their own insights to discover the need for changes and modification, for example, to discover that alignment might need correcting or some modification required after an insight on the part of the student that their knees joints are constantly sore and irritated after practising Tai Chi. It is posited by advocates of the Discovery Learning Method that students are more likely to remember concepts if they discover on their own than by direct instruction from the teacher. Not only is this akin to "re-inventing the wheel", but there is no empirical evidence to support this claim, quite the contrary in fact. Kirschner et al (2006) suggest that fifty years of empirical data does not support those using unguided instructional methods of Discovery Learning. They call for those using these techniques to explain their actions in terms of empirical data. Moreover, some educators have produced evidence that Discovery Learning is a less effective instructional strategy for novices than direct instruction (Tuovinen and Sweller, 1999). While Discovery Learning is very popular, it is suggested that it is often used inappropriately to teach novices (Kirschner et al, 2006). Learners should be given some direct instruction first, and then later be allowed to apply what they have learned.

1.43   Teaching Image - Teaching Image is the direction an instructor faces in relation to the participants. The complexity of deciding different tools and techniques for different circumstances means that a teacher needs to have several teaching image choices to use in any one class situation.

(a)   **Mirror Image** is where you face the participants and use opposite moves to them. At the same time you cue them to do the opposite to what you are doing. This is of course cueing them to do what they will be doing next. If you begin with a L STEP to the side, they will do a R STEP. You also need to verbally cue them (opposite to what you are doing). This means when you are stepping out to the L you are saying "R foot ready". If people have good vision, there is no need to say "right foot" – just "get ready". To indicate which leg will become full stance on the "sink", the instructor can briefly pat the supporting leg to indicate the side where the sinking will occur. This is very simple and very efficient.

This way of teaching certainly does take some time to become competent. The best way is to look at a student and know that you want them to step to the R – so tell them to – "Get ready to step to the right". You then look at their foot and put your L foot out to match – after you have made the verbal cue. It will only be a fraction of a second behind and is about the same time as it takes them to hear you, process it and begin the action. You don't have to tell them every step of the way "right" or "left". This is where consistent use of cue words come into force – "get ready", "travel", "balance" and so on. Mirror teaching is a little bit like massage where the masseur's hand should never leave the body even to change actions. Mirror Image keeps the connection with the student and helps to hold the focus.

(b)   **Reverse Image** is where you have your back to the class, use the same leg and travel in the same direction. This is commonly known as the "Follow Copy Method".

(c)   **Combination Image** is a mixture of both mirror and reverse image within the one segment eg. Showing front view and back view – "watch me".

(d)   **Participant Image** is where you mix with them as a participant - in a circle, or actually with them in the class while some one else leads out the front. Note: All teachers should work towards being thoroughly proficient at Mirror Image because it allows the teacher to
- look at the participants and be safe
- watch for strain or difficulty with moves, changes in colour or expression
- motivate with your face and achieve better verbal acuity and clarity
- make a connection with your students
- keep yourself focussed on the group (and not away with the fairies on your own journey!)

After they have learned the new work, you can step to the side and get right out of the picture altogether. If you are happy with the level of competency, you may decide to teach a new section next lesson. If not, you can still be happy for their effort and teach it again next lesson without saying anything. Many people will be grateful. If there are students who have grasped the new work, they can focus on a principle.

1.44   Teaching Positions - The highest priority apart from program design is good visibility, which means –
- Instructor must be able to see all participants
- Participants must be able to see instructor

This will make an immediate connection with everyone on the floor and is most important when teaching movement and especially so with Tai Chi because some people will be able to pick up more knowledge than others. Everyone should have equal opportunity to learn (and see) at their own pace.
Your teaching position will depend on the class format.

CLASS FORMATION - There is some choice in this. Teaching in front of the class does not have to mean taking the central place in the middle. Consider the following (thanks to Judy Morwood, Brisbane):

1.   LINE FORMATION

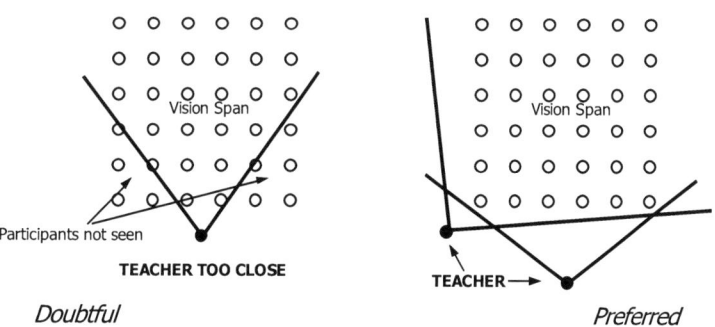

2.   CIRCLE FORMATION

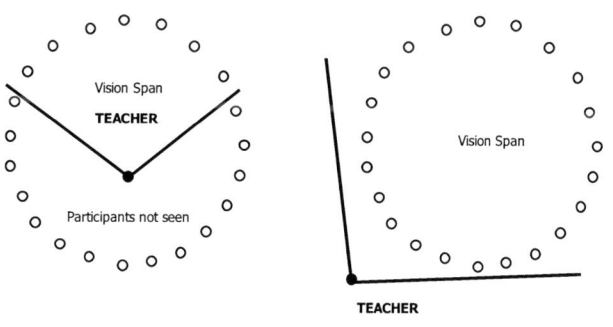

3.   FREE SPACING OR PIGEON HOLES

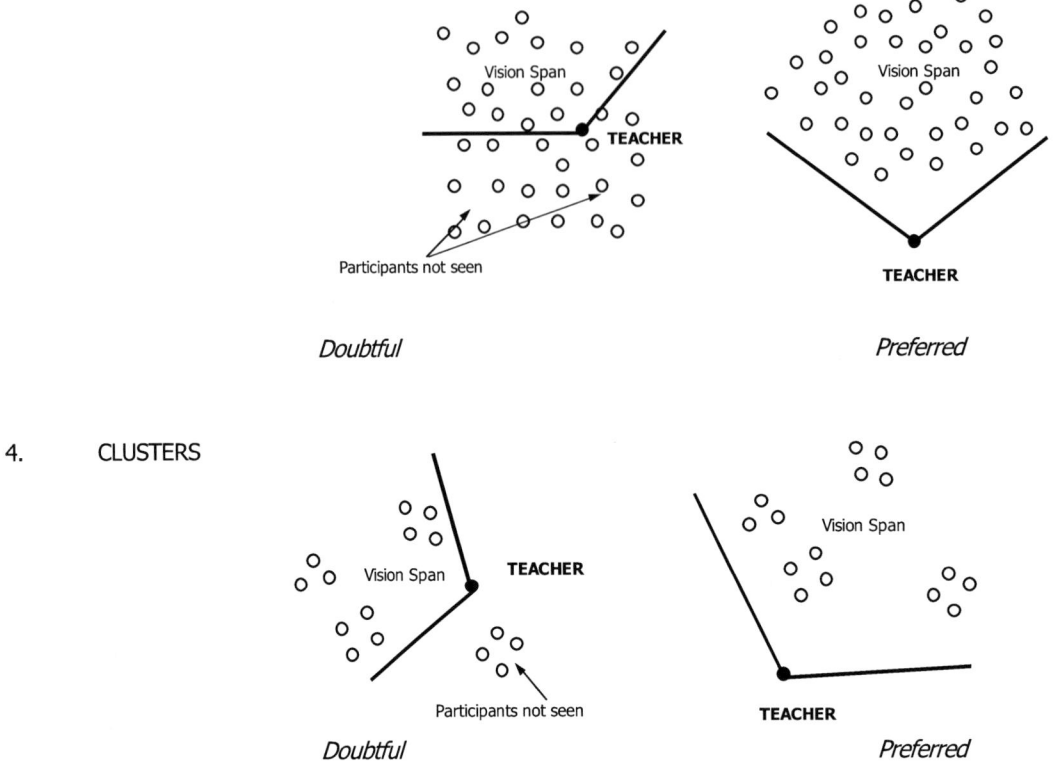

Doubtful   *Preferred*

4.   CLUSTERS

Doubtful   *Preferred*

1.45   Constructive Caring - Tai Chi instructors will inevitably have contact with persons who have been excluded from other forms of exercise not because they have some life threatening illness but because they have had some difficulty with communication such as hearing or visual impairment. Some might have a congenital disability, but others may have developed a disability through disease or accident and others may be in rehabilitation.

How can we assist these people in the communication process and allowing them experience a group class or session in general class? We can help them with "Constructive Caring" which can be summed up by - "Help the person to help herself or himself". As a general guide, if a person has a disability:

- Resist the temptation to do everything for the person concerned. They already will have a health or medical clearance to attend and need to participate at their own level.
- When frustration occurs, offer assistance if appropriate and avoid completing the task through impatience. Encourage the person to finish it and have some dignity and accomplishment. In fact just being a participant in the class in a normal way can be a wonderful experience.
- Encourage safety and discourage over-protectiveness.
- Relate to the person as you would to any one and don't single them out as being different. They will know the difference and appreciate it.
- Allow time for the person to talk about how they are feeling and allow emotion to show and be accepting of this by not being dismissive but not prolonging it either.

Most importantly, follow your instinct. Think carefully before you utter words which may be far from appropriate or even offensive. Ask yourself, "If I experienced some disabling illness, how would I want people to relate to me? How would I like them to offer me assistance?"

Be aware that sometimes people communicate their attitudes and emotions by means other than speech, for example eye contact, facial expression, body posture or gesture. Our unspoken body language confers an immediate response and is often easier to understand than our spoken words. It is therefore not surprising that many people with hearing impairment attend Tai Chi classes with great success.

A common problem for elderly people is failing eyesight and/or gradual loss of hearing. In hearing loss, usually high frequency sounds such as bells ringing are lost first but progressively the lower speech frequencies become affected and the person has difficulty hearing people talking. This is especially so in crowded places but a Tai Chi for Health class will not have this frustration. Some participants with considerable hearing impairment remove their hearing aid during a class and rely totally on the communication with the instructor for their performance cues. An Instructor who is proficient in verbal and visual cueing is a great advantage for the hearing impaired.

For those who do wear a hearing aid, some orchestrations and background noise becomes very irritating. If participants show signs of frustration ask them about the music or volume and attempt to rectify it on the spot. Do not wait till the conclusion of the lesson. Mostly Tai Chi music is so soft it does not cause a problem for the hearing impaired because they don't hear it at all.

In communicating with people with mild to moderate hearing loss don't shout, speak slowly and clearly, sit or stand at the same level, don't turn your head away as you speak. Don't give eye signals to others nearby indicating you're inability to be a successful communicator. Not only is this "bad form" but is insulting to that person. Try to position them close to the front if they feel comfortable. The nature of a gentle Tai Chi for Health class will automatically draw to it persons who have communication impairment.

People with loss of vision need not be excluded from Tai Chi. However, for safety reasons several points need careful consideration:
- As the Instructor, you will need to know the sort of vision loss, for example, if images are blurred, if the person has tunnel vision, if the person has peripheral vision, if the person has no vision. Many people who have limited vision also have problems with balance. Vision impaired people need extra precautions for movement because they do not have the visual cues or the proprioceptive cues that a sighted person has to aid balance and knowing their place in the world around them.
- For safety, all visually impaired people need to consider working in the chair to learn and consolidate some of the work. Much work can be done on a chair such as is part of the Tai Chi for Back Pain program (Tai Chi Productions, 2009) and the Tai Chi for Health & Falls Prevention program (Exercise Medicine Australia, 2009). However, standing work with visually impaired people is still possible though not without special techniques and training. Broadly speaking, these people learn their forms by holding onto another person and mirroring their movements and weight change. Visually impaired people are very sensitive to movement and movement change and they usually have a high level of focus and sensitivity. At first they stand behind their guiding person, holding on with both hands around the waist. Later they stand beside them holding onto their shoulder. This is not the sort of work that is done in a normal class situation – but it is clearly possible on a one to one basis. Keep in mind that the TCA form Advanced 6 Movements can be done very successfully straight ahead instead of turning.

1.46 Cueing - Cueing are clues for the student to train the memory. Often teachers cue too much and for too long, which means the students never get to think for themselves or they tune out altogether. Not to cue at all is at the other end of the continuum and is not helpful for students starting Tai Chi for the first time. Beginner's minds are often cluttered and jumping all over the place. Cueing beginners, tells them what to think and when to think. A lot of teachers make the assumption that people should be able to do this straight away, but this is not the case. If chronic pain, depression, lack of confidence etc are added into the equation it is even more reason that people need some guidance for how to think to do movement. Having a quiet, ordered, disciplined mind when you start Tai Chi is not the norm. Cueing can be one of those short cuts that greatly assist with learning. It is not a matter of indiscriminately calling out a verbal cue to assist the student but a highly useful tool that relies on experience to be truly successful. The Instructor has to read the non-verbal cues to see what is needed and sometimes the teacher is mistaken in this interpretation.

Cueing should be timed so that the utterance is made just before the action is required. But it should not be used every time and should decrease as the amount of repetition increases. By the time the student is showing the move independently of the teacher no cues should be necessary. Good cueing techniques are vital so that class participants can follow directions and perform without mishap or confusion.

Cueing is a skill that everyone can improve. Even very experienced instructors can often find ways to enhance their cueing. Sometimes a class can be well prepared and managed and planned, music choice is excellent, timing perfect but the class doesn't gel - because the cueing has been inadequate. In time the only cueing going on in a Tai Chi class are the non-verbal cues and communication between student and teacher – hopefully smiles all round.

If an instructor's cueing is inadequate or overbearing:
- frustration increases
- stress increases
- enjoyment decreases
- motivation decreases
- enthusiasm decreases
- effectiveness decreases

Cueing can be neatly slotted into two categories - verbal and visual.

Verbal Cues – One of the most important things to remember with verbal cueing the concept of the **Reference Point (RP).** Make sure to introduce and highlight this concept to the student early for the sake of consistency.

The RP is the starting point of each section for practising. The end of the previous section will most often become the RP for commencing a new section (see Unit 3.15 for example of RP).

Be consistent with such movement cues such as:
- Begin
- Get ready
- Travel
- Balance

These are working cues for control of movement flow

Also be consistent with such concept words such as:
- Float
- Sit on the perch
- Feather Touch
- Sink

Always cue "just" before the action. It is too late to cue once the movement has started. The whole idea of cueing is to let the participants know what is coming up and to give a memory cue for them to activate themselves. In time your input with verbal cueing should be unnecessary. As you become more experienced, it is the non-verbal cue, which for many take on the greater significance and has the most value. It is also important to know that not all students are "aural "in their learning capacities. Some students may "hear, but appear to not be listening". They may be so busy trying using other learning strategies.

Visual Cues - The visual cueing of the instructor is for many the main focus. (This is why it is so important that every participant can see you and you can see them). These are non-verbal cues. The music might be familiar, or at least pleasurable, there might be an awareness of who is standing beside them, there might be an awareness of being hot or tired – but the main focus will be on looking at the instructor. When the focus is on the teacher, it is therefore of some importance that the teacher is groomed and has a pleasant and welcoming expression. The appearance of the teacher has a lasting impression on the student. He or she is the focal point when the student reflects on what the form looked like when they go home. Visual cues are delivered through facial expression and body language. Also many students "may be looking but do not see" and do not make the adjustments through visual cueing or copying because they have not yet processed the information.

Facial Expression - aids motivation, make eye contact, smile, nod head

Body Language - can lift the mood of the class and make a lot of fun- or the opposite.

Props - Some people might benefit from using a balloon to learn to feel the concept of the resistance. Older people could use a large woollen pom-pom to feel how to hold the ball, or "turn the waist". Generally, props are not required for Tai Chi. Having a piece of golden thread to remind them about being "held up", pressing the head towards the ceiling is a powerful metaphor. Children also respond well to props, for example, dropping a feather to the floor can demonstrate empty stance very well.

Participant Cues - WHAT SORT OF cues do participants give the instructor?
- facial expression
- skin colour or pallor
- sighing
- gasping
- frowning
- slumping shoulders
- talking
- gestures

Cues are two way processes. Even when verbal cues are no longer required, when the class is able to self cue, then eventually perform their Tai Chi "on auto pilot" being able to focus on one thing to improve – cues still happen. Students learn to cue from their nearby fellow students and they wait for the approval from the teacher when they are finished. Giving them something to improve if it is offered very lightly as a suggestion rather than a fault is a wonderful way to motivate the very willing and enthusiastic student. It is not the role of the teacher to find fault and correct ad infinitum but rather to bring out the person into their Tai Chi and see where it goes.

Student cueing with teacher following: After students have some familiarity with the choreography or principles, the teacher can challenge students (not all students feel comfortable with this straight off). The challenge is to encourage each student within the group to verbalise "what comes next" using whatever cueing words have been agreed upon by the group. Where the movements have been broken into "numbers", with each number representing a transitional RP, the student can verbalise what should be happening. This method greatly accelerates the memorising of the movement, but is not for the student who only likes to follow, in particular, the "Inflexible student" (see Unit 1.83).

1.50   IMAGERY & CONCEPTS OVERVIEW
   1.51   Introduction
   1.52   Visual and Verbal – Picture & 1000 Words
   1.53   Body Analysis - Biomechanics of Movement
   1.54   The Traditional - Martial Imagery
   1.55   The Modern – Imagery & Imagination

1.51   Introduction - One of the techniques central to the effectiveness of Tai Chi for Health (TCH) is "concept imagery". While Tai Chi is viewed by some as a martial art, the reality is in the modern age there are many students who commence Tai Chi who do so exclusively for health and fitness reasons and who do not wish to engage in "martial", "combat", or violent forms of imagery as part of the learning process. We need to respect and understand those wishes by these students and through the special training of the TCH Instructor using appropriate "concept imagery", this should not present any problem. The idea of "concept imagery" simply put, is to find some constructive way to help the student "make the right connections" by finding the appropriate metaphor, verbal and/or visual, for the student in front of you, a metaphor that assists the student in trying to remember how to move and co-ordinate the body and most importantly, a metaphor coupled with encouraging the student to use the "mind" as a key part of the learning strategy. The "mind" will only be receptive if the metaphor is understandable, accessible and culturally acceptable. Culture, gender, social class, age, legal and ethical principles are all variables which need to be factored into the process of finding the appropriate "metaphor". While knowledge of the "martial" metaphor may be of some value to some students in the learning process, this knowledge is not a prerequisite for the delivery of the Tai Chi for Health program as a highly effective form of exercise for all people in a modern age.

Teachers need to be mindful that many parts of the brain play a part in movement such as fine motor control, gross motor control, balance, muscular response to stimuli, monitoring of glucose levels and carbon-dioxide levels, calcium and hormones, vision, memory, co-ordination and many others. Some of the neurones in the body have more than 100,000 connections to other neurones and may be as long as 1.37 meters (as in the motor neurones from the spine to the big toe). How neurones connect is unique in every person. The massive complexity of making a movement is therefore uniquely wired resulting in a unique action. For this reason a teacher expecting uniformity in a class is an unreal expectation. This is why it is so very important for students to have permission to do their Tai Chi in their own comfortable way under the informed guidance of a competent caring and accepting teacher.

Some teachers feel that new students should learn the shape of the movements first. That is, they learn the routine of the forms (12 Form Sun Style, 24 Form Yang Style). Then they begin to learn Tai Chi. Perhaps under ideal conditions, if the teacher encourages upright posture from the beginning, explains about "comfort" and gentle and relaxed breathing and continuous movement when they are learning the forms – slowly little piece by little piece – the student will be exposed to the many health benefits of Tai Chi long before they formally learn and apply the principles themselves in the form.

The beginning student does not have to know the principles and how they work for Tai Chi to benefit their body from the first lesson. In fact, the idea of the KISS principle ("keep it simple, sweetheart) minimising the knowledge component of teaching has a much better result for the motivation and encouragement of the student than those who are overwhelmed and confused and misled by too much information and detail too soon.

1.52   Visual and Verbal – Picture & 1000 Words - We live in an age where international influences of the "visual" sign are being increasingly used to transcend the limitations of a culturally specific language. Many of the road signs, safety signs, signs for direction, toilets, accommodation and the colour codes of traffic lights are based on cross-cultural conventions that enable the international traveller to navigate the hazards of unfamiliar territory. These "visual" signs are translated back into the culturally specific language of the reader of the sign to make sense of and navigate the unfamiliar terrain. These particular forms of "concept imagery" are not only for international travel but of course also function within any particular cultural and language group.

What we are looking to understand here is the semiotic relationship between the "visual" sign and the "verbal" words within any particular language group and how meaning, purpose and intention are derived from this relationship. This semiotic relationship can be simply termed – "concept imagery" where words in themselves function as signs in their own right generating a "visual" image of the word or cultural concept. In this regard, "concept imagery" within Tai Chi for Health facilitates a communication process whereby the TCH Instructor is more efficiently able to assist students to effectively navigate their way through the unfamiliar, seemingly simple forms of slow controlled movements of a Tai Chi for Health exercise program for the purposes of health improvement.

In Unit 3.10, we discuss the context of Tai Chi knowledge relating to "yin-yang" theory the contemporary social science of semiotics. Semiotics like "yin-yang" theory is well positioned to facilitate a greater understanding of the relationship between "things" or "signs" that involve "verbal" and "visual" metaphors, which combine into the idea of "concept imagery". Simply put, this semiotic relationship between the "visual and verbal" is best characterised by the well-known expression of "a picture is worth a thousand words". The discipline of "semiotics" identifies the communicative power of "concept imagery" in terms of "word objects" and "visual objects" – where words can be converted into visual objects or images and vice versa. The TCH Instructor does not need to become an expert in semiotics, however, but does need to understand that the Eastern philosophy of "yin-yang" theory has its equivalent in contemporary scientific forms of knowledge where empirical based evidence and logical forms of reasoning are the base-line for a modern approach to a Tai Chi for Health.

Before we address "concept imagery" in more specific terms, we need to challenge the claim made by the Confucian approach to Tai Chi as a Martial Art [2] which suggests that martial "concept imagery" is the only legitimate form to be used in the delivery of the Tai Chi for Health exercise program, that choreographed sequences and the principles of biomechanics and functional movement can only be explained in martial concepts. If we accept that the main purpose of Tai Chi for Health is not to facilitate martial and combative prowess, but is to exercise and to enhance health, fitness and well being, then we are free to disengage from the Confucian claim. In other words, the TCH Instructor is not limited to martial imagery of any specific Chinese martial art, but is essentially free to examine and utilise alternative ways of expressing "intention" of movement and exercise as part of the modern approach to the Tai Chi for Health activity. For the enterprising TCH Instructor, the limiting factor in the use of "concept imagery" that can be brought to bear to enhance and facilitate the transmission of knowledge is the imagination itself facilitated by a semiotic or "yin-yang" understanding of "concept imagery".

1.53   Body Analysis - Biomechanics of Movement

"We look but do not see, we hear but do not listen.
Our conscious mind is focussed on nothing and everything" Anon

The modern Tai Chi for Health Instructor is a teacher of movement, and as such needs to have a reasonable knowledge of "Body Analysis" of posture and movement and how this relates to "concept imagery" as an important strategy in the effective teaching of movement. Teachers of any form of human movement (whether dance, Tai Chi or sport) who require the student to only "follow me" thus do not utilise skills of "Body Analysis" as they do not find the need to explain, describe and communicate their actions and performance. Regardless of any particular teaching style, all students, however, are actively engaged in the process of observing movements either from their own teacher, or from DVDs or books, in order to study the detail of movement of the various forms and postures. The technique of observing structure and detail is a learned skill and therefore can be accessible to all teachers who are interested in a modern and efficient ways of teaching. Through a strategic and informed approach to teaching using "Body Analysis" as the "concept imagery", the student will greatly benefit through this teaching/learning approach. How the student responds or "picks up" on the detail always relates to practise, to experience derived from focussed practice. The more the focus is on using the conscious mind to look, see and analyse through acceptable forms of concept imagery that relate to the physical body, the more effective will be that practice.

Each of the body parts or components relates in some way to the whole body – the posture, the placement of the arms and hands and fingers, the amount of knee bend, the placement of the body weight, the body alignment and joint alignment, the position of the gaze. A person new to Body Analysis will recognise a general image and have a reasonable representation of the movement. An experienced teacher will see at a glance, in an instant that something is not where it could be or should be. The experience and attitude of a good teacher will be able to decide whether it is the right time to make the correction or if it is important enough to correct at this time. However, there is more to it than being the right time to make a correction. It is also about knowing your students, their readiness, their willingness, and their abilities to know when it is appropriate for that correction.

When looking at a movement the teacher has to know either through experience or instinctively that movement is a co-ordinated system of pulleys and levers. The skeleton is the frame and the soft tissues cling to it and around it. Some joints act as a fulcrum such as the knee. When the muscles contract and shorten their length, the tendons pull on where they insert on the lower leg causing the knee to straighten. Being able to not only look but also see the position of a hand or degree of turn in the wrist defines the ability to make a mental connection from a visual image to reproducing this image in a physical form and with words describing the action and position. The advantage of having a real image or a real teacher (as opposed to a digital image) is the possibility of there being interaction, a connection between the student and the teacher at any particular moment. Biomechanics of movement involves posture, weight change, delivery of force, accuracy (from experience), involvement of the senses, muscular strength, flexibility, ability to gear up the right amount of energy to not only achieve that goal but to manage the stability of the body and maintain control.

---

[2] The Confucian dialectic as a part of the conceptual framework for the traditional martial art of Tai Chi Chuan is discussed in detail in Unit 3.11

POSTURE is simply the static position of the body. In Tai Chi the static posture of each form or part of a form is considered to be the "ideal image" for the related movement to occur and be modelled upon. Most postures in Sun Style are upright, but some are required to have a slight degree of forward inclination. This is so in the preparation for the Double Jump in the 73 Forms as an example to be able to generate enough force to get off the floor. In more physically demanding movements there has to be some freedom of movement in the upright position simply because of the shape of the human body, individual differences in the human body and the momentum of forces which spiral and lead the position of the body to change. Some styles have a deliberate forward posture, such as Wu style, and this is correct for this style. Generally, if the posture is not ideal, it compromises in some way the biomechanics of the movement required. The student will have to work much harder than is necessary if the posture is not where it should be. When out of alignment, other body parts are less functional – always. Either the joints are out of alignment (vulnerable to injury) or the muscles need to work much harder than is necessary thereby wasting energy. Even the body organs can be forced into positions, which is not natural or conducive to good health and wellness. Ingrained and incorrect postural habits will over time compromise good health and fitness.

Training and developing ideal posture within the movement of the form often takes months and sometimes years. As we age, loss of bone, muscle atrophy and trauma, illness and depression can have a significant impact on posture. Some students need specialist assistance from a health professional to help to improve posture and it is a role of the Tai Chi for Health teacher to be able to refer such students for appropriate therapeutic assistance.

Biomechanically, posture of the body may be thought of as a long lever passing through the centre of gravity of the body. The Tai Chi term - "Loosening of the waist" allows the postural line to rotate around this axis of the lower Dan-Tien or centre of gravity like a rotating shaft in a mine or a maypole. When the postural line leans away from the centre it is less strong, less functional unless counterbalanced in the lower body in the opposite direction. Also think of a horizontal axis passing through the centre of gravity (or Dan Tien) and the hips. When this axis tilts away from the horizontal, the spine will tilt also.

WEIGHT CHANGE - How the body manages weight change has a great bearing on stability. As soon as we begin our Tai Chi the weight is constantly changing until we finish. At least this is what we hope for. In reality of course we stop and start many times. This principle of movement is not unique to Tai Chi and all movement sequences do this to a lesser or greater degree of continuity building and expending forces and energy through momentum. Sometimes Tai Chi teachers fail to realise the significance of the importance of teaching students how to feel where their body weight is and when to shift it. They need to know clearly what is "full stance" and what is "empty", what it feels like when it is safe and balanced and when the body is ready to shift the empty leg.

Many people with chronic conditions (as well as people in good health) now use the Sun 12 (Tai Chi Productions, 2009) to assist their improvement for health. If teachers are interested particularly in teaching balance for falls prevention and building confidence for fear of falling, it is the principle of being able to differentiate full and empty stance as well as learning the technique of weight change which need early work and focus. First teach about the posture, then how to change the weight.

STRENGTH - Muscular strength plays a significant role in the biomechanics of movement. It is not only the muscles that need to strengthen but also the ligaments, tendons, fascia and bones. Muscles that are not strong will more likely tear and rip, ligaments will overstretch and detach from bone, tendons will snap and bones will break. Without muscular strength, doing the smallest movements may cause damage to a de-conditioned body while others in more robust health can manage incredible feats of strength and endurance.

When the tissues of the body are strong, people are able to do more physically. They can live more productive and more satisfying lives. Holding up the body to stand even without movement requires muscular strength. Propulsion forward, sideways or backwards or upwards requires a force on the tissues to overcome inertia and direct the force of the body weight in a particular direction. The bigger the movement, the greater the force required.

If the tissues are strong and balanced and are able to work a whole co-ordinated unit of the body, the range of movement will be greater. This means the body can balance, kick, leap, bend, jump, push, pull and so forth. If the tissues are weak, the movements will be limited, small and weak. As teachers we can see that facilitating improvements in strength even in "apparently" small increments and what might seem "apparently" insignificant ways will improve functional movement. The link of course is that any improvements will impact on quality of life. It is important for the Tai Chi for Health Instructor to be aware that one of the great myths of Tai Chi practised as a martial art is that there is no need for muscular strength. This is simply wrong as this misrepresents the fighting ability of the efficient martial artist to be able strategically relax in order to maximise the explosive moments of a strong and powerful body structure co-ordinated in the delivery of force as demonstrated in certain movements through the Tai Chi form. (see Davies, 2006)

FLEXIBILITY - Having freedom of movement around the joints changes the dynamics of how we move. There are many factors that may impact on flexibility (see Unit 2.21). In its very simplest form each movement requires an optimal flexibility for the desired action. Some movements require a little flexibility, some require a lot. If the flexibility is too much for the desired action, the movement may be compromised and damage may occur. Imbalances in the strength of the muscles, in particular the agonist and antagonist muscle groups, may cause problems for some movements. If the shoulder is flexible and the hips are not, some actions will be less able to generate the force necessary for the actions and injuries may occur to the back, spine or knees.

Improvements in flexibility need to be accompanied with increased body temperature and muscle strength through mind-body focus and hard work and practice. Aristotle once wrote "We are what we repeatedly do". He probably had a much deeper meaning – but it does very well for flexibility also. If the body is tight and inflexible, gradually with patience and work it will become more flexible and strong.

LOADING UP - means "getting ready" for action. It involves a pre-condition for practice because you need a "memory of the action" to prepare for it. Loading up involves accuracy and this means if you gear up too much energy the force will be too great. Similarly if you gear up too little, the delivery of the force will be weak and the movement or action you are trying to execute will not be successful.

Loading up for a movement sometimes borrows from the previous movement using the momentum of its action to fuel the next movement. This is one reason why the principle of continuity can be so important. Another reason is that it keeps the energy distribution process smooth and even. Keeping the continuity smooth will minimise muscular stress and minimise wasted energy. Getting ready for a movement does not mean having lots of energy available. It means preparing the exact amount of energy you need to control and perform the movement as required by your conscious mind. Continued practice and focus, with more practice, more practice and focus, will eventually place this action on automatic and its action will require very little conscious effort.

CENTRE OF GRAVITY (CG) (Dan Tien) – Apart from the brain, the most important aspect of movement mechanics comes from the centre – the CG of the body or what is referred to in the Chinese literature on the subject as the lower "Dan-Tien". We are talking here about balance and equilibrium of the body. Movements can be done without a conscious focus on the CG because most movement occurs in this way automatically as an automatic response to memory. As a baby toddles and begins to walk the movement patterns are laid down. As adults we move in this way in a co-ordinated balanced way via the CG and the muscles and connective tissues around it. If however we wish to do a difficult or relatively unpractised move such as a spin or kick or jump, we have to focus on the CG. We need to lower it to become more stable to be able to control the action with increased focus on controlling other body parts. This requires a conscious adjustment to control the dynamics of the force.

The accuracy of our actions comes directly from memory not only from the brain, but also from the tissues themselves. Accuracy involves repetition and practising with focus, not practising with an empty mind. Accuracy and gearing up energy requirements involve not only the preparation for the movement but also the timing and the control of the amount of force to be generated. To illustrate, when executing a spin or a turn, there has to be correct technique involving a pure central line, a lifting through the spine and head, and a lowering of the CG for stability and when spinning on the toes the raising the CG. Spinning requires an additional technique to control the force, and that is, the position of the arms or leg whether close to or away from the body. This positioning determines the spinning force generated. If the body judges it wrongly, the result will be a flawed move. The more accurate the preparation in the understanding the structural biomechanics of the movement, less energy is required. Once again, this relies on memory - experience through practice. Other factors affecting the execution of a movement are – fatigue, lack of focus, strength and general health.

POSTURE-OF-THE-EYES - The orientation of the eyes plays a very important role in the biomechanics of movement. The most important role is that of proprioception – that is where the body is in relation to everything else. If we cover our eyes, it is much more difficult to move. Our eyes pick up messages about distance and depth perception, which help us to balance and move in a smooth co-ordinated way. The eyes also focus sometimes close and other times distant. If the eyes are cast down or too high, the position of the head will more often than not be positioned out of the central line of the posture.

BODY STRUCTURE - Many students believe that a movement is simply - parts of the body moving in sequence. It is much more than this. Any action requires the co-operation and integration of the whole body all the time. Teaching movement correctly is best achieved by understanding this concept of the whole body working in unison. Learning tiny pieces of movement step at a time is how this is best achieved because of the mental focus that is required. This means that upper and lower do not have to be learned together. Breaking it up in small pieces and then putting it together works even better for complicated or new movements. But it is the whole body including balance, energy systems, blood, nerves, strength, flexibility, accuracy, memory senses that make the movement.

1.54   The Traditional - Martial Imagery - The "concept imagery" associated with Tai Chi as a martial art quite legitimately refers to the concept of martial force and martial power. As we have outlined elsewhere, the division of the martial arts into "external" and "internal" finds its mirrored expression in the use of the dichotomy of force being split into "internal" and "external" forms of power, energy, chi or ki.   As a martial arts concept, "external force" is based on those "concept images" which directly relate to muscular and physical force and strength whether gentle or brute. The martial concept of "internal" force is related to technique, biomechanics, leverage, co-ordination, posture, mind-focus and martial concepts of "borrowing" the opponent's force through yielding, deflecting, sticking and "push-pull" techniques. Accordingly within the context of Tai Chi as a martial art, there is nothing mystical or magical about "internal power" as part of this involves learning how to use "mind-body" connections to maximise the use of combination of technique for the intention of defeating or neutralising the opponent using a strategic amount of external or muscular force.

Within the training regime of Tai Chi as a martial art in the modern age, "internal martial power" is considered the key "concept imagery" used to evaluate the solo performance. It is the main metaphor to describe a range of techniques designed to increase leverage, to limit the use of "external" effort or force for the strategic purpose of achieving a successful outcome. A smaller person properly trained thus is potentially able to defeat a larger, much stronger opponent in combat, by using sufficient physical "external" force and power, but through the leverage of the smaller combatant's superior skills, referred to as "internal" force. Within the context of Tai Chi as a martial art, the effect of defeating an opponent thus demands a combination of physical power with an appropriate level of skill and technique sufficient to neutralise or defeat the opponent's combined use of so-called "internal" and "external" forces.

The Tai Chi for Health Instructor, however, needs to be aware that within contemporary approaches to Tai Chi there is what is termed the Confucian approach to Tai Chi as a martial art. This approach ascribes mystical, extraordinary and even supernatural powers to the Tai Chi for Martial Arts Master. This takes the extreme form of the "master" being able to move an opponent without any physical contact, at a distance, to fling the opponent (invariably the senior student of the Master), effortlessly and obediently flying across the room. The power of "internal chi" is given as the explanation, which is considered to have no reference or regard for principles of biomechanics or leverage or muscular strength (see Montaigue, 2007). It is this "faith" in this particular concept of the power of "internal chi" that not only invokes a healthy scepticism, but unfortunately becomes the basis of rejecting all forms of the martial arts by those who view this "faith" in power of "chi" as something anathema to their own religious views. What is relevant for the Tai Chi for Health Instructor is not to be intimidated by the Confucian view of Tai Chi as a Martial Art in its extraordinary claims to superiority and monopoly on the "WAY", the only way, which Tai Chi should be practised. What is needed is to be able to differentiate Tai Chi for Health as something fundamentally different from the Confucian approach to Tai Chi as something devoid of an empirical or scientific basis for health benefits of Tai Chi as a form of exercise. Moreover, it is also important for the Tai Chi for Health Instructor to be able to articulate this difference, to be able to position Tai Chi for Health as being fundamentally different from all forms of Tai Chi practised as a martial art, whether traditional or Confucian.

1.55   The Modern – Imagery & Imagination - As suggested above, the only limitation as to what non-martial forms of "concept imagery" can be used is the imagination itself. There are many ways to describe the concept of force and power without needing to rely on martial images of violence. For example, we can analyse the biomechanics of the "brush-knee push" movement by examining physical or sporting activities that use the same biomechanics to maximise co-ordination of all parts of the body and delivery of force and how the mind is instrumental to focussing on maximising the technique for the desired effect. These activities include - baseball pitching and hitting, swinging a golf club, serving at tennis, throwing a ball or stone. The TCH Instructor therefore has a specific challenge in teaching this form in such a way as to enhance co-ordination between the upper and lower body. This is significant area of difficulty for many students.

As TCH Instructors, the use of accessible and constructive forms of "concept imagery" will significantly speed up the process of learning to co-ordinate facilitating the movement of the whole body as a unit, and thus fast-tracking the student's feeling of well-being and health enhancement, and sooner than later beginning to feel more relaxed, have more energy and deriving more health benefits. In general terms, what is important is to make the right connections with the students in order to more effectively transfer to the student the knowledge about Tai Chi for Health which is aimed at enhancing health and fitness. While there is absolutely nothing wrong with using martial concept imagery, the TCH Instructor who values and respects the wishes of students in their class, will need to be responsive and find suitable non-violent "concept imagery" to facilitate and enhance the so-called "internal power", that is, the techniques of co-ordination, posture, biomechanics all within the ethical and legal frameworks of safety, mutual respect and the sharing of knowledge.

IMAGINATION as METAPHOR - An important part of being efficient in our teaching is to use our imagination to find a comparison with something in the everyday experience of the student – a metaphor to help convey another dimension to the functional concept of "Body Analysis". If an image, a conceptual idea of what is trying to be learned is added to the learning process, it can significantly aid the learning process. The brain is quite capable of making another connection with the movement of the body with something that is familiar. It is merely linking an image to a movement. Some suggestions of concepts or images to facilitate the teaching of movements are as follows:

Co-ordination of Upper & Lower Body - Puppet on String - Consider the relationship between the fist (upper body) and follow step foot (lower body) in the punch from the TCA 12 movements. For students familiar with the concept imagery of a "puppet" and the string from the top to the bottom, this is easy to "SEE" in the mind's eye, so to speak, and is immediately recognised and processed by the student. The concept imagery of the "Puppet" can also be used almost everywhere where upper and lower body co-ordination is required. What is important, however, for the TCH Instructor, is to ensure that the concept imagery is agreeable to and understandable by the student.

Relaxing the muscles around Joints – Concept of Song [3] **– Cotton Reels** - to let go of tension - Imagine two cotton reels touching – or make two fists touching and lightly pressing together. Pulling them apart means you have to let go of the tension. This can instantly relate to the elbow, shoulder, fingers and other joints and immediately a lengthening and loosening can be felt in the muscles. Even the knee on an empty stance can be softened and lengthened.

Relaxed Lifting & Lowering – Balloons - When Opening and Closing using an actual balloon or imagining one will give the feeling of adding the resistance. Students can actually feel this and can make a connection with the amount of resistance and what it feels like to do this. It can then be added to other forms.

Grounding - Biscuit Cutter - Lowering of centre of gravity - Using mind-body focus on even pressing of feet into ground, to avoid or be conscious of not gripping with toes. Biscuit cutter outline of the base of foot solidly pressed into floor, like cutting a biscuit. Americans use the term "rooting" to mean the same thing as "grounding".

Resistance - Water - Resistance can also be conveyed by remembering or visualising the feeling of moving through water.

Thrusting - Jewel Box - The image of handing a jewel box or a music box to someone is basically the shape of the hands at the end of Form 1 in the Sun 12.

Upright Hand - Toby Tall - This is a little children's rhyme that helps people remember to keep their fingers pointing upright in the Sun Style. Using the fingers of one hand start with the thumb. Good for a laugh.

> *This is Mister Old Tom Thumb, he is round just like a plum*
> *This is Mister Peter Pointer, h e is such a double jointer*
> *This is Mister Toby Tall, he's the tallest one of all*
> *This is Mrs Ruby ring, she's too smart for anything.*
> *This is little baby one – hmmm hmmm hmmm*

Keeping "Toby Tall" pointing to the ceiling and the hand gently curved keeps energy in the hands is a short-hand expression and a reminder for specific Sun Style posture of the hands for such forms as Open and Close hands, Brush Knee push, Single Whip and others throughout the form.

Transfer of Weight - Feather Touch - This is the "touch down" for the heel (or toe) in any movement. It clearly is empty stance – as light as a feather. First "touch down", then lower the toe (or heel), align the knee first and then transfer the weight.

Transfer of Weight - Testing the Water - This is used for side stepping Sun Style to encourage people to step onto the toe. First test the water with the toe (empty stance). If the water is nice, proceed to commit the weight until the whole foot is in the water. If it is good, bring the other foot in too, toe first then heel.

Transfer of Weight – Stepping on Ice – Stepping on Hazardous Floor without sight (power blackout at night) – This provides an immediate visual image of the need to step lightly otherwise you will crash through thin ice, or trip on hazards on floor.

Lowering Centre of Gravity - Avoid Jumping off the Cliff – This is to highlight the feather touch principle above to not fall into empty space.

Balanced Stances – Avoid walking the tightrope – This is to visualise the need for hip or shoulder width stances and to achieve stability with the front foot in alignment with the hip to avoid the mid-line.

Lowering Centre of Gravity - Sitting on the Perch - If you can imagine a metal rail you can perch your seat on, let it be placed at the top of the back of the leg. Try not to sit on a stool as it will be too much. Just sit on the edge like a little bird on a perch.

Crossed Hands – Butterfly - This is the Block before the Close in Form 9.

---

[3] Song or sometimes spelled in English as "Sung"

Delivery of Force - Pitch the Ball, Golf Swing, Tennis Serve, Throwing a stone - This will convey the movement of Brush Knee and the biomechanics in co-ordination of upper and lower body, in utilising power in the hips, and in importance of body structure.

Parry and Deflect - Pat the child on the head and take off the glove - Parry arms are always difficult to grasp initially. The turning of the hands actually go together, but initially the pat will happen first and then the second hand will have to turn to take off the glove. Eventually they will be co-ordinated especially when the student begins to "turn the waist" (hips and waist together).

Preparation for Movement in Yang Style – Holding the Ball or Beach Ball – This prepares the student for relaxed shoulders and elbows pointed downwards – followed by movement and change with focussing on turning the beach ball upside down without dropping it. There is no "holding the ball" image used in Sun Style.

Posture of Body - The Golden Thread - This of course could be any type of thread, an invisible thread, string, or a cord. Remind students that they don't have to stand tall like a soldier but that they are being held up or suspended. This gives the added permission to relax the muscles of the upper back, chest, arms and legs while pulling up through the central line of the spine and out of the top of the head to "above". Remember also, that the string needs to pull down as well stretching two ways at once.

Follow-Step – Riding a scooter – This highlights the need for downward pressure for the rear foot, not on toe but on the ball of the foot.

Looking Ahead – "Look Eyes" from Karate Kid – To encourage students not to look down, to focus on intention of move, and to improve posture and stay alert.

Gentle Neck stretch - Nodding peacock or nodding pony - gives a strong image of a gentle head movement for stretching the neck and relieving neck stiffness.

Close, Carry The Tiger & Push the Mountain - Waves roll over and gently roll back on the sand - These are Forms 9 and 10 of Sun 12 Form and can be used for chair work and breathing.

Top hand of Waving Hands in Cloud - Tiger looks through the jungle – to highlight the need to keep hand lower than eye level.

Lower hand of Waving Hands in Cloud – Hand floats on water - To highlight the need for softness.

There are of course many metaphors that can be used if appropriate to the learning situation. The substitution of concepts or images is only limited to the skill and imagination of the teacher. Different images may be more appropriate for different groups and for different forms. Anything that will enhance learning and processing is worth a try when the usual names and language fail to convey the message.

Many health professionals are now working with people with chronic conditions. Among these the older aged surely must be recognised as one of the most marginalised groups needing physical activity. Improved appetite and sleeping patterns, enhanced mood, improved flexibility and enhanced social interaction are reported outcomes for appropriate physical activity with the aged.

The modification of Tai Chi using the 12 forms here has a huge base of evidence already reported for safety and efficacy as a physical activity suitable for the aged and these other groups. Also, many people in these groups do not respond well to the harshness or the descriptive terms such as "block and close", "parry and punch" and respond much better to a softening of these terms to make the movements more acceptable and easier to perform – such as "over the hill and push the mountain", "pat the boy on the head and take off the glove".

In addition there are several arm and hand movements that have a strong image component. Many people find this sort of imagery work very soothing and this lends itself to deep abdominal breathing. For example see Australia Dreaming see Unit 5.50). The following imagery with words and action has been provided by Nancy Kiefer (Master Trainer with Dr Lam's Tai Chi for Arthritis program):

Spinning the Silk
- Take hands up Sun Style to front, fingers pointing straight ahead, palms facing each other, raise the fingers to open prayer position in front of the chest. Breathe in, breathe out (open/close)
- Extend arms to the front, fingers pointing straight ahead.
- Select index finger and thumb of both hands and press lightly together as if holding onto a thread of silk.
- Keeping the other digits pointing straight ahead, gently draw the hand back towards the body as if pulling the thread of silk between the thumb and one finger.
- When upper arm is vertical, release the thumbs and index fingers (open/close). Reach forward again, fingers pointing straight ahead.

- Repeat using the middle finger, then the ring finger then the baby finger remembering to keep the other fingers uncurled if possible with open/close between each thread.
- On the last movement reach all the fingers straight ahead, close arms, fingers pointing up, open/close. Finish by resting the palms on the knees.

All of the movements should be smooth and gentle and continuous. Each thread can be visualized as a different colour. The last movement has a bunch of coloured threads. Over time, add resistance, Song (loosening of the joints) as principles and add extra open/close Qigong movements.

Focus entirely on deep, relaxed and quiet breathing throughout

Imagery as Practice
Many Tai Chi practitioners use imagery both as a way of practising their form and as a very effective method of enhancing performance. Students remember an image from class that helps them remember what they wish to practise. If the student's mind is "busy" they will have difficulty in drawing up an image because of distraction during the lesson. Being able to conjure up an image mentally may sometimes be a difficult task. But people do improve their ability to image by having enough memory laid down. Being able to imagine the whole form can be an aide to performance simply because it is so efficient. Some people actually imagine themselves doing a difficult move and keep imagining it until they can perform it successfully. In addition, the physical body can rest and the brain can continue to practise. Imaging reduces the risk of over-practice which is often the cause of unnecessary injury and fatigue.

This is not to say that the body itself does not receive benefit from this action by resting. It is known that the mind can imagine performing the movement better than the body is physically capable of. The improvement to performance is estimated to be around 10%. Lying down and resting or sitting on an aeroplane can be another way to fit in a practice in a busy life. Add the breathing to the practice and the body will soon relax.

It is not important to try and achieve instant "perfection" of the "correctness" of the form and posture as it may happen that some students may only be able remember the metaphor and not the "correctness" of the movement when practising. Some students unfortunately believe that they should achieve "perfection" immediately. Patience is one of the lessons Tai Chi teaches to those who are willing to learn. Distortions of the "correctness" of the form may arise. The overriding factor here is always safety as to the timing of when to correct and how to make corrections. In time, the student will become more skilled in using "Body Analysis" techniques, through mind-body focus and will be able to incorporate more detail into the movement and form beyond the basic shape. This is the layering process with new imaging being superimposed on the established layer.

1.60   MUSIC
      1.61   Introduction
      1.62   Music and Mood
      1.63   Music in Class

1.61   Introduction - Music is something that is familiar to many if not most people from all cultures across the world. Everyone has a response of some kind to music and it involves the emotions to a lesser or greater degree. People either like it or they don't like it or they are indifferent to it. They can like some forms but not others. They can be deeply moved by it or irritated by it. Whether it is a drum or a Stradivarius, music has many forms each of which is received with just as many different responses, varying from person to person and from culture to culture.

Music appears to be a universal human competence. It is suggested (Cross, 2001) that "music, like speech, is a product of both our biology and our social interactions; that music is a necessary and integral dimension of human development and that music may have played a central role in the evolution of the modern human mind". All "cultures" have music. From our perspective we think of music as something that is made electronically, or by instruments. It can also be something produced by humans through their voices when they sing or soothe, croon or hum. Music can be a drum, clap sticks, the pluck of a string. Pitch, tempo, loudness, softness, melody and cacophony are all qualities that describe music. It can be rain on the roof, wind in the trees, a bird's song, a bubbling stream or the gentle waves on the sand. Because music is sound it is immediately linked to one of the human senses and it is for this reason that music involves the emotion and the deepest and oldest part of the brain.

Music is an important social component of the ceremonies and societal rituals that are an integral aspect of the "rites of passage" for many cultures – birth, marriage, death. Music can be either a private pleasure or a social shared experience for enjoyment. In any respect – music has an emotional connection with people of all ages. People use music to express their feelings, songs of praise, songs of love, songs of despair, soothing lullabies, stirring songs for battle, laments, ballads, songs of passion and courage. To produce musical sounds requires memory and focus and a particular attitude and involves hearing, resonance, breathing, posture, timing and technique.

This section will provide some basic ideas around the purpose and value of Music being part of the Tai Chi for Health class or activity.

1.62   Music and Mood - Does music influence mood and if so, what are the implications of using music in Tai Chi practice?

(a)   Scientific research - With more than a million references on research on the effects of music on mood on the internet, there can be no doubt that observational studies and proper scientific studies make a very strong case for music effecting mood in humans. Many studies show changes in mood occurring using many different types of music such as grunge, hip hop, relaxation, classical. McCraty et al (1998) is just one study which investigated the impact of different types of music on tension, mood and mental clarity finding significant increases with relaxation, mental clarity and vigour and significant decreases in hostility, fatigue, sadness and tension. He found that grunge music increased hostility and tension and reduced relaxation and mental clarity while pan pipes and rain forest sounds produced significant increases in relaxation, mental clarity and vigour.

Lai (1999) found significant differences in physical output for heart rate, blood pressure and mood states after music intervention.

The significance for Tai Chi teachers involved in research is that music should be treated a variable to be controlled and not ignored. This would mean that the music would have to be exactly the same and should be played at the same volume or deleted from the session. In addition, because music can have such an effect on mood, any experiment involving health outcomes for Tai Chi should also control for the segment in the class when music should be played. For example, should it be played for the warm-up? Should it be stopped for most of the conditioning phase and only played again at the end of this phase?   Should it be played for the cool-down? Should it be played throughout the whole lesson? Should it be omitted altogether?

In the class situation, is the music only important for beginners or are experienced Tai Chi students soothed emotionally by the addition of music? Should the music be played for the whole lesson? Are more experienced students happy to use music very intermittently during the lesson or is their learning and lesson enhanced or interrupted by playing music?

At the very least it should be recognised that this variable cannot be ignored with scientific studies. It has to be omitted or controlled.

(b)   Relaxation - Certainly there is much evidence to suggest that music does effect mood. For teaching purposes, the very first question for a beginner class should be "why is the student here". The answer to that question can be related directly to the inclusion or exclusion of music in the program or at least consideration of when it is played, choice of music, volume etc. It should be recognised that if music dominates the lesson, learning will not be as efficient because it interferes with the focus. However, in many situations, the choice of music is extremely important and is one of the reasons people actually attend or are willing to be part of a class. The music is soothing and it makes them feel less stressed. Maybe the student will not even recognise the impact of the music.   It is simply a pleasant feeling they have when they do Tai Chi, a combination of the music, the gentleness of the activity and the non-threatening environment created by the teacher.

An important reason cited by many students and also the main reason students are referred to Tai Chi by their medical advisers is "for relaxation" and music is more often than not a significant part of the mood of the class.

(c)   Tool for Practice - In any setting of Tai Chi learning, music does not always have to involve the familiar CD collection. It can be
- Drum
- Sticks
- Guitar
- Piano
- Band
- Singing

1.63   Music in Class - When considering what sort of music would be most suitable for Tai Chi, any of the following could be used:
- Relaxation /mood music
- Traditional Chinese music
- Music specifically composed for Tai Chi
- Indian music
- Reiki music
- Culturally specific music
- Class specific music

3 aspects of Music to keep in mind in the class
(1) choice of music
(2) volume of music
(3) frequency of playing during the session

(a) **Choice of music -** Relaxation or Reiki music for beginners is sometimes so slow and dreamy it puts the students to sleep! Teachers need to listen to the music on the CD and choose quiet yet bright tracks. Tai Chi is certainly slow and gentle and relaxed, but the mind should be alert and sharp – not half asleep.

Many new students also like to do Tai Chi to popular tunes such as "Tears from Heaven", and other popular and familiar songs. Occasionally this works but mostly only for a special performance or for fun (which is a good enough reason). Sometimes tunes such as "Pachelbel's Canon" having a more distinct beat can be played softly for training exercises such as Parry, Parry or Tai Chi walking where repetition is required. The gentle rhythmic sounds compliment the movements and consolidate the patterns and timing. It certainly reduces the feeling of chaos when everyone is keeping an even beat – but it doesn't allow for students listening to their own balance and being ready or not ready for the change of weight. After the repetitive training, turn off the music and let them pace the movements according to their own strengths. This sort of music is often ideal for demonstrations but not for refinement.

There should be some consideration given for culturally specific music being played in appropriate circumstances. With careful selection it would give a sense of familiarity and relaxation and in some circumstances would be more appropriate as classes are being established eg Maori, Indigenous Australian, Greek, African etc. As Tai Chi is from the Chinese culture, traditional Chinese music can be gradually introduced until it is familiar and acceptable.

(b) **Volume of Music -** In most teaching environments the music should be just audible. If it is too loud it interferes with the focus for training. If it is missing, beginners particularly miss it and need it to help reduce the stress they put on themselves trying to be perfect on their first lesson. Not understanding these demands and believing that music interferes with focus are the reasons that many teachers don't allow music.

Many new students have some level of anxiety either from their lifestyle conditions or from the stress of starting something new and feeling awkward. As the evidence shows, soft music effects mood positively. Even classes held out in the open have the environmental setting washing over them, soothing their anxieties and helping the mood also.

When students begin to focus on principles and concepts or are practising in a session, music is usually not required. In fact, as students absorb and understand the principles and deeper aspects of Tai Chi, the music will indeed interfere with their focus and many will find it unnecessary. By now these students are feeling a sense of achievement and accomplishment, which expresses itself as pleasure or satisfaction or contentment. These students already have learned to relax and let go and to focus and to clear the mind.

Generally music is usually used for public performance and demonstration but not for competition within the traditional Tai Chi as Martial Art.

(c) **Frequency during class -** Beginners need music. It is soothing, comforting, pleasant and helps to make them feel more comfortable. In these circumstances the music should be played softly throughout the class.

When students are more settled, the music can be turned off during the learning/practise phase of the lesson and turned on again towards the end for the "show me" phase and the cool-down and finish.
Advanced students usually do not need or want music – unless performing.

1.70 **MODIFICATIONS IN TAI CHI FOR HEALTH**
1.71   Introduction
1.72   Principles of Modification
1.73   Modifications to Sun Style 12 Forms – Bed & Chair
1.74   Modifications to Sun Style 12 Forms – Standing
1.75   Modifications Sun Style 31 Forms

1.71 **Introduction -** Within the framework of a modern Tai Chi for Health, modification is a necessary change or adaptation that can be made to a form, or training activity, to find the safest way to adapt the movements to the capabilities of the individual student.   The overriding concern in regard to modification relates directly to a matter of safety, to do no harm. This arises from the legal Duty of Care that the Tai Chi for Health Instructor has towards each student within the class where it is not the choreography of the "Tai Chi Form" which dictates the movement, but the capacities of the individual student as identified in the Tai Chi for Health Matrix of Performance (see Unit 3.40).

A vital part of this Duty of Care is to understand that responsibility for how movements are to be performed in a safe manner rests primarily with the Tai Chi for Health Instructor. It is not sufficient for the Instructor to give a blanket statement to the class saying: "Everyone work within their own comfort zone" assuming that "everyone" knows how to and will modify safely and sensibly for themselves. Moreover, the lack of responsibility may be further compounded where the Tai Chi Instructor turns the back asking the class to follow, oblivious to safety factors in the performance of the Tai Chi Form. Moreover, the Tai Chi Instructor should not assume that everyone is comfortable and not hurting or feeling pain. This is a confirmation of the idea of the Tai Chi Instructor to encourage students at all times to communicate.

Learning to modify the "Tai Chi Form" is perhaps one of the most challenging aspects of teaching and learning Tai Chi for Health. It is difficult for not only the teacher but also the student who fails to recognise the difficulty and potential danger of certain movements and attempts to perform these without regard for any need to modify. The focus of Tai Chi for Health should not be on striving for excellent performance in accordance with Wu Shu competition standards of Tai Chi for Martial Arts, but on maximising the health benefits of exercise derived through safe and effective application of Tai Chi principles within the "Tai Chi Form" and related activities. Both teacher and student need to accept this contract of safety as a necessary precondition for performance of any "Tai Chi Form" or related activity.

1.72   Principles of Modification - With imagery practice students can improve their ability to perform a movement. However, in the meantime it is more important to encourage the student to focus on performing a movement that is comfortable and does not cause muscular tension or worry. Maintaining a relaxed posture, breathing gently and keeping a gentle flow of the movements are more important to health than performing a movement in its original form.

Knowing what is comfortable is certainly something that may have to be taught by the instructor. Students often perform their forms with the alignment of the body – particularly the back and knee – not in the best position. Allowing students to look at backs, work in partners, having the "no touch" rule, looking at their own knees in relation to their feet – are all worthwhile exercises to learning what is comfortable.

Students are often very resistant to change (as are teachers sometimes). When the teacher says "are you comfortable" – they may be because they have spent many years of their life in that position. Making small suggestions to change, showing and looking at alignment, feeling (mind to body) what the body feels like, making little adjustments and deciding if that *feels better* is all part of not only being comfortable, but *being more comfortable*. How does the student know if it feels better? When posture and alignment are improved for the student, there is a subtle change in the comprehension of the working level – and that is that the movement is easier to do - it is more efficient. The body is then in a position to be able to relax more and let go of excessive muscle tension.

Being comfortable with a form does not mean that a student does a modified version of the original form forever more. Some people will always need to modify some moves according to their capabilities, but others will improve with practice and perseverance. With better alignment of joints and strength increments modification can be reduced and the forms will look more like the original form.

It is important that students realise that the Tai Chi they are doing is to be adapted to their body at any particular time. No two students perform their Tai Chi in exactly the same way and any one student does not perform their Tai Chi the same way every time they practise. If the aim is to improve health (which we know happens because we are practising Tai Chi) then the real skill is trying to achieve a high level of Tai Chi in the most efficient way we know and to feel well. This will occur through good techniques and understanding and application of the principles over time. To accomplish this may mean adjusting the movements to reduce tension in the body. Modifications are a very efficient way to improve health. With time and patience the need to modify may reduce.

Many people now understand that if they practise Tai Chi they can feel better or they can have an improved sense of well-being. Fortunately Tai Chi has very wide arms embracing the discipline. Tai Chi can be practised with very positive outcomes in many different circumstances. Tai Chi can be viewed anywhere in a continuum from the very basic position of lying flat on a bed   visualising the form to performing a set in its original structure. Any time that the mind focuses on the movement is practise and is therefore worthwhile.

Below are some suggestions for describing modification. Directions are given as for the face of a clock. For example – looking straight ahead is 12 o'clock. Directly behind is 6 o'clock. 3 o'clock is immediately to the right and so forth.

1.73   Modifications to Sun Style 12 Forms – Bed & Chair: People who are well often practise their Tai Chi forms in their minds whilst lying on a bed as a way to relax and to get to sleep. However, some of the basic exercise movements of Tai Chi can also be performed on a bed by people who are de-conditioned or recovering from ill health. It is important to be aware that any form of exercise might be contra-indicated for certain health conditions and it is for this reason, that such modification has the approval of their health adviser.

Health professionals are in a ideal position to introduce all or part of the 12 Forms for therapeutic purposes during recovery. Below are some suggestions:

(i)   **Bed – supine position – Adapted from Dr Lam's Sun Style 12 Forms**

Flat	1	focus on breathing in, breathing out
Flat	2	visualise movements
	3	visualise movements with Qigong
	4	visualise a movement or set with focus on a principle

Pillows	1	posture of opening and closing
	2	posture of raising and lowering
	3	waving hands in cloud (from centre of thigh or less as Reference Point)
	4	single whip right and left
	5	basic 6 right and left
	6	parry, parry arms
	7	close, and push mountain

(ii)   **Chair - sitting position (no use of legs)**

1	posture of opening and closing
2	posture of raising and lowering
3	basic 6 right and left
4	advanced 6 right and left (brush knee 12 o'clock)
5	12 forms and reverse
6	5 element Qigong

Note: In sitting position the arms should not go beyond the alignment of the thigh for "Cloud Hands". This means that the arms do not wander to the side risking twisting of the spine, but stay at about 10.30 and 1.30 (or less). With the hips fixed on the chair, try to press the head towards the ceiling, to elongate the abdomen, keeping the chin tucked in.

(iii)   **Chair - sitting position (limited use of legs)**
Modifications for legs
Starting Position (SP) hips, knees and ankles aligned at right angles and comfortable

Form 1- Opening Form
- Lift and lower arms
- Lift L heel. Anchor R leg. Lift foot
- Feather touch L heel to floor, on the spot (OTS)
- Roll onto ball of foot. Press to floor
- Pick up R foot
- Place down OTS toe first

Form 2- Open, Close
- Press R foot to floor
- Press L foot to floor

Form 3 - Single Whip
- Lift R heel, then toe, feather touch R heel slightly side R, foot angled to 1.30
- Lower toe (roll) to floor
- Press slightly on base of foot. Check knee alignment over mid toe

Form 4 - Wave Hands in the Cloud
- Press L foot to floor, bring back R foot to SP
- Press R foot, Press L foot, Raise R heel
- R toe, R heel OTS, L toe, L heel, OTS
- Repeat R toe, heel and L toe heel two more times

Note: If this group/student will be progressing to standing Tai Chi, it is helpful to use the same cueing terms. For example "get ready" "travel" "balance" "change weight". Using visual cues such as "feather touch" will be the same terms of reference for the standing work. Learning will be faster.

Form 5 - Open, Close
- As for form 2

Form 6 - Closing Form or Beginning of the Advanced 6 – Brush Knee
- Press R foot to floor
- Lift L heel, lift foot off and feather touch to 12 o'clock on heel OTS
- Roll onto ball and follow step R ball OTS

Form 7 - Playing the Lute
- Pick up R foot again and roll back slightly turned out, anchor
- Follow step with L ball OTS

Form 8- Deflect to Parry and Punch
- Feather touch L heel, toe to 11.30 OTS
- Feather touch R heel, toe to 12.30 OTS
- Feather touch L heel 12o'clock, roll to toe and follow step R in hip line

Form 9 - Block and Close
- Roll back R toe 12.30
- Anchor R and follow step L

Form 10 - Carry the Tiger and Push the Mountain
- Feather touch L heel, roll, anchor
- Follow step R

Form 11 - Open and Close
- R heel, toe to SP
- Adjust L foot to SP

(iv) **Chair Standing -** Chair can be used as an aid in two ways:

a. To assist with support for change of weight learning technique first holding two chairs (or a rail) then holding 1. If the student is de-conditioned and has poor balance, chairs are not really stable enough. In these circumstances, it is safer to use a rail for walking practise and learning transfer of weight. Here the student can hold onto a fixed support with two hands. Fatigue can be a safety factor and standing work should be introduced gradually.

b. To give psychological support to maximise confidence and minimise fear of falling

Note: Begin training by standing feet apart in front of chair and practising form arms only. Then add changing weight and sinking slightly without moving feet at all – just weight change, lowering centre of gravity to find full stance or partial stance, pressing the sole of the foot gently to floor. This is ideal for first stages of transfer of weight. Student learns the patterns, co-ordinates mentally transfer without actually moving away from the chair. Later:

Form 1 Use 2 chairs. Only take a small step to minimise loss of posture. Hold on with both hands.

Form 2 Hold with one hand if transfer of weight is insecure.

Form 3 Begin this form only when forms 1 and 2 are stable.
Place chairs in front, holding on with both hands; or
Leave legs in open position and Form 3 arms only
Practise legs holding on with both hands

Form 4 This form can be practised legs first.
Hands can be practised separately.
Using hands and legs – only use one hand at a time, holding on with the other

Use a rail or bench to practise side-stepping holding 2 hands

Students with limited mobility or limited visual ability should not be encouraged to do Advanced 6 (Standing) Form. Practice time would be better spent learning the 12 forms seated, arms and legs separate then together seated and being taught how to relax the joints, how to breathe and some of the principles which are most appropriate. Encouraging more controlled movements with focus would not only be safer but would afford achievable health benefits such as mental quietness, flexibility, breathing, enjoyment, improved circulation, better sleeping, pleasure and so forth.

For more mobile students, practise the Advanced 6 to 12 o'clock. Gradually try at an angle to the corner so there is some degree of turn and variety. Eventually, the direction change will be of great benefit for balance and stability and falls prevention. Initially, the follow step can be replaced with a rocking movement. After Playing the

Lute, simply lower the heel, weight to front leg for first Parry keeping both heels anchored, rock back onto R for second Parry, rock onto L for punch, rock back for Block and Close, rock forward again for Push Mountain etc.

1.74   Modifications to Sun Style 12 Forms Standing Position:

Basic Six - Forms 1 to 6 need not be modified except to make the movements comfortable. Students with limited flexion for knee, hips, and stiffness in shoulders should be encouraged to perform the forms in normal or close to normal standing position and normal stepping length. Arms can be quite bent and soft until strength begins to build.

Students who are unable to stand on one leg and lift the other hip to make the feather touch for the heel touchdown for stepping forward can modify by sliding the foot along the floor in the early stages especially in form 1 and form 4. Even though the foot should "pick up" it is better to glide across the floor than to allow the spine to tilt away from the centre alignment. This is especially helpful for people with reduced sightedness or reduced confidence.

Advanced Six - Form 6   Segment 1 of the Brush Knee is better turned to 10.30 by lifting the R heel and placing it on the diagonal. This means the turn is decreased from a 90 degree turn to a 45 degree turn. This will be easier to achieve a bow stance before the transfer of weight. Many students prefer to put the weight on the L hip and lift the R toe in to 10.30 rather than turn the heel. Making this modification ensures that the students can put their weight safely on the R hip, knee and ankle to adequately prepare for the bow step of the Brush Knee. This careful placement will do much for safety, strength and ultimately falls and injury prevention. Also making the step "short" is safer and less stressful.

Form 11: The transition after Push the Mountain to opening the R hip to change direction for Open Close often is a problem for hips and knees. Try rolling back the follow step of PM on the R foot to a full transfer of weight until the L foot flexes. Turn L foot to 10.30 front, bring the R heel to touch L heel.

1.75   Modifications Sun Style 31 Forms -Any part of the 31 forms can be adjusted to suit physical ability. Modifications should always be made to ensure that performing the movement feels comfortable and does not cause stress to the student. The main reason modification is made is to improve safety. Remembering the overall precaution for teaching Tai Chi is "to do no harm", if there is any doubt on the judgement of the instructor that the student is attempting something they are not capable of – that is a safe, aligned, comfortable execution of a movement or part of a movement it must be modified. This will allow time for the body to adjust and strengthen enough until it can cope with the demands on the body the movement requires. Sometimes it might be necessary to eliminate some moves all together for overall safety.

Any improvement will rely on repetition and cognitive awareness. The amount of repetition required is something that cannot be measured because it relies on individual adjustment and each micro-environment is unique. Similarly, the level of awareness, recognition and sensitivity is individually matched to each student. Teaching the student to "listen to themselves" is an integral component of improvement.

Form 21: Brush Knee and Twist Step Right & Leisurely Tying Coat - Begin with weight on R hip, adjust L foot by lifting heel to align to 1.30 then Brush Knee as usual. Only half step back with L foot, small step forward R. Take next step back L slightly wide and accept weight on hip in sitting position with R arm outstretched in front of shoulder. Reduce size of R arm swirl to minimise the potential for the twisting of the spine.

Form 25 - Punch Underneath Elbow - First step is same, but back follow step is taken to 7.30 – on the diagonal back for alignment of R foot. This ensures the bow step to six o'clock and avoiding stepping onto the tightrope.

Forms 26-28 - If change of directions for Repulse Monkey is dangerous, leave Form 25 same as in original form without modification but do the Repulse monkey R and L to 9.0'clock. Then Left leisurely Tying Coat as usual.

1.80   WORKING WITH SPECIAL PEOPLE
      1.81   Introduction
      1.82   Understanding Personality Theory
      1.83   Who Is In This Class Today
      1.84   Conclusion

1.81   Introduction - Everyone at a class is special. As they relate to each other everyone plays a part to a smaller or greater degree. The relationship of the teacher to each student and the relationships of the students with each other all knit together hopefully in a cohesive way that has good outcomes for all the people involved. Some people will enhance the atmosphere of the class with their personality and attitude to others. Others will be important also in that because of who they are and their life experiences, their personality can negatively impact on the atmosphere and learning outcomes of the class.

Very briefly, we will take a glimpse at personality theory in everyday life and then we will focus on identifying specific personality types who may be present at our classes and whose right to be there is every bit as important as the keenest most affable member of the class. Some strategies will be offered to help the TCH teacher work to maximise the benefit of the learning experience for everyone.

We can:
- Make the class a pleasant experience for everyone
- Use participants as a resource
- Minimise negatives by turning them into positives
- Reach the objectives of the learning experience

1.82   Understanding Personality Theory - Students at Random - Teachers who teach at many different venues will tell you that the classes are all different – and this is so because of the different class dynamics – or how the different personalities relate and interact with each other. Classes work well when people get to know each other and when the students begin to feel comfortable with the teacher.

The "random mix" of the class is also constantly changing both as students come and go over time and also as people begin to relax and feel safe. The very nature of Tai Chi should be non-threatening - people work at their own level, people do their Tai Chi as their body dictates. People are really unconcerned about how other people's bodies are working. They are trying very hard to understand and learn about their own body. In any Tai Chi class there will be a number of health conditions, chronic conditions, good health, poor health, all ages, male and female. There is enormous potential for differences in the atmosphere created by the random mix.

The method of introducing the students that works very well because of its informality is done as part of the warm-up when people walk around meeting and greeting each other. Having their name on a badge helps new students feel that they are not alone in a room of strangers and it identifies who they are. It also gives the more experienced students the opportunity to give a friendly personal welcome to the new ones. They very well know the first class "feel". There is also the method of sitting everyone down and introducing each other in a friendly and relaxed manner which works very well too. This method has the added advantage of helping the teacher discover not only who is in the class and why they are coming, but gives an idea of the personalities he/she will be working with. This can give an insight into identifying basic personality types to the teacher. Identifying why a student is coming to class is not always the most obvious reason and can be a mindful reminder to the teacher why the students are actually there.

There are many methods of classifying different personalities. Riso & Hudson (1996) outline nine personality types listed as follows: Reformer, Helper, Motivator, Individualist, Investigator, Loyalist, Enthusiast, Leader and Peacemaker. For our purposes today we can look at one of these personality types – "The Helper" and we will profile someone in everyday life who may be described as the "classic helper". They would be – "Empathetic, compassionate, feeling with and for others. Caring and concerned about their needs. Outgoing and passionate, they offer friendship and kindness. They are thoughtful, warm-hearted, forgiving, and sincere; encouraging and appreciative, able to see the good in others; dedicated and supportive of people, bringing out the best in them. Service is important: they are nurturing, generous, and giving – truly loving people. At their best: deeply unselfish, humble, and altruistic, giving unconditional love to self and others. Feel it is a privilege to be in others' lives. Radiantly joyful and gracious". (Riso & Hudson, 1996) The person with these qualities is hard to find, but many people have some of these qualities.

Most people tend to classify others in terms of their personality rather than any specific attributes. We say people are "bright" or "funny" or "complaining" and how we observe them and categorise them has an effect on us. In our target working environment in the class, we will extend from personality to include behaviours. People can be draining, frustrating, confronting, co-operative, responsive, helpful, and sometimes threatening. Taking a look at cognitive-behavioural theory may help you to understand how people behave, how they respond and how they learn. [4]

How we view others and how we respond to our students' personalities can be learned and trained just as we learn the "123 Step Method" for teaching practise. By observation, we can modify our responses to their personalities and behaviour and significantly enhance the learning environment of the class. Every lesson can be a learning experience with regard to recognising, understanding and working with the personalities and behaviours of our students.

However, people rarely are classified as one personality type or another. Rather we are complexes of what I would consider to be "substantial and insubstantial" properties of all of the basic types.

X..X   (continuum)

---

[4] for a comprehensive list of texts - see Mulhauser, 2009.

Whether it is done consciously or subconsciously, people who work with large numbers of people do categorise the people they need to work with – it is a tool we use to assess the dynamics of our group at that present time and how we best use their personalities and behaviours to achieve our objectives as teachers.

The methodology of teaching should be mostly the 1,2,3 method as it works the best for efficiency. The other methods – following and sectional teaching can be used as required. No two classes should ever be taught with exactly the same strategies for working with students. How teachers draw from their own skills and knowledge, their own personality and work satisfaction parameters, their teaching skills and people skills and their knowledge of managing the various personalities and behaviours make each class and even each lesson a little bit different from another. However, it is the personalities and experience of the participants, which will have the greatest potential to make the difference between a good lesson and a great learning experience.

From the teacher's perspective, teaching should be all about the student. The teacher and the student *together* make the teaching. Managing individuals and the group as a whole will result in what the students take away from the workshop or class – their knowledge, their understanding, their desire to improve and their confidence and motivation. How well this is achieved will have a significant bearing on the interactions between the TCH Instructor and the specific types of personalities you will find in any group of people working together.

1.83   Who is in this class today - We will now briefly look at a selection range of specific types of personalities and characteristics that can present at a Tai Chi class.

The Administrator -The administrator is undoubtedly one of the most important people at any class. If the class is not small, the administrator always puts in a lot of effort to make the organisation of the paperwork workable and not intrusive to the rest of the class. As the Greeter, this person sets the tone of the class and the welcome is always a sign of acceptance. If the welcome is poor, the student will have some reservations. When the greeting is warm, students relax and feel part of the group. As the teacher, you need to maximise the little spare time you have before and after the lesson. Performing "book work" will take up your valuable time and opportunity you have to communicate with your students and form a good level of understanding of the class dynamics with your students. Most good organisers are motivated by their desire to help and they see the value and worth of having a Tai Chi class available in their community.

Their skills and friendliness oversee the roll, the registration of new students, the giving out of medical clearance forms and class information, and they will manage the financial requirements. Their valued role in service to you and your students means that you will not have to deal with administrative duties or financial aspects while teaching and will have all your available time to talk to and be available to your students.

Class Assistants - These people are those in a position of influence and responsibility in your class environment. Most assistants will be students who are highly motivated with their Tai Chi but who are also gentle and undemanding in the class situation. They can be most useful in an emergency situation and it is advisable that the class assistant is trained and current in First Aid and CPR. Some TCH teachers are lucky enough to have assistants who have completed the TCA or TCD basic training and have some understanding and competency in teaching method, safety and precautions. This is an ideal situation, but careful consideration should be given when your students actually help with the group teaching. If they are not trained, other students resent them to a degree and this is justified. On the other hand, the class assistants need nurturing as well with their own development with Tai Chi. In this situation, the teacher needs to provide another class at an advanced level, or include the general learning part for everyone the same only giving added tasks for those who have been training longer – so that they may grow and develop as well.

The personality of the assistant will be willing, informed, respectful to the teacher and the teacher's desire for how the class is run. This person needs all the qualities of kindness and helpfulness that will make them approachable by the students. The students will trust them and not feel incompetent or humiliated when working with them. Hopefully, they will know how to have fun.

Helpers - Helpers are truly an asset to the class as well. Their role is usually "someone to follow" or being friendly enough that new people will want to ask them questions – or stand next to them. They are also people who can be a friend to new people and make them feel comfortable and accepted. These people are usually easy going and friendly. They generally keep a low and modest profile and can see a need often before you think of it yourself. Strategy: Be clear in your request and this person will get it right for you. For example if you want the chairs in a particular way, don't say, "Can you fix the chairs?" Rather, "Would you place the chairs in two rows in a semi circle?" They also make good helpers for talks and do not need to be scene-stealers.

Delights These people lighten your load and give you a chance to relax. It is easy to spot this type of person – they give good eye contact, smile readily, are organised, ready and waiting, on time, polite and considerate, interested and are often competent students (into the bargain). They will be attentive and, answer when you speak, they will be responsive and come up with an answer when many are reluctant to answer or even respond verbally. You always hope there are two or three delights in your class to make it flow happily. Strategy: All you will need to do with this person is make eye contact and they will oblige. They frequently make excellent leaders of small groups and are reliable and exact in their response to you, not requiring special attention and approval from you or the group generally.

Shadows - This personality can be described as sticky. They are basically good people though they are often thick skinned and seem insensitive to the signals you and others are giving. They are unresponsive when you look to other students and demand your exclusive attention at least once in every lesson. They often have black/white aspects to their personality and do not accept change or new ideas readily. However, many of these people have other sides to their lives that cause them great hardship either now or in the past. They are fighters and need recognition and support not criticism. They often grate other people so they need to be controlled. However, their journey is as important as any of the other "easier" personalities in the group. Strategy: Do not feel obligated to give this person too much of your time during the lesson but try to find time to support them perhaps for a few minutes before or after the lesson. Try not to have favourites and try not to avoid people either. Every student should have equal value of your time and effort.

Expert - Exposure to this type of personality can be confronting. This person is at pains to show your lack of depth or knowledge or technique or teaching skill by espousing their superior knowledge to anyone who will listen. This type of person is often aggressive and fortunately they are not common in the class scene. Look kindly on them. Their confidence is fragile and their behaviour is flawed. Often they are very fixed in what they believe and are sorely pressed to think beyond what they already know.

Their rigid performance in front of others gives them an audience to reinforce their statements and put you "on the spot". Their tone is often aggressive and the overall aim of the behaviour may be to attempt to devalue you (the person) and what you are teaching. More often there is a prejudice – you are a woman or you are a Chinese person (or you are not a Chinese person). They could be ageist, or fattist – or anything they dislike. Strategy: Look on their behaviour as a flaw. They have a need to boost their own confidence. Remain calm and confident in your knowledge. Do not allow this person to dominate the valuable and brief time you have with other students. Tell them that you are interested to expand on what they are saying and that you would like to hear more. Suggest meeting at the next break to discuss their issues further. Bring the group back gracefully and confidently to the current task.

Inflexible Student - This type person is not common to Tai Chi classes. Most people are there because they want to learn and be with other like-minded people. Such a person will display a resistance to change from characteristics of their own understanding and do not feel confident about embracing new ideas. The teacher needs to know something about why this student is attending. Perhaps they know they need relaxing but "forget" themselves in class. They may also be rigid and unresponsive to the principles of Tai Chi, such as posture and differentiating between insubstantial and substantial and other more exacting principles of movement. This personality is threatened and insecure with change. Their attitude in the class is often nothing to do with the teacher or the other students but rather where they are themselves with other aspects of life. Strategy: Make light of their inability to change and develop. The fact that they are there is enough. Don't ignore them but don't give them overt correction either. This type of person is in a wonderful position to relax and enjoy doing Tai Chi. Ignoring them is not the way to be their teacher. When you get a chance and in an informal moment, ask them "How do you feel about the follow-step" and so on. You can acknowledge subtly in the practice sessions when they respond to the changes they have made. We are not there to change their personalities but to find ways to teach that are acceptable to them. Do not be offended by them or feel angry – go with the flow and enjoy the experience of finding a way to reach them. Some you can never reach – but they can enjoy themselves doing Tai Chi helping them improve their QAL.

The Silent Type - The shy or silent student exhibits all of the characteristics of the helper. They do not always lack confidence but often do not have good people skills or the need to be social. This person has wanted to learn about Tai Chi and has paid to be there. Because they are not overt personalities, does not mean they are not enjoying the class and moving forward with their health plan. Strategy: Respect this person's feelings by not drawing on them openly. She/he will need to feel unthreatened and relaxed enough to focus on the class and not be conspicuous or in fear of being put in the spotlight. Begin by making some sort of eye contact or smile to this person to give approval at a personal level. It won't take much – just being aware of her/him. It would be a shame to lose a valuable caring gentle soul doing a lot of good in a comfortable and safe environment simply because the teacher did not respect their need for anonymity.

Perfectionists - These people are obsessed with detail and can be very demanding of your time. Early in their training, their constant interruption can interfere with the flow of the teaching environment and they can be frustrating to you and other students. Know that their meticulous behaviour spills over into many aspects of their social, business and private lives. Again it is a way of getting recognition and acknowledgement for their good work. Their biggest enemy is themselves as they put demands on their own expectations that they would never expect of others. Somehow, they are not what they appear to be – that of the importance of being "right" but their own needs are actually less important to them – otherwise they would care more about their own welfare. They expect that they should be able to do things that other humans would not be expected to do, expecting less time for integration, less time for consolidation, no permission to make errors and so forth. Strategy: The most efficient way to handle this person is to whisper: "I can see that you are very interested in getting all the details correct" and then say: "Take particular notice in the 'watch me' section when I demonstrate the move. Really focus in the "follow me" because I will do it exactly the same each time". A nod or smile is enough for them. You are still nodding and smiling at everyone else as well – but they don't see that. They are self-focussed.   In time they will relax.

Husband/Wife – Mother/Daughter etc - This combination is often a great advantage because one encourages the other to attend and for practice. It is an activity they can share and get much enjoyment from over the years. Very rarely is this dynamic a problem. Occasionally people in a relationship compete at some level with each other. Strategy: stay well away from interfering unless it causes a concern to other students.   You can't play matchmaker at class. It is always possible to put them into different study groups and come back together for the cool-down and close. Their ways of sorting this problem is best left to them. The subtle problems created by working together will not give either of them the best outcome for the lesson. Drawing attention to it only makes it worse. The easiest way is to leave them alone. Place them in separate groups if possible. It is a difficult situation – but stay out of it.

Use your ears and your eyes and your heart – especially use your instinct.

1.84   Conclusion - Just teaching your knowledge is not always enough. You might be very dedicated yourself and believe strongly that Tai Chi teaching is what you want to do. Learning how to work with people is something you can work on and improve with experience.
General Strategy: Remind yourself that everyone at the class is important to you. Without them there is no teaching. You are going to work extremely hard to reach your teaching goals and your reward will be if helping these people to understand and develop Tai Chi to improve their quality of life. Your wish to teach them sincerely, competently and enthusiastically will succeed. Recognise that the world is made up of all sorts of personalities – not just the ones that you are drawn to.   Learn about personalities from further study and by observing how people behave.

Train yourself to always focus on their good points as this will lift them and encourage them more than anything else. Never, never embarrass people or humiliate them in any way. Not only it is hurtful to them, but also it is extremely bad form for the leader of a group and de-values your role as "teacher". If you feel really angry, turn away and take a deep breath. Smile and say something like "let me think about this for a moment". Do think about it, because this situation may come up again and you will need to handle it better next time. Make a rule to deliver corrections generally ie to everyone and only make a point of correction if you think it is an unsafe move.

How you conduct yourself, how you speak, how you handle people, how you listen, how you eat, the intonation of your voice, your punctuality, how you behave generally, your ability to be unruffled will be what people see. Always assume that people notice everything. Stay with your values but be mindful that the world is made up of all sorts of personalities and circumstance. Stay flexible and be happy.

UNIT 200
ESSENTIAL KNOWLEDGE OF HUMAN BODY

Unit Overview	**2.10**	**Anatomy & Posture**
	2.20	**Stretching**
	2.30	**Physiology & Breathing**
	2.40	**Safety & Health Management**

2.10   ANATOMY & POSTURE OVERVIEW
2.11   Introduction
2.12   Posture - General
2.13   Posture - the Muscles
2.14   Alphabetical List of Muscles
2.15   Knees & Neck
2.16   Age and Posture
2.17   Alexander Technique

2.11   Introduction - A basic scientific knowledge of human anatomy and function for the Tai Chi for Heath Instructor is essential for a variety of reasons related to Safety, Secular and Scientific aspects of a modern Tai Ch for Health. The most important is maximising safety in the Tai Chi for Health exercise and health management activity. Tai Chi for Health Leaders who already have some knowledge of human anatomy and function - such as accredited physiotherapists, nurses, medical doctors, exercise physiologists, fitness trainers and marital arts instructors - are significantly better positioned to link the Tai Chi for Health activity to a scientific knowledge of human anatomy and function and to a more informed understanding of safety as part of a modern Duty of Care. However, Tai Chi for Health Leaders who have little or no knowledge of human anatomy and function and the relationship to a modern Duty of Care – such as non-accredited martial arts and Kung Fu Tai Chi Chuan teachers - present a significantly greater risk in relation to safety factors in the delivery of the Tai Chi for Health activity.

Another important reason is that a scientific knowledge of human anatomy and function provides a common language and understanding between the Tai Chi for Health Instructor and the Health Professional who has a Duty of Care responsibly to assist the patient in having informed consent about the integrity and safety of the Tai Chi for Health exercise program (Appendix 2). In Western society, the educational and professional training of the Health Professional operates within a secular and scientific framework of understanding human anatomy and function and does not include concepts of "Chi", "Meridians" and the "Dao of Nature" as is frequently articulated within certain traditions of the Chinese martial arts and Kung Fu Tai Chi Chuan.   Moreover, the Tai Chi for Health Leader/Instructor is expected to have some understanding of the scientific research and literature relevant to safety and health management of the Tai Chi for Health exercise program.   Without some basic scientific knowledge of human anatomy and function, such an expectation is at best problematic and at worst potentially harmful.

What does scientific knowledge of "human anatomy and function" mean? Anatomy is the study of the structure of the body, which includes the study of bones, muscles, nerves, systems, cells, blood, lymph, and organs. Anatomy can be studied at a developmental level, a microscopic level, a comparative level and a functional or movement level. Physiology is the science of function, that is, it is the study of how the body works. (Crouch, 1972, p10) There is of course overlap between both disciplines. This Unit will examine only a very small portion of this enormous field of study and is offered as an introduction to a Western and scientific understanding of human anatomy and function specifically pertinent to safety and health management issues of a Tai Chi for Health exercise program.

2.12   Posture - General - Consideration of posture is central to all Tai Chi teaching and should be the central focus when teaching beginners. The focus from the teacher's perspective is with regard to (1) safety (2) speed of the body's efficient response to physical activity and (3) ultimately better health for the student.   Optimal alignment should be considered as important to health and well-being as Strength, Flexibility and Aerobic Capacity and Absence of Anxiety as positive changes to body alignment can improve body function profoundly. As a precaution for Instructors, remember when teaching posture that to touch another person in any way, even by the touch of a fingertip – is not only too much but in most cases is totally unnecessary. Improvements and changes have to come from the person themselves, their cognitive effort and hard wiring and may take years to improve. Instead of touching suggest looking in a mirror or asking someone to film them. In this way they can clearly see malalignment even though they feel their posture is upright. Self-correction also helps to connect the mind to the body. With advanced students, the teacher may touch with the fingertip but only after asking permission from the student. For the older aged, staying upright and balanced is enough.

Ideal posture is important for the following reasons:
• Body mechanics are working optimally when alignment is correct

- Everyday activity is efficient and less restricted
- Fatigue is minimised
- Muscles will function well because power can be generated
- There is reduced risk of falls
- Breathing can improve
- Improvements in gait can be dramatic
- Body organs sit in their anatomically ideal position

Posture refers to how the body is positioned. We may talk about lying posture, supine or prone or foetal position, and sitting posture slumped or straight. "Posture" can also refer to body parts such as "the posture of the arms" or "the posture-of-the-eyes". Position or posture of the body, or parts of the body, determines a large part of how the body works. Small positive changes in posture can help the body to work more efficiently and more safely. For our purposes, "Posture" here indicates upright standing position.

What society accepts as an aesthetic posture consists of having:
- A relatively straight back with no increase of natural curvature at the thoracic or lumbar
- A flat abdominal wall
- No rounding of the shoulders
- Head straight

Posture Check Suitable for Tai Chi Movement and Postures
- Look at the chin. How far does it protrude forward, or upward or downward?
- Look at the inward curve of the cervical spine? Is it excessive?
- Look at the thoracic spine (upper back). Is it excessively curved outwards? Does it show a hump anywhere?
- Look at the lumbar spine (lower back). Is there excessive inward curving? Is it flat?
- Look at the muscles of the buttock. Are they strong or do they sag, or have they disappeared?
- Look at the abdominal muscles. Are they strong and flat or do they protrude and sag downward?
- Look at the pelvis. Is it tilting forward or backward?
- Look at the level of each hip (viewed from the back). Are they level?
- Look at the level of each shoulder (viewed from the back). Are they level?
- Look at the scapula. Are they even? Is there any winging?
- Look at the knees. Are they locked back or are they sightly bent?

One can draw an imaginary straight line falling through the middle of the head, in front of the ear, through the anterior cervical spine, through the centre of the chest, through the lumbar spine, through the centre of the hip, through the knee and slightly anterior to the ankle joint. This is the ideal posture through the centre line of the body going through the centre of gravity behind the umbilicus. Many people try to improve posture by lifting the sternum and sticking out the chest, often lifting the head and tilting the chin "like a soldier". Much is achieved by elongating the spine by imagining the head is suspended from the sky, gently sinking the upper chest, softening the upper back and gently tucking in the chin and keeping the eyes straight ahead. Understanding the position of the head, shoulders and trunk is fundamental to efficient Tai Chi practise.

The sensation of good posture is achieved by gently pressing the top of the head towards the ceiling, forming a strong central line down the abdomen and then pulling down from the waist and gently tucking the pelvis slightly under allowing the limbs to relax and the knees to soften. This is an ideal posture for practising Tai Chi. This position where every thing is in absolute balance (before the "yin and yang" of movement) is known as Wu Chi. Improvements in posture often take a long time. With the aged skeletal structure improvements may only be small but never insignificant. Remember the guidelines concerning touching. Try to encourage change to posture via accessing the mind of the student to correct themselves.

PLEASE note that many of the spinal and other skeletal changes in the aged are permanent and all will have a degree of osteoporosis and soft tissue degeneration in both men and women. Some conditions will be extreme. Any attempt to "change" posture can do enormous harm by anyone not properly qualified. Best practice would be simply to ask, "does that feel comfortable" with the student managing their own body for balance and stability awareness. Optimal posture for any person is only gained by practicing the correct alignment of the body and will only be achieved with improved flexibility and muscle strength. Incorrect posture causes problems with many of the body's functions. These problems will be increased in the ageing or ill body or through continued poor habits.

2.13   Posture - The Muscles - The place to start improving posture is to gently lift the top of the head towards the ceiling. Tuck in the chin, allow the sternum to sink and muscles of the upper back will relax. Perhaps the most important segment in maintaining the ideal erect posture is the position of the pelvis. Because the pelvis joins the immovable portion of the spine (the sacrum) to the mobile portion, deviations from its normal position are reflected the full length of the spinal column. Ideally the anterior and posterior superior iliac spines should be in a straight line.

Examining the posture:
- Which posture type?
- Is the neck curved inwards?
- How far is the chin forward?
- Is the upper part of the spine humped? All of it or just at one place?
- Are the abdominal muscles protruding and sagging downwards indicating weak lower abdominal muscles?
- Is the curve to the lumbar region too far inwards or is it flat?
- Are the buttock muscles strong or are there "no" buttock muscles?
- Are the knees locked back or bent more than natural?

A posterior tilt straightens the lumbar section of the spine (while a downward tilt accentuates the lumbar curve). Some of the muscle groups involved in upright posture of the pelvis are:
- Abdominals
- Hip flexors
- Gluteals and hamstrings
- Erector spinae
- Shoulder girdle

Abdominals: Well-toned abdominals (both the rectus and the obliques) are necessary to pull the interior pelvis up towards the ribs and to compress and support the internal organs. The transverse group play a vital part in the integrity of the lower spine and greatly assist lower back strength.

Hip Flexors: The iliopsoas in particular which attaches to the top of the femur and to the lower half of the vertebral column and sacrum needs to be able to stretch sufficiently to allow for placement of the pelvis. These muscles have a tendency to shorten the more sedentary we become.

Gluteals & Hams: These major muscle groups are important in anchoring the posterior pelvis down in the correct position. They are also important for walking and balance.

Erector Spinae: The action of these muscles should align the spine into a vertical position and allow the sternum to re-orient itself away from the spinal column.

Shoulder Girdle: The best functioning of the internal organs calls for an erect position of the chest and neck, and a moderate adduction of the shoulder girdle. The muscles which extend the neck and spine and which pull the scapulae closer together (such as the rhomboids) need to be strong. The anterior chest should be flexible enough to allow shoulders to be maintained in an open position.

Lumbar Spine: The lumbar spine needs to be flexible to allow the downward pull by the gluteals and hamstrings and also to prevent tight hamstrings. Also the sacro-iliac nerve is partially stretched. When the hamstrings are too short, they pull on the pelvis tilting it posteriorly. This causes the buttocks to tuck under, bending the knees which in turn limits the lifting of the feet and the frequently seen "shuffle" of the aged. Compound this with the anterior movement of the neck and head and the sunken chest – and this is the stereotypical posture of ageing.

Caution: *When thinking about and trying to alert students to their posture think about the concept of two trees. A young tree will be able to load up with incredible weight and bend to contain that load, but an old tree is often fragile and hollow and will snap with the smallest load. As teachers, remember that we cannot see into the body, and in your enthusiasm to build muscular strength remember too there is real risk of bone damage and causing great harm. Trying to "improve" posture to your ideals is strongly contraindicated. Gently ... gently!! Keep your intention to no harm as your first priority.*

Having a good understanding of the musculature of the body will help you as the teacher become more aware of the role of muscles in posture and movement. Having an understanding of muscles does not mean you become an expert or take on the role of a therapist, but rather it means having an awareness of the function of the muscles, having a working knowledge of functional anatomy will help you to focus on what is important in the training you offer and noticing when improvements have been accomplished. It is important to have some awareness of the ramifications of muscle atrophy (Rolf, 1998; Rosenberg, 1989, 1997; Iannuzzi-Sucich et al, 2002; Lexell, 1997) and the functional capacity of muscle with disuse (see Baumgartner et al, 1998; Daley et al, 2000).

Muscles that are especially important for posture are: muscles of the neck, all the musculature of the spine, the abdominal groups, the gluteals, the hamstrings, lower leg and foot. Students always wonder about why the abdominals are so important for back strength. Explaining how they work can be very useful in helping students make the mind/body connection. When students press the head gently towards the ceiling (sitting or standing with relaxed knees) the abdominal group should be activated and can actually be felt naturally – albeit minimally – about 5%. Any forced activation of the abdominal muscles could interfere with breathing. Explain that the deepest of this group (Transversus abdominus) wraps across the abdomen like a girdle and supports the back and spine. When arms and legs begin to move the stability of the spine comes from activation of these deep muscles, and the deep muscles of the back which act as anchors. This would explain why falls and injury are so prevalent when the core strength is weakened through inactivity or a more sedentary life style and through ageing.

The famous FICSIT study in Atlanta in 1997 first drew world wide attention to the value of using Tai Chi as an intervention for reducing falls. Part of the whole picture of how Tai Chi works is that this type of physical activity uses the whole body as a co-ordinated unit with muscle strength gains being an integral factor of falls prevention. Other studies looked at gains in strength in relation to balance with Tai Chi as the intervention training vehicle (Wolf et al, 1997; and Wolfson et al, 1996). Skeletal changes that have an effect on posture are: degeneration of the neck, changes to the curvature of the spine, dropping arches of the feet, position of the heel, changes to the knee, osteoporosis and disease/condition of the bone eg Paget's disease, arthritis (see Lam and Horstman, 2002). Also, many chronic diseases such as Parkinson's disease and Multiple Sclerosis effect posture as well because of cognitive changes throughout the nervous systems which effect gait. People working in the health and fitness areas are well aware that muscle loss and inactivity do have an impact on falls and injury (see Rantanen et al, 1997; Mahoney, 1998; Fransen et al 2007; Voukelatos et al, 2007), and studies show that increased muscle strength is one of the factors that helps to reduce the number or falls experienced by people who participate in Tai Chi as a form of physical activity. An understanding of some of the more important muscles and functions in the teaching of Tai Chi for Health are summarised as follows:

2.14 List of Muscles and Function [5]

MUSCLE	Function
BICEPS BRACHII - Long & Short Head	Flexion of arm and supination of the hand
BICEPS FEMORIS Long head	Flex leg and extend thigh and lateral rotation of leg
BICEPS FEMORIS - Short head	Flex leg and extend thigh and lateral rotation of the leg
DELTOID Anterior; Middle; Posterior	Whole muscle abducts arm; in part, may flex, extend, and rotate arm
ERECTOR SPINAE	Extend spine
EXTERNAL OBLIQUES	Works with int. oblique on opposite side to flex trunk laterally and rotate
FLEXORS OF TOES	Flex foot digits
GASTROCNEMIUS	Plantar flex foot, assist to flex leg
GLUTEUS MAXIMUS	Extension and lateral rotation of thigh, braces the knee
GLUTEUS MEDIUS	Abduction of thigh and medial rotation
GLUTEUS MINIMUS	Abduction of thigh and medial rotation; weak flexor
HAMSTRINGS - (see biceps femoris)	
ILIPSOAS (see Iliacus & Psoas major)	
INFRASPINATUS	External rotation of arm; may assist in both abduction and adduction of humerus
INTERNAL OBLIQUES	Works with ext. oblique on opposite side Compression of abdominal viscera; flexion of vertebral column
LATISSIMUS DORSI	Extension, adduction and medial rotation of arm. Draws shoulder backward and downward
PECTORALIS MAJOR	Flexion, adduction, and medial rotation of arm
PSOAS Major	Flexion and medial rotation of thigh; flexion of lumbar region of vertebral column
QUADRICEPS (see Rectus Femoris, Vastus intermedialis, Vastus lateralis Vastus medialis	
RECTUS ABDOMINUS	Flexion of vertebral column compression of abdominal viscera
RECTUS FEMORIS	Flexion of thigh and extension of leg
RHOMBOIDEUS MAJOR	Adduction of scapula and slight rotation. Depression of shoulder
RHOMBOIDEUS MINOR	Adduction of scapula and slight rotation of shoulder. Depression of shoulder
SEMIMEMBRANOSIS	Flexion and medial rotation of leg, extends thigh
SEMITENDINOSUS	Flexion and medial rotation of leg; extends thigh
SOLEUS	Plantar flexion of foot
SUBSCAPULARIS	Rotation of head of humerus medially, aids adduction, abduction, flexion and extension.
TENSOR FASCIA LATAE (TFL)	Flexion of thigh, medial rotation, abduction
TIBIALIS ANTERIOR	Dorsiflexion and supination of foot
TRANSVERSUS ABDOMINUS	Constriction of abdomen
TRAPEZIUS	Draws head back, rotates scapula, draws head to side, braces shoulder, adducts scapula
TRICEPS BRACHII Long head	Extension of arm and forearm. Longhead also adducts arm

---

[5] For a complete list and further detail - see *Crouch, 1975, pp 260-76*

Lateral head	Assists to extend arm
Medial Head	Assists to extend arm
VASTUS INTERMEDIUS	Extension of leg
VASTUS LATERALIS	Extension of leg
VASTUS MEDIALIS	Extension leg

Muscles are categorised as smooth, skeletal and cardiac and all are specialised and all have a contractile property. Smooth muscle is involuntary, being under the control of the autonomic nervous system. Cardiac muscle is highly "automatic" and is also controlled by the autonomic nervous system. Skeletal muscle is under the control of the voluntary nervous system and is somewhat dependent on the will of the individual though much happens "automatically" through habit. Unlike cardiac muscle, skeletal muscle fatigues easily.

The role of skeletal muscles is to support the skeleton but listed below are some of their features:

Skeletal Muscles
- Are 40% of body weight
- Provide voluntary movement
- Maintain posture
- Breathe
- Chew and swallow
- Eliminate
- Articulate speech
- Communicate – smile, wink, frown, kiss, snarl
- Give shape to the body
- Play a role in preservation – turn head, sniff, see, protect
- Used for locomotion
- Store nutrients

It is important also to understand the role of Fascia and its relationship to muscles. Each muscle and muscle group is encased in a sheath-like connective tissue membrane. There are specialised stretching cells in some fascia that have a protective role in preventing injury. The fibrous texture of Fascia joins together at the end of the muscle to form a tendon. The tendon knits into bone and facilitates action. The health of the muscles and fascia at the sides of the legs is very important in falls prevention. Biomechanically, complex movements such as "Waving Hands in Cloud" and "Single Whip" play a significant role in keeping these tissues healthy and strong.

A feature of muscle that is relevant for physical activity is that muscle has properties of contractibility and extensibility. The balance of how much muscles contract or extend is related to the balance of the muscle groups which is related to posture. Nothing with muscles works in isolation. Having an imbalance in the muscle groups that work together has a direct effect on posture and gait and can have implications with health including frequency of falls and injury. Tai Chi uses the whole body in a unifying manner and muscle balance is a feature of how the movements work together effectively and efficiently.

Understanding the Bigger Picture of How Muscles Work - Sometimes when we think of the action of muscles we tend to think of a particular muscle doing a job – eg the quadriceps in front of the thigh straightening the knee. However, most of the muscles that are responsible for movement work with other muscles together in a group and are called Synergists. For example, the action of straightening the knee involves not only the quadriceps but also the hamstrings at the back of the thigh. The Agonists at the front cause the leg to straighten increasing the angle of the knee. The Antagonists then at the back of the thigh control this action and lengthen to accommodate the stretch.

The balance between the groups involved in a movement should be such that the movement is co-ordinated and smooth allowing easy co-ordinated mobility. This requires a good balance of strength of the muscles. When the muscles are uneven and not balanced, injuries occur. Over time, even small imbalances caused by poor habit or injury impact on posture and balance. Muscle imbalances can have such an impact that the entire alignment of the body can be compromised. For example, the hamstring group at the back of the thigh are a powerful group with the tendons originating on the lower pelvis. If the hamstrings are shortened due to lack of mobility or lack of normal stretching with activity, the tendons are powerful enough to influence the alignment of the pelvis. Here the pelvis is tilted posteriorly as the "bottom" disappears.   The alignment of the pelvis has an effect on the thoracic spine and neck and also limits the ability to flex the ankle for toe clearance. Over a period of time this results not only in the shuffling gait typical of some elderly people but in the increased likelihood of falling. The significance of this is that balanced use of muscles and continued mobility has a significant effect on the quality of life for many people.   In the elderly these problems may be exacerbated by general loss of strength, poor balance, loss of eyesight and appetite, diminished cognitive function and the added complication of medications.

When researching anatomy the TCH Instructor needs to understand the planes of reference:
- Median or Midsagittal – dividing the body into equal parts

- Sagittal - any plane parallel to median
- Frontal or Coronal – divides the body into Anterior and Posterior
- Transverse or Horizontal – divides the body into superior and inferior

To communicate intelligently with health professionals you should at least know that
- Plantar – on the sole
- Palmar – on the palm
- Medial – towards the mid-line
- Lateral - away from the midline or on the side or edge
- External – on the outside
- Internal – on the inside
- Posterior - back
- Anterior - front
- Proximal – nearer to the body
- Distal – away from the body – or end
- Dorsal – back
- Afferent – conveying to (nerves)
- Efferent – conveying from (nerves)

2.15   Knees, Head and Spine

(a)   Knees - The knee is being highlighted as the single most important joint except for the spine requiring special care and awareness in the study of movement. A basic understanding of the importance of the functioning knee joint is an essential aspect for safe teaching of Tai Chi for the motivated instructor. The knee functions as a pillar to support the body weight when standing and moving and to give structural support for mobilisation. It has cushioning between the thigh and lower leg to protect the joint from friction and the rolling action of the joint, but it is also subject to wear and tear due to overuse and injury or from direct pressure from excess body weight. It also has a little bone in the front called the patella which acts as a fulcrum for the large muscles of the thigh. It too is subject to injury mainly from falls and when it is damaged impacts on the ability to bend the knee. Strengthening the muscles of the thigh and leg support and stabilise the knee joint.

Teaching Points

1. If a student has a chronic condition of the knee, it is vital that doing Tai Chi does not aggravate the joint and lead to more pain and injury. A worsening will inevitably occur if excessive forces are placed on the joint holding the body on one leg or changing weight from one leg to another. Further injury can occur if (1) the knee bends too deeply or if (2) the knee is allowed to go beyond the alignment of the feet, making an acute angle at the patella. In biomechanical terms this means that there is a degree of shearing force along the line of the femur to the apex. The momentum of the force will go beyond this point and increase the risk of injury. For example, the danger for injury is greatly increased by having too much weight and being too far forward on the forward leg in the "Single Whip".

2. An overweight body places an increased load on the knees causing damage over time. Added to this are the degenerative changes caused by a congenital condition, by an injury or by arthritis and it is easy to see that the knees are vulnerable.

    Teaching any movement for the knee safely is achieved by:
    - Having good alignment between the middle of the foot and the middle of the knee joint
    - Keeping the body weight over the hip, knee and foot alignment when changing weight i.e. when the bulk of the body weight is carried by one leg and hip
    - Keeping the spine long in optimal posture position to lighten the load on the lower back and knee
    - Adjusting the depth of bend to a comfortable working level – even if this is almost normal stance
    - Not allowing the bended knee to go beyond the alignment with the foot
    - Adjusting the weight supporting knee and foot to turn in to 45 degrees when executing a directional change
    - Lowering the toe first (after the feather touch of the heel in the stepping movement) to align the knee and foot *before* transfer of weight

The large muscle groups in the front and back of the thigh in large part determine the quality of the action of the knee joint. Studies reveal that there is a significant loss of function and loss of skeletal muscle due simply to ageing (see Rosenberg, 1997). Muscle atrophy will have a significant effect on the strength and integrity of the joint. Thirty minutes or more a day of continual weight bearing movement will undoubtedly have a beneficial effect of maintaining as much muscle as possible.

In practising Tai Chi not aligning the centre of the knee with the centre of the foot, or not adjusting the foot when changing direction may be shown to contribute markedly with pain and damage to the knee.

The posterior muscles of the thigh (Biceps femoris, Semitendinosis and Semimembranosis form the "hamstrings". Failure to lengthen and stretch this muscle group contributes to a posterior tilt of the pelvis, a flexing of the knees and the limited ability of the tibialis anterior to lift for toe clearance – all of which contribute to falls and injury. Added to this the abdominals are compromised and silent. Practising Tai Chi increases the flexibility and strength of the muscles of the leg which in turn pull less heavily on the pelvis, allow more free movement of a "step" and allow the toes to lift. The improvement of the posture, even if slight gives some work to the abdominals and strengthens the back.

- How important is muscle lengthening or stretching?
- How important is strengthening leg muscles for quality of life?
- How important is knee alignment and base of support?
- How important is learning how to change direction safely?
- How important is upright to the optimal position for that individual?
- How important is teaching the student how to execute movement comfortably and unhurried? How important is patience, gentleness and encouragement?

Many teachers are unaware of the importance of stepping into the hip line when changing direction. Too frequently students perform a "Brush Knee Push" movement stepping onto the "tightrope" along the mid line of the body. In no way does this help to prevent falls and is in fact a dangerous move for students who are physically unstable particularly with balance. Every "Brush Knee Push" should be performed in the "bow stance" for the wonderful health benefits of stability and balance that are so frequently taken for granted at a younger age. In addition, modification of the supporting leg in changing direction may be necessary in changing direction in order to protect the knee joint from being stressed by not being in proper alignment.

Practising Tai Chi in and unsafe and therefore potentially damaging way is contrary to the ideals of Tai Chi for Health in a modern setting – that is to do no harm, to improve health and quality of life.

(b) **Head** - Some mention should be made with regard to the placement of the head in Tai Chi. The warm-ups comprising of the stretches for the major components of the body – neck, shoulders, spine, hips, knees, ankles, hands teach the correct placement for the moving and still body in Tai Chi. The stretches for the neck clearly ensure that the top of the head is lengthened and the chin is tucked in, eyes level before the stretches commence. Yet, when students begin their Tai Chi practice many droop their spine and hang the head or look down. Some students are in fact shy and are in the habit of the downward glance.

When a student lowers the head it more often than not over-sinks the chest and compromises breathing to a lessor or greater degree. Also jutting out the chin causes strain in the neck and upper shoulder muscles. By consistently saying "tuck in the chin" before either lowering the head or turning the head in the warm-ups soon become a habit that is transferred to the practising of the forms. Leaving students to "feel comfortable" without showing them how does nothing to help the student in the long run.

In the warm-up set, it is an important teaching point to re-align the chin before each stretch.

(c) **Spine** – The spine can be classified into five segments of the Vertebral column with abbreviations:
1. Neck - C1 to C7 – Seven Cervical vertebrae of the neck
2. Chest – T1 to T12 - Twelve Thoracic vertebrae joining the ribs to the vertebral column
3. Low Back – L1 to L5 – Five Lumbar vertebrae which support the body weight and the forces of the body
4. Pelvis – S1 to S5- Five fused Sacral joints
5. Tailbone - no abbreviation – Four 4 Coccygeal joints

A spinal vertebra has two main parts – 1. Vertebral body cushioned by the discs (except for the fused joints) face anteriorly; and 2. Neural arch from which spinous processes protrude posteriorly (which can be felt on the surface of the back) and transverse processes aligned to the side. The deep muscles and ligaments attach to the "processes" and other surfaces of the bone and move the spinal column. Between the vertebral body and the processes lies a canal or tube-like structure which carries the spinal cord for most of the length of the vertebral column. Also, the spinal vertebra provides the protective structure for the spinal cord from which all the nerves leave the protective conduit of the spine for other parts of the body. This basic knowledge will help the Tai Chi for Health teacher to understand the structural characteristics of posture and the importance of lengthening the spine to activate the deep muscles. It is the deep muscles that anchor the body to allow the limbs to action movements away from the base of support. If the structure of the spine is not strong or properly aligned, then movements become compromised with a risk of injury. [6]

---

[6] For further information and detail on this topic, refer Crouch (1975) or access through an internet search under the key words – "vertebral column", for example see Emory University (2009) and Human Biodyssey (2008).

2.16   Age and Posture - Our skeleton appears to be stable but throughout life it has very many different forms. The spine of a baby and toddler are different from a young child, a teenager, a young adult. Throughout life many people sustain traumas and injuries, but also as we age our habits of how we move, sit and stand have a direct effect on how the skeleton supports us. Many of these habits have a detrimental effect on health. During adult life, the skeleton is in a constant state of change building bone and resorbing bone. With the process of ageing, the spine shortens due mainly to shrinkage of the discs and crushing of vertebral bodies. In the aged, the effects of osteoporosis may be seen in a lateral curvature of the spine known as Scoliosis and/or in altered anterior/posterior alienation of the entire vertebral column.

Listed below are the most common presentations of postural problems. Usually a problem in one area of the body may lead to or result from a problem in another area, as the body adjusts to gravity.

1. **Rounded Upper Back** (Dorsal Kyphosis) - Change in the normal curve of the thorasic spine in a backward direction. Sternum is depressed and the rib case is lowered

2. **Round Shoulders** - This often accompanies 1. The shoulders are positioned forward, tips of shoulders anterior to normal gravity line. Shoulder blades more separated than normal, and chest is sunken.

3. **Hollow Back** (Lumbar Lordosis) - Exaggeration of the normal lumbar curve. Pelvis tilts forward, abdominals stretched as abodomen protrudes.

4. **Swayback** – A forward tilt of the legs from the hips and backward inclination of the trunk at the hips allow the pelvis to be in front of the gravity line.

5. **Flatback** - This presents as a decrease in the normal forward curve of the lumbar spine until it is practically flat or may even have a slight backward bulge.

6. **Lateral Curve** (Scoliosis) - This is an abnormal curve usually accompanied by abnormal rotation of the vertebrae. Cause of the abnormality is largely unknown and is often detected during rapid growth in adolescence. In the aged, osteoporosis and chronic conditions of hips, knees and other injuries have a direct bearing on the spine.

2.17   Alexander Technique - The Alexander Technique is a method of improving an individual's posture and movement, based on the idea that there are 'correct' and 'incorrect' habits or methods of standing, sitting and moving - which vary according to the person. Use of the correct method, which mainly involves keeping the neck and spine in alignment or at an optimal angle for movement (such as standing from sitting position), is said to benefit physical and mental health. The reason it benefits is because, if people move in a biomechanicaly safe way, they have less wear and tear, fewer injuries, less fatigue and more efficient breathing.

The technique is not an exercise program, but requires practice and experimentation on an individual basis with the guidance of a tutor. Nothing in the technique conflicts with orthodox medical opinion, and it has the respect, though not the unqualified approval, of doctors and physiotherapists.

Frederick Matthias Alexander (1869 - 1955), a Shakespearean actor who developed his technique when he lost his voice due to poor posture and over-use. He made a study of the body musculature and how the body moves and developed the technique, which is named after him.

The technique itself teaches the student how to feel where the curves of the spine begin and end and how to isolate and hold the spine for efficient movement. It studies how to sit, how to lie, how to walk up and down stairs, how to get out of a chair, how to walk and so forth.

The most obvious visible malalignment in adults especially older persons occurs with the thoracic spine and neck. As a consequence of this, the other main support areas such as the lumbar spine, hips and knees are thrown away from the centre of gravity producing the typical stance of an aged person.

For many people the curvature of the spine is a consequence of osteoporosis and disc degeneration but many younger aged people can benefit from some form of posture re-alignment before habit changes the alignment of the spine permanently. It is not unusual to see poor posture in asthmatics and in people who suffer severe depression. But it doesn't have to be. Some asthmatics are superb athletes, and many severely depressed people present a healthy persona. People who live a sedentary life style also frequently exhibit poor posture and other health conditions that are often self-imposed.

Except the very old aged, almost everyone responds to a gentle lifting of the sternum. This has the immediate benefit of opening up the rib cavity, lengthening the abdominals and drawing the dorsal muscles into a neutral position. Once this is achieved to a lesser or greater degree, the head is placed back on the spine instead of the usual forward position. Be aware that on lifting the sternum, the head is not tilted back but sits level with the eye-line in horizontal position.

In many people the pelvis leans back and the groin area is thrust forward. As a consequence of this the knees are bent or locked in. In addition to the mal-alignment of the spine, two factors contribute to poor stance in the lower body - loss of muscle and loss of flexibility. Lack of exercise mainly from lack of walking and incidental physical activity of daily living means reduced musculature - weak gluteals, weak quads and weak hamstrings. A reasonable stride length means that the hips are fully extended. Without proper stretching of the hip, the 'break of the leg' at the top of the thigh (where the hip flexes) will always be bent. Long periods of sitting without stretching add to the limited mobility. The knee too will also be bent and the ankle will not flex. In the aged this is typical of the shuffling gait so often a factor in frequent falls. It is not only older people, but many younger people do not "pick up" their feet and shuffle when walking.

The Alexander Technique also teaches how to sit more efficiently by positioning the body on the ischial tuberosities or "sitting bones" rather than slumping back on the chair. When the head is adjusted to tuck in the chin and the posture-of-the-eyes is straight ahead this is not only an ideal posture for Tai Chi Chair (or Tai Chair) but is also excellent for breathing practice.

As a teacher, try to remember that poor stance in others may not always be self-imposed such as laziness. Some people are in so much pain or they have loss of cognitive connection and are unable to walk and their loss of function may become a spiral downwards for quality of life. A person with longstanding grief will not consider good posture a priority. A person with chronic severe asthma will lean forward to shallow breath to get ANY air in or out. A person with osteoporosis will be extremely fragile and as with all aged persons with poor posture and pain they must be handled with caution and patience. Usually the smallest correction can make a great improvement to the quality of life. Again, the improvements have to come from the student in very small increments as there will be limitations. However, even a small change such as tuck in the chin will assist greatly with neck strain. In the younger aged or chronically ill person, the changes may be truly significant and will make a considerable difference in the prevention of many unnecessary consequences of ageing.

2.20   STRETCHING OVERVIEW
   2.21   Understanding Stretching
   2.22   The Preparation Phase
   2.23   The Conditioning Phase
   2.24   The Recovery Phase
   2.25   Priority Muscle Groups

2.21   Understanding Stretching

What is Flexibility? FLEXIBILITY is the range of motion (ROM) possible around a joint or set of joints. Like other components of health and fitness, flexibility varies considerably between individuals.

WHY STRETCH? All movement involves an element of stretch. The more the muscle can be elongated, the greater force will be generated for movement or action to occur. Flexibility is an essential motor quality. Some motor qualities are a greater part of genetic inheritance such as speed (power) and endurance – both of which can be enhanced through training. Balance has to be developed early for elite performance but can certainly be enhanced and retrained to an excellent level in adult life. Strength, endurance and flexibility can be trained to a high level at any time.

What is Stretching? STRETCHING is normally referred to as the technique(s) designed to increase or maintain flexibility. Stretching is tissue elongation from the resting length. There is therefore a continuum of stretching throughout the entire ROM of a joint.

The fitness industry recommends stretching 1 – 2 times per week for the maintenance of ROM and 2 – 3 times for further adaptations and improvements. Increases in ROM will occur regardless of duration of the held stretch, but holding for 20 seconds is recommended to accommodate maximum muscular effort. In Tai Chi stretching occurs both isometrically and isotonically. Practising daily and learning how to relax properly and then learning how to loosen the joints will gradually and more importantly safely improve ROM. How long it takes depends on the person's body composition, their attitude and how often and how they practise.

Which tissues are involved in Stretching? MUSCLE - has elastic property that rebounds back when stretched. CONNECTIVE TISSUE - Fascia which forms about 30% of the muscle bulk is the specific connective tissue we aim to stretch. Fascia is an opaque glad-wrap like substance that not only covers each muscle fibre, but also each muscle fibre bundle and the entire muscle. It wraps around muscles like a thin blanket keeping it together and contained. Facia can tear and become scarred through injury causing some degree of stiffness. Inflammation can also seep along the muscle sheaths and cause pain.

Fascia has what are known as visco-elastic properties. The elastic part is like a rubber band - it returns to its original length after being stretched. The viscous or plastic part is similar to plasticine - if it is stretched, it assumes the new position. Therefore, it is possible for fascia, with its plastic component, to alter its length "permanently".

OTHER TISSUES - such as ligaments and tendons MAY need to be stretched under specific clinical conditions. Mostly, these tissues remain firm to maintain joint stability. These structures have a high component of plastic properties and minimal elasticity. Consequently, these tissues do not return to their original length once stretched. Since ligaments are vital for joint stability and tendons for motor control, work on these structures is usually only performed by physiotherapists and other qualified health professionals.

It might be noted that when a ligament is damaged around a joint (eg. at the ankle) it is relatively easy to hurt the ankle again as the ligament has the plastic property. Ligaments are similar to tendons, but the cartilaginous fibres are not so regularly arranged. There may be some elastic present (eg in the ligamentum nuchae of the neck), but usually the function of ligaments is to secure the skeleton. Where tendons join muscle to a bone, ligaments join bone to bone and repair to a damaged ligament may take a surgical intervention or may take many months to knit back into bony tissue.

Limitations to Flexibility

1.	Bone Structure	8.	Activity level
2.	Muscle Bulk	9.	Inflammation or Fluid Retention
3.	Fat	10.	Scar Tissue
4.	Fascia	11.	Lack of blood flow
5.	Skin	12.	Muscle Temperature
6.	Age	13.	Muscle Reflexes
7.	Gender		

Reflexes

The Stretch Reflex: This is a protective mechanism to prevent over-stretching and its associated injuries. It is an automatic response to the rate of change in the length of a muscle and the ultimate length that the muscle reaches. When muscle length is rapidly increased, the response is rapid muscle contraction.

The Inverse Stretch Reflex: This is also a protective mechanism. When substantial tension is built up in the muscle-tendon unit through either contracting and/or stretching the muscle, this inverse stretch reflex causes the muscle and its associated muscle group to relax to avoid rupturing. The mechanism is a body of Golgi Tendon Organs, which are found in the tissue where muscle and tendon combine.

There are two kinds of stretch receptors to respond as reflexes: one detects the magnitude and speed of the stretch and the other the magnitude only. According to Kurz (1994) static stretches improve static quality and dynamic stretches improve dynamic flexibility – which is why it doesn't make sense to use static stretches for dynamic action. There is a considerable but not complete transfer to dynamic flexibility by executing movements similar to the task gradually increasing the range to facilitate neural pathways that will be used later in the "workout".

Factors affecting flexibility in older persons

1. *Age* - with advancing age most people reduce physical activity for any number of reasons
2. *Activity Level* - moving through small ranges decreases flexibility.
3. *Arthritis* and *other degenerating conditions* - chronic conditions of inflammation and/or oedema and deformity.
4. *Body Fat* - in younger aged particularly at hips and buttocks and abdomen. Often accompanied by muscle atrophy. In the Frail Aged "fat" is usually not a problem as it offers some protection for falls and offers some reserve during illness.
5. *Muscle Atrophy and weakness* - particularly extensors of the back, glutes, hamstrings and quads- radically altering the body alignment.
6. *Dorsi and Plantar Flexion* of the toes affect balance and gait.
7. *Shortening* of finger digit tendons limits manual dexterity, strength and grip.
8. Reduced *body temperature* reduces flexibility. Older persons usually lose some control over thermoregulation, compounded by inactivity.
9. *Adhesions, scar tissue, prostheses & bony outgrowths and pain* limit flexibility.

Why is understanding stretching important for Tai Chi for Health?

1. To improve the ROM about joints -
   - To increase the ability to absorb shock
   - To help resist or cope with trauma
   - To maximize independence

- To maintain smooth gait
2. To facilitate a balance of opposing muscle groups
   - Unbalanced muscle groups are a factor in falls and injuries
   - Good balance of muscle groups means good control of movements
3. To decrease muscle tension and improve muscle relaxation
   - Aged persons are just as tense as younger people
   - Tension reduction improves well-being
4. To improve and maintain optimal body alignment
5. To "feel free"
6. To decrease muscle soreness for those able to enjoy walking and improved functional wellness
7. To promote blood flow through the muscles helping waste removal and tissue repair

Teaching stretching - Basically there are two ways to stretch - through movement by DYNAMIC stretching and through holding positions or postures or STATIC stretching.

Dynamic stretching is adequately achieved by gentle movements, such as in slow rocking moves of legs and feet or sways and arcs made with the arms. Tai Chi and moving Qigong are perfect examples of this type of stretching and is well known to be a very safe and effective way to stretch. Everyone who practises Tai Chi improves their flexibility – some substantially so. Improvements in flexibility allow the body to function better for daily activities which in turn has a significant effect on mental health and quality of life.

The impact of loss of flexibility is often underestimated. As with activity generally, declines directly relate to loss of health, loss of function and an ever increasing spiralling downwards in wellness and confidence. The beauty of stretching with Tai Chi is that it is barely noticeable to the practitioner. The overriding question when practising Tai Chi is "is that comfortable" and the person assumes a relaxed and acceptable position. Stretching becomes something that happens naturally as a consequence of doing this sort of physical activity, gradually increasing the "what is comfortable" range.

Ballistic Stretching is categorised under Dynamic Stretching but is generally not taught as part of Tai Chi for beginners. In some of the Intermediate and Advanced forms, ballistic kicks are part of the set and should be trained just as carefully and safely in the warm-up phase of the class. Care and attention should be given to starting at 70% effort or less and doing six or more repetitions for each leg gradually increasing the range and taking care with the alignment of the spine and hips. A relaxed attitude for ballistic practise is much more successful than practising with tension forcing the muscles into a potentially damaging range.

Static stretching, sometimes known as passive or assisted stretching, involves slowly moving a muscle group into position to 70-80% of the maximum stretch and holding it without movement up to 15 seconds or longer. The muscle group will slowly relax and thus stretches slowly until mild tension is felt. In practising the form, there is an interplay between dynamic and static forms of stretching.

As in "Rate of Perceived Exertion" rule from Fitness, the control and level of stretch is left entirely to the self-reporting of the participant. A stretch "too little" is always better than a stretch "too much". Slowly, gently, regularly is safe for all students and particularly so for aged persons. If a participant reports "pins and needles" or pain - reduce stretch immediately and teach them to look for this sign. This means that the student is stretching to their maximum. It is the responsibility of the instructor to teach correct and safe technique, being mindful of the 70% rule, gradually increasing this level, but never to a "full" stretch of 100%, and thus locking the joints. Locking the knee or elbow to achieve a static stretch should not be attempted as this not part of Tai Chi for Health.

An essential part of Tai Chi for Health is teaching personal responsibility to participants to learn to know their own body and how to read it and also to know what to expect with the feeling in and around the joints. Pushing to maximum level implies a kind of self bullying and a forceful expectation of a level of achievement. The kindest thing about this attitude is that it shows "ambition" and that in itself has a small positive aspect. It is knowing how much to stretch and learning to have patience and persistence that is the lesson. Forcing a movement – such as bending the knees too deeply too soon will hinder the rate at which the knees will be more strong and flexible. Flexibility is more than the angle of the joint – it is muscle strength, tendon, bone, ligament, fluid and a whole micro-environment. Flexibility will be a consequence of patience, relaxation and persistence.

Another type of static stretching often used by elite athletes and martial arts practitioners with special flexibility needs is Proprioceptive Neuromuscular Facilitation (PNF), which is a stretching method developed by two physical therapists Knott and Voss (1968) in the United States. They described complex movement patterns aimed primarily at training people with cerebral or spinal injuries. This method is where the person applies an isometric contraction against an increasing force applied by the practitioner. Laughlin (1999) has adapted the PNF approach to stretching called Contract-Relax (C-R) Method and CRAC (control - relax with agonist contraction) in the fitness industry but this method is not part of Tai Chi especially with de-conditioned or aged persons. It can however be successfully used with fit and active students and senior students under proper supervision. However, it is not part of Tai Chi for Health Instructor Training. Encouraging people to relax is an essential component of improvement of flexibility.

A note to etiquette: Be mindful as a Tai Chi for Health Instructor not to advertise or "show-off" your own flexibility as this is not what teaching Tai Chi for Health is about. The focus is and should always be on the student. Gear your level to the same as or just a little more than the student.

Flexibility and Breathing - Holding the breath or shallow breathing is one of the body's responses to stress and is a protective mechanism for part of the "fright/flight" response or other health related issues. This means that when threatened or in pain people tend to hold their breath and the muscles of the trunk in particular have elevated tension. According to Laughlin (1999) electromyographic studies have shown than tension in the muscles is slightly elevated with every in-breath and that this decreases with the out-breath. This suggests that any stretching effort requiring a relaxation component will be enhanced if it is performed on an out breath. This is also an important technique and principle of yoga training. By taking a deliberate breath before stretching, the effect is heightened, as it will mean more air and a longer out-breath phase. Perhaps more importantly is that the body will become attuned to exhaling with relaxation and once learned and consolidated will help to stay more relaxed and flow over to general living.

It is very difficult to relax the body while the muscles are tense. This doesn't mean that the body has to be floppy – a mistake made by many Tai Chi players. We need some muscle tension or tonus – otherwise we would fall over. In fact, good posture and muscle tonus is "controlled falling". The degree of muscle tension varies from person to person. Western thinking to reduce muscle tension is to take a walk or take prescription medication. The relaxed rhythmical patterns of abdominal breathing go hand in hand with relaxation. A relaxed body can improve flexibility.

2.22 The Preparation Phase (Warm-up & stretching) - This initial phase of the Tai Chi class prepares the body for activity. Physiological goals of this phase include increasing muscle temperature, blood flow, oxygen delivery, lubrication of the joints and to improve muscle contractile abilities. This phase is also important for preparing the individual psychologically. This will mean that the student has a mindset that focuses on the task closing off the outside worries and concerns. This change of focus which is task driven has the bonus of drawing attention away from pain. People who practise Tai Chi have been shown to reduce pain by about one-third (Song et al, 2003)

"Warm-up" means many things to different physical activities. Certainly for Tai Chi, the warm-up phase is very important. It not only prepares the heart and vascular system for work by increasing body temperature, increasing the flow of blood and oxygen to the muscles setting the focus, but it also provides a series of gentle stretches for the major components of the body. Several minutes of slow, static stretching DO NOT fulfil the aims of the warm-up, neither does s brisk walk or jog. Gentle sub-maximal ROM isotonic movements around major joints combined with selective light static isometric stretches of large muscle groups of the thighs and buttocks are most effective. The slow controlled movements of the Tai Chi warm-up gently flowing in a continuous way are ideal for invoking slow relaxed diaphragmatic breathing.

Muscle fibres have a strong elastic component and they are connected functionally to the less elastic fibres of the tendon. When muscles are not stretched by lack of movement or exercising within less than full range of motion shortening will occur eventually. This then impacts on the body structure to which they are attached. Often the warm-up is extended to include a mini version of the conditioning work performed slower and up to about 70% of the normal sub-maximal range. This is an ideal way to "brush the cobwebs" and prepare for the main body of the class activity.

What is achieved in the Warm-up?
- There are two different stretches for the neck, shoulders, spine, hips, knees, ankles performed three times. In performing the warm-up like Tai Chi form ensures that the elbows wrists and hands also stretch.
- Focussing on the body part to be stretched ensures the desired range is achieved efficiently and in the safest way.
- Muscles move isotonically and isometrically throughout the 10-15 minute phase
- Slow abdominal or diaphragmatic breathing is readily incorporated in the set
- Opportunity is made for posture correction and improvement throughout the set
- There is ample time to correct alignment and learn self-body placement and awareness
- The set allows ample time to focus on transfer of weight and improvement of balance
- The warm-ups can be the vehicle for teaching how to lower the centre of gravity and be more stable
- How to relax the joints can be taught in the warm-up phase
- Learning how to sink the shoulders and the elbows can be taught throughout the set
- Placement of the gaze and position of the head and chin can be readily taught in warm-ups
- The whole warm-up set can be performed as a Qigong by linking stretches with transmission movements
- Focussing so intently on specific body movements and concepts will reduce pain
- Having repetitions in stretching means the person can relax without worrying about "what is coming next"

- Working in a relaxed manner without stress ensures improved flexibility
- Working for 15 minutes in a gentle and even way will elicit a mild cardio-vascular response

What are the goals of the warm-up?
- Increased focus and awareness
- Improved co-ordination
- Improved elasticity and contractibility of the muscles
- Greater efficiency of the respiratory and cardio-vascular systems

After a general preparation, the student can target specific movements as a drill in preparation for the training section of the lesson. In the Sun 12, stepping forwards and backwards with the follow steps, stepping sideways with the follow step under the hip, parry arms, continuous walking, cloud hands can all be practised in a series, purely as a biomechanical preparation for the form practise. The training and preparation of flexibility should always proceed from the general to the specific.

2.23   The Conditioning Phase - This component is the work phase of the program. During this phase much stretching is going on. Every movement requires components of stretching and relaxing. It is during this phase that the student is more likely to stretch a little further when learning and practising a complete or part complete set. Repeating a set is not only having an effect of improving endurance but is also improving flexibility. A student is more likely to relax and enjoy the movement if it is familiar. When teachers teach moves too quickly, there is a corresponding level of anxiety or tension with unfamiliar and unlearned movements. Moves have to be co-ordinated, and controlled for both gross motor and fine motor skills. These moves become "learned" when the many aspects of movement have been "wired" into the brain and body memory.

Learning new work is challenging, but slow relaxed repetition enables the body to improve flexibility under ideal conditions. Learning new work before it has been consolidated will be inefficient in the long run. A lesson that appears to have nothing new but is achievable without effort will not hold interest for a long period. Work which seems impossible because it is beyond the capability of the student causes frustration and sometimes annoyance and certainly disappointment. Striking a balance is something that is learned by communication and co-operation between participants and instructor. As with many other aspects of teaching it takes time and persistence.

2.24   The Recovery Phase (Cool-down & Stretching) - The aims of this phase include returning the body functions to resting levels, preventing venous pooling, dissipating waste products, and maintaining or developing flexibility. The recovery phase of the Tai Chi class is a time for letting go of any tension from the learning phase and reminding students to return to abdominal breathing. The gentle shaking of hands and feet releases tightness in the muscles and helps to bring everything back to a pre-exercise state.

Generally, older persons respond very well to stretching and improvements are seen on most joints but not all. Seniors love stretching because it frees their joints and makes them feel less stiff. Significant improvements to flexibility to the upper body, knees and feet can be made by persons who are limited to chair exercise. Hips are difficult to stretch in the chair. For chair work, the main precaution is that the teacher should not touch the student to try to improve alignment or stretch muscles. Students are encouraged to always feel comfortable with any move. Teaching stretching movements to people with cognitive impairment is best left to health professionals.

Being familiar with the muscles of the body and their origins, insertions and actions will always be of great importance to teachers who teach Tai Chi. And in the design of their programs. The focus of Functional Fitness and Wellness is an essential consideration for all classes. If the training has been moderate to intense, stretching facilitates recovery by relieving cramps, muscle spasms and tension, and by releasing good blood flow to the muscles.

2.25   Priority Muscle Groups

Stretch Hip Flexors by - Holding onto the back of a chair or a bar. Extend one leg as far behind the body as is comfortable. Ensure that leg is directly in line with the hip and not crossed over the midline. In the Tai Chi Warm-up this stretch is achieved in the (forward and) backward stretch for the hips combined with opposite swings for the arms and stretching in the shoulder area. This stretch is the main stretch to counteract long periods of sitting and inactivity. It also assists with improvement to gait.

Stretch Hamstrings by - sitting with good posture. One leg at right angles at the knee and ankle, knee joint in line with the hip joint. Other leg straight in front, heel on floor, ankle flexed. Place hands on the bent thigh about half way between the knee and the groin. Pull up through the head and bend very gently forward from the hips keeping the back straight, the ankle flexed and the knee extended. Hold still then try to relax the muscles above the knee while in stretched position. After the stretch, place hand underneath the stretched knee and lift back into feet flat position.

This stretch is achieved very well in the Tai Chi for Health stretch for the hip. As the leg comes forward the heel is placed lightly in line with the hip. With the toes pointing toward the knee, the Achilles tendon receives a great stretch as do all the muscles at the back of the legs. Stretched hamstrings improve gait considerably because they originate at the pelvis. Tight hamstrings will be powerful enough to tilt the pelvis posteriorly. A disappearing bottom is often a clear sign of shortened hamstrings. Practising the concept of "feather touch" when transferring weight will help to maximise the stretching of the groups on the back of the leg.

Stretch Calf Muscle - The sit hamstring stretch will also stretch the calf muscle. In addition -

Stand near a post or doorway in normal posture. Flex the ankle against the wall or post. Heel will be on the floor, toes on the post. Lean the whole body in alignment towards the post – gently.

More easily, the simple heel/toe stretch in the warm-ups not only stretches the muscles of the back of the leg and their tendons but strengthens the tibialis anterior which is so important in toe clearance and the prevention of falls.

Stretch Quads by - Standing on the floor, holding onto the rail. Place leg, two steps above keeping posture upright. Participants should always hold on when performing this stretch. Quads can also be stretched from the floor, lying on the side, knee bent and thigh slightly back. However, alignment of abdomen needs to be perfect and this stretch is contraindicated with any problems with the knee joint and is simply not safe for older persons for many reasons. Perhaps the most simple quad stretch is to stand upright, bend the knees and tilt the pelvis posteriorly (tuck the tailbone under).

Quads are adequately and safely stretched in any backward movement. As the participant becomes stronger and can keep posture upright, backward movements are an ideal way to stretch. Sun Style especially is a composite of forward, sideways and backward movements and very good levels of flexibility about the hips can be attained with practise.

Stretch Lower Back and Gluteals by - Sitting on a chair feet flat on the floor, hips, knees and ankles at right angles. Place hands on thighs and gently lean forward slightly from the pelvis, keeping head in the same alignment as the spine. Keep back in position as the bend progresses forward. Starting position is upright. Hands on thighs can help to push the abdomen up against gravity for the recovery of the stretch coming back to neutral.

A much more efficient way to stretch the lower back is to achieve correct posture. The White Crane Stretch or the first spinal stretch is executed from about the waist up through the spine to the neck and from the waist down and slightly under.

Many students bend their knees more that they are capable of at this time in their development. In Tai Chi the back should be held upright. Leaning forward and displacing the pelvis posteriorly, will allow a deeper bend but the upright posture is lost. When posture is improved so much it allows the student to work with an ideal posture, the muscles of the back and legs are not strained. The relaxing will enhance stretching and strengthening. Combined with breathing and control of the pelvic floor the lower back will be functional and strong.

Stretch Pectorals by - sitting on a chair. Place right hand on inside of right knee. Hold onto back of the chair with left hand. Keeping the shoulders and hips facing the front, ease the elbow towards the back without twisting the spine.

Finding ways to correct the distension in the upper back groups and reduce tension in the shoulders and neck by letting these muscles deflate will allow the pectoral group to stretch and sit in their best functional position. When the muscles of the back are rounded or distended it also impacts on the flexibility of the shoulder and the shortening of the pectoral muscles. Working in an ideal posture over time will improve the functioning of these groups.

Stretching in Practice - Most of the muscle groups of the body respond very well to the gentle strengthening and stretching that happens with Tai Chi. A great advantage of learning and practising Tai Chi is that it is self regulating. Tai Chi is both static and dynamic and occasionally ballistic. It requires a warm-up phase to prepare the body for work, a conditioning phase to improve strengthening and flexibility and endurance and a cool down phase to bring everything back to normal. It is not common to injure by overstretching in Tai Chi. If this does occur it will be because the student has been too ambitious.

2.30   PHYSIOLOGY & BREATHING
   2.31   Energy Systems – Aerobic & Anaerobic
   2.32   Science of Breathing
   2.33   Anatomy & Function
   2.34   Training Breathing
   2.35   Abdominal Breathing
   2.36   Relaxation and Mind-Body Focus

2.31   Energy systems - For the Tai Chi for Health Instructor who subscribes to a modern Duty of Care, it is important to have a basic understanding of the science of breathing and energy systems other than the traditional explanation of Tai Chi as expressed in metaphysical terms of the power of "Qi" linked to Chinese medicine, Daoist and Confucian philosophy.   The following is a basic outline of the classical scientific model of energy systems accepted within the modern approach to the physiology of exercise, fitness and health. The student is encouraged to research this topic further, in particular, to examine evidence based research which links the Tai Chi for Health Matrix of Performance to health science research.   In other words, the Tai Chi for Health Instructor engaged in teaching specific populations or Special People needs to understand not only the complexity of different populations and different levels of health and abilities but also the specificity and currency of evidence based knowledge of each population.

The human body can be viewed as a number of different systems that are interconnected for the body to function as a unit.   These systems include – skeletal, muscular, integumentary (skin), nervous, endocrine, cardio-vascular, respiratory, lymphatic and immune, digestive, urinary, reproductive (Colbert et al 2007).

There are three broad categories of energy sub-systems that are used for the purposes of muscular effort. (see Marieb, 2006; and Brianmac Sports Coach, 2007) All three systems use the chemical substance called Adenosine Triphosphate (ATP) to create muscular power.   Since ATP is the only energy source that can be used to directly power muscular activity, ATP must be regenerated continuously if contraction of the muscle is to continue.

Each sub-system operates in different ways in relation to the demands on the body for muscular power:

(a)   Direct High Energy Immediate Reserve – Required to kick start all muscular activity but the necessary chemical to provide this activity is quickly exhausted (in about 20 seconds).

(b)   Aerobic Respiration – At rest and during light to moderate exercise, some 95% of the ATP used for muscle activity comes from aerobic respiration.   This sub-system is fairly slow in the chemical reactions in the conversion of glucose to power muscular energy and requires continual delivery of oxygen and nutrient fuels to the muscle to keep it going.

(c)   Anaerobic – Literally meaning "without oxygen", this sub-system switches into play when muscular activity is intense, or oxygen and glucose delivery is temporarily inadequate to meet the needs of the working muscles. The sluggish aerobic mechanisms cannot keep up with the demands for ATP.   Under these conditions, lactic acid is produced.   The chemical reaction here within this sub-system is nowhere nearly as efficient as the aerobic systems using huge amounts of glucose for the muscular activity, accumulating lactic acid promoting muscle fatigue and soreness.

In the year 2000 this classical model of energy systems was questioned in regard to limitations this model had when it came to explaining fatigue (see Sports Fitness Advisor, 2007).   The critique challenged the general concept as overly simplistic that fatigue develops **only** when the cardiovascular system's capacity to supply oxygen falls behind demand, therefore initiating anaerobic metabolism.   It is argued that fatigue is a complex subject that can result from a range of physical and psychological factors.   In an attempt to produce a more holistic explanation, Noakes (2000) developed a model that consisted of five sub-models:

i)   The classical 'cardiovascular / anaerobic' model as it stands now
ii)   The energy supply / energy depletion model
iii)   The muscle recruitment (central fatigue) / muscle power model
iv)   The biomechanical model
v)   The psychological / motivational model.

Essentially, it is argued, this new model of energy systems recognizes what coaches have witnessed for decades - that performance and fatigue is multifactorial and complex. It adds strength to the synergistic and holistic approach to sport usually found in the most successful athletes (see Sports Fitness Advisor, 2007). For our purposes as Tai Chi for Health Instructors, this new and complex model draws immediate attention to our Duty of Care in the face of the complexity, the permutations and possibilities embodied in the Tai Chi for Health Matrix of Performance (see Unit 3.40) with different populations of Special People.

2.32   Science of Breathing - This sub-unit is aimed at creating a basic understanding of the physiology and anatomy of how breathing functions and how this knowledge should be integral to a modern Tai Chi for Health. Intuitively, we know that breathing itself is the lifeline for the body and that when we are alive we are breathing, and when we die breathing ceases. However, a modern Tai Chi for Health needs much more than this, it needs to be properly informed about how certain environmental factors can be dysfunctional to breathing patterns and thus can adversely impact on the health and well-being of the individual. In addition, we need to understand how dysfunctional posture contributes to dysfunctional breathing and in turn impacts negatively on health and well-being of the individual   In this sub-unit, we briefly examine how "training breathing" and how abdominal breathing techniques can contribute towards enhancing health benefits of practicing Tai Chi for Health.   A large part of staying well is ensuring our breathing activities are working as well as possible. Through the practice of Tai Chi for Health it is possible to enhance the quality of breathing, which is widely recognised to improve the quality of life.

In our everyday life, we experience a wide range of stressors to which we have an immediate emotional response, where the nervous system responds by stimulating a number of physical responses hard wired into the human psyche and habitual practices. For example, we are walking down a street and unexpectedly there is a loud explosion. Physiologically, the heart rate increases, breathing becomes rapid and shallow, body temperature increases, we perspire, and our muscles begin to prepare us to the initial "fright" for an anthropologically speaking "fight or flight" response. We are now programmed and prepared for action - to do battle or retreat. There have been a myriad of chemical responses that have accompanied these physiological activities resulting in increased stress and possibly physical and mental distress.

Over a prolonged period, continued stress has an accumulative effect on the body where the instinctive "fight or flight" responses now have become hardwired into our habitual forms of going about our modern life, always on strategic alert waiting almost consciously but instinctively for that "loud explosion". Our posture deteriorates and has become compromised, we are tense, shallow breathing - fatigue and anxiety invade our sensibilities. What do we do to remedy this? Apart from relying on substances to reduce stress, many turn to physical activities. Some play squash, run a marathon, swim a channel, climb tall mountains, or many more conveniently go to the gym, pump iron and gaze at the shiny muscles and physique of others reflected in the mirror while thrashing the bicycle machine that interminably goes nowhere.

As Tai Chi for Health Instructors, what can we offer to address the stressors of modern living that might have significantly fewer side-effects and risks of injury such as narcissistic necrosis, [7] cardiac incidents, torn tissues, herniated discs, exhaustion and so forth? Properly practised deep breathing exercises using abdominal or diaphragmatic breathing may well provide some relief for any form of stress, with chronic stress taking a bit longer to overcome ingrained patterns of poor posture and poor breathing habits. Tai Chi regularly practised as moving soft Qigong (see Unit 3.15) can readily facilitate focussed deep breathing, slowing the heart beat, oxygenating the body, reducing the breathing rate, inhibiting perspiration and relaxing the muscles and thus enhancing the feeling of well being. A better quality of life will follow.

2.33   Anatomy & Function - Throughout our life, the main function of the respiratory system is to provide continuous exchange of oxygen and carbon dioxide to and from the body.

The *respiratory tract* is more than the lungs. It includes the nose and nasal sinuses, the mouth, the pharynx, the larynx, the trachea, the bronchi and the alveoli where the exchange of gas (oxygen and carbon dioxide) takes place. Briefly:
- The nose and oral cavity warm and filter the air
- The pharynx is dependent upon the tone of the tongue muscles, the soft palate and the pharyngeal walls.
- The larynx lies about the level of C4-6 (see Spine under Unit 2.15 [c])
- The trachea is held up by a strong cartilage and bifurcates into the bronchi at about the level of T5-6 (see Spine under Unit 2.15 [c])
- The right lung is divided into three lobes and left lung has two.
- The bronchial walls contain smooth muscle and elastic tissue and cartilage.
- Gas movement occurs by tidal flow in the large airways, but in the alveoli gases exchange by diffusion.
- The pleura is a double sac surrounding the lungs and lining the thoracic cavity
- The alveoli provide an enormous surface area for gas exchange averaging 160 square metres

The Diaphragm though not part of the respiratory tract plays an important role in breathing. It is a large muscle sheet dividing the thorax with the lungs and heart from the abdomen – the peritoneal cavity and extends to the pelvic floor - liver, spleen, stomach, kidneys, bowel and sexual organs. It is attached to the lower six ribs and the lumbocostal arches of the lumbar vertebrae with innervation from the phrenic nerves (from C3-5 – see Spine under Unit 2.15 [c]). There are three large openings in the diaphragm for the aorta, the vena cava and the oesophagus.

While the lungs themselves are passive organs in the breathing process, there are also several other physiological roles that the lungs contribute to such as a blood reservoir for emergencies, filter, metabolic activity and immunological production via an immunoglobulin (IgA) secretion and so forth. When the pleural cavities are closed, the lungs are open to the atmospheric environment and are subject to pressure. When the breathing muscles (diaphragm and intercostals) contract it causes the internal pressure to fall and the lungs enlarge causing the outside air to rush in to fill the partial vacuum. When the breathing muscles relax, the intercostals soften and the diaphragm rises forcing the air out.

Respiration (or breathing) is under both voluntary and involuntary control. It should be noted that this subdivision of the nervous system does not suggest that the control of nerve impulses is anything but a continuous functional network with many of the structures overlapping and interrelating. Under normal circumstances breathing occurs without awareness and is handled by the brain to automatically and effortlessly adjust to the needs of the body. This control can be overridden by voluntary intervention via the cerebral cortex. The respiratory control centres in

---

[7] Self-inflicted injuries or even death caused by significantly unrealistic expectations of the limits of the human body and psyche.

the brain are located in the medulla oblongata, in the 4th ventricle and in two other sites in the brain. It is in the medulla that the level of carbon dioxide concentration in the blood is determined. Apart from miniscule deposits of dust and water the inspired air contains 21% oxygen, .03% carbon dioxide and 78% nitrogen. Expired air contains 16.4% oxygen, 4% carbon dioxide and 78% nitrogen.

Often respiration is described by rate, volume, oxygen and carbon dioxide exchange, airway reactivity and mast cell activity (Fried, 1993; Wientjes, 1993). Healthy people mostly breathe in a smooth regular way when asleep or at rest. Sometimes sleep patterns are erratic and respiratory patterns are anything but smooth and even paced. These patterns also slip over to daily recognizable breathing patterns, which are reflected in the language, which describes it. Everyday expressions such as "breathe a sigh of relief", "like a fish out of water", "we can all breathe easily now", "all puffed up", "she's an inspiration", "breath of fresh air", "full of hot air", "don't hold your breath", "gasping for breath" reflect how the conscious mind relates to the normal functioning of the body.

When we think of normal function of breathing we think of a smooth in-breath (inspiration) followed by a smooth out-breath (expiration). However, normal breathing can include - gasps, sighs, rapid breathing or panting, breath-holding, chest breathing or shallow breathing. As well, the breathing rate and volumes automatically adjust to match the demands of the tasks required. When does normal breathing switch from being functional to dysfunctional and impact on the well being of the individual? According to Pepper (1994), this can be explained in terms of the acquisition of bad-habits. Breath patterns are covertly conditioned to common or habitual activities. These conditioned patterns include breath holding when the telephone rings, shallow thoracic breathing when entering data at the computer keyboard, and gasping during speech. These responses are components of the alarm reaction which were probably evoked and then conditioned during initial skill acquisition (excessive striving) and were never unlearned. Hence, the dysfunctional breathing patterns have become part of the physiological response during task performance.

An individual in good health breathes from three to five litres of air per minute. The tidal volume (av.500ml) multiplied by the respiratory rate (14 breaths/min) is the minute volume (7.000ml/min). Not all of the tidal air is involved with the diffusion of the gases in the lungs, as this process does not start until it reaches the bronchioles and is roughly one third of the tidal volume. The part of the tidal volume, which does diffuse multiplied by the respiratory rate is known as alveolar ventilation and is approximately 5,000ml/min. Peper and Tibbetts (1994) states that effortless diaphragmatic breathing consists of a slower respiration rate of up to 8 respirations per minute with a large tidal volume of up to 2000 ml occurring. He also notes that the exhalation time including the exhalation pause is significantly longer than the inhalation time.

The significance of this is that effortless diaphragmatic breathing elicits internal quietening (mindfulness) and relaxation. For students who practise Tai Chi, slow abdominal or diaphragmatic breathing is at the very core of what happens with their breathing and hardly without knowing they can expect the very useful and healthful benefits that come with stress reduction.

2.34   Training Breathing - The training of effortless breathing through Tai Chi for Health using soft Qigong (see Unit 3.15) can begin with the first lesson. It can be seen as a beginning in the retraining of old habits to hard wire effortless natural breathing to be the breathing of choice in most circumstances. Before training can begin MacHose and Peper (1991) advise that many clients suffer from "designer jeans syndrome" and will need to loosen their clothing to limit abdominal displacement as well as the habitual bracing of the upper thorax as a habit of stress and conditioning. Excessive efforts of breathing mostly involve the scalene and trapezius groups, which are the accessory muscles involved and the common site of muscular stress induced pain.

Role modelling as suggested by Shaffer et al (1994) should be what happens in a Tai Chi class. Rather than leaving many questions unanswered concerning breathing, a quick survey of any class will uncover a "need to know" component about breathing. Breathing is the lifeline and people are aware of the value of good breathing techniques and are hungry for assistance. Physically putting the hand to the chest and abdomen or at the sides of the lower ribs is a very "hands on" approach to teaching breathing as well as making the mind/body connection real instead of something on the periphery of what they think it is. Using their own hands for this process at once makes an awareness connection with their own body.

Peper and Tibbetts (1994) suggest the following strategies for assisting with mind/body connection for breathing:
- Place hands on lateral side at the waist touching the lower ribs. Press towards the centre of the body during exhalation. Pull hands outward during inhalation
- Place hands on abdomen and apply pressure to abdomen during exhalation
- Rock shoulders gently during exhalation and inhalation to reduce bracing
- Teacher exhales audibly at the same time and slightly longer than when the client is exhaling
- Guide exhalation with imagery such as exhaling through straws or pipes

When thinking about the breath it is important to be objective in how one looks at what is happening during breathing. Being introspective, or blaming or self-judging calls on an emotional response and reaction. To achieve an objective analysis of breathing asking the following might be helpful:

- What can I feel as I breathe in
- What can I feel as I breathe out
- What is moving with my breathing
- Does my throat feel obstructed
- Is my breathing jerky or smooth
- Am I forcing or am I calm
- Is there a pause
- Am I emptying
- Do I have enough air to feel comfortable and relaxed

For teaching, some of these points could be written down as a reminder to the teacher to focus on one of these points each class and by repetition and practice the mind-body connections can be taught and developed by the student.

There are other imagery concepts such as breathing in through a pipe to help relax the throat or imagining breathing through a straw for people whose lungs are hypersensitive. If it is a stressful exercise have the students sit. Feel free to discuss what they are feeling so that they have the confidence to know they can understand and feel this really happening in their bodies. To empty more completely, each student whispers "ha ha ha ha ha ha ha" to encourage a longer expiration and complete emptying. Sometimes, this will make the students laugh which is exactly the method of emptying and is fun too. Focussing on breathing in and failure to empty out properly will result in hyper-ventilation and this is to be avoided.

At no time should a student be aware of "air hunger". Learning breathing should be a non-invasive gentle connection by the student with their own body. Being aware, listening to their breathing is both comforting and calming. There are no absolute respiration values as every person has their own biological needs. Each person therefore needs to adapt and vary breathing to suit their unique circumstances. Keeping focused and keeping "comfortable" always offers a safety margin and a chance to improve.

2.35   Abdominal Breathing
- An increased supply of oxygen is available to the body
- Enhanced movement of the diaphragm gives a gentle massage to the internal organs
- Conscious deep breathing affects the nervous system, calming emotional response reactions in the body
- It is a more efficient way to breathe

All of this means more simply that the body is "more-well". Daily living in most circumstances brings its share of mental and physical stress which impacts severely on health. Abdominal breathing should be quiet, smooth, slow, deep, continuous and relaxed. Like posture, think of Abdominal breathing as a "work in progress" improving and strengthening with time and patience. How to start teaching abdominal breathing:
- Whether sitting or standing, release the tension in the shoulders and neck by focussing on posture. Press up gently through the head, feel like being suspended from a thread, allow the shoulders to let go and relax with the chin gently tucked in
- Spend some minutes in this quiet space doing nothing but focussing on posture and relaxation.
- Keeping elongated in the spine allow the abdomen to relax. Focus on the belly and observe the movement of the abdomen
- Being continually focussed and staying calm will be the strongest assets for training breathing. Students need to learn to become their own coach and concentrate on posture and relaxation until the mind begins to focus on the breath. If the mind wanders, simply return the focus back to breathing.
- Quiet relaxed abdominal breathing will enhance energy. Just stay as long as is comfortable and gradually over time the period spent in this relaxing exercise will increase and will become easier.

Breathing can be introduced from the first lesson with Tai Chi Form but only if it is not made too complicated. For the intermediate and advanced students who have learned the Tai Chi Form, it is a very special experience to apply the mind-body strategy of focussing on breathing and discover what is happening with the body with the focus on the breath. Often times the forms quieten down considerably and a "Song" quality can be experienced. Another focus with breathing is to match breathing to the movements and keep a steady even relaxing pace and rhythm. Yet another is to match the intention of the movements (martial intention) with the breathing. Here the breath alters to match the energy requirements of the form. Performing a set at a quick pace or slowing it down to a very slow pace can feel very different. The Sun Style has the Open/Close concept throughout the form. The very upright posture built into the Sun Style with the follow step ensures an excellent posture for Qigong breathing – and a very pleasant and healthful way to exercise (see Unit 3.15 for detail).

2.36   Relaxation and Mind-Body Focus - A certain amount of tension and stress is vital for everyday life.
Basically our body is well designed for coping with acute stress - the "fight or flight" phenomenon. However, we are not meant to cope with chronic stress, where this becomes "distress". In modern times, stress is often loaded psychologically so that the body is not physically exhausted. After the event, the body is still in a state of tension and the body does not always recover quickly.

Common signs of stress overload may be seen in the following:
- Overreaction to minor problems via excessive anger, impatience
- Increased use of alcohol, drugs, coffee, cigarettes
- Overeating or loss of appetite
- Reduced work efficiency and reduced decision making ability
- Headaches, indigestion, teeth grinding, skin conditions, heart palpitations and so forth

A Tai Chi for Health class is an ideal environment to teach technique to reduce the detrimental effects of stress on the body. Teaching relaxation is a method of teaching self-management to participants enabling them to have the skills to reduce the harmful effects of stress and achieve a more tranquil lifestyle.

STRESS - The "fight or flight" response produces a chemical cocktail to activate the body when under stress. With the assistance of the hormones of the pituitary, thyroid, adrenal and pancreas, the response in the short term can be lifesaving, but in the long term over-response may be damaging to the body.
- The brain becomes stimulated
- The glands begin to secrete hormones
- The involuntary nervous system becomes innervated
- Decreased digestion
- Increased metal alertness
- Increased rate of breathing
- Increased sweating
- Increased blood pressure and heart rate
- Increased blood clotting ability in case of injury
- The liver releases sugar, cholesterol and fatty acids into the blood for energy supply to the muscles

Many people, in particular, the older adult often suffer from loss of function (due to disease and inactivity) and intermittent or chronic pain. The effects of stress occur through frustration, worry, depression, grief and loneliness and may be manifested and reported to the teacher as follows:
- Feeling unable to settle down and relax
- Explosive annoyance/anger at minor irritations
- Anxiety or tension lasting more than a few days
- Inability to focus attention on a task
- Sleep disturbances
- Tension headaches
- Aching neck and shoulder muscles
- Indigestion
- Loss or increase of appetite
- Diarrhoea or constipation
- Heart palpitations
- Asthma attacks

Some class participants will arrive in a less than ideal state to benefit most from the Tai Chi for Health program. Tai Chi for Health can include as part of the warm-up segment, visualisation (focus), controlled breathing and gentle movement with complementary alignment. Participants will be warmed and their joints and muscles prepared for stronger work.

Teaching Tai Chi for Health as Relaxation Techniques - Within the Tai Chi for Health class, there are a number of well-recognised relaxation techniques – which include standing, seated and lying down Tai Chi (see Modifications in Unit 1.73) meditation, visualisation, deep breathing, listening to music. Using different methods and suggesting alternatives to the specific activity will allow people to find an approach to learning how to relax that suits their individual physical and emotional needs.

Locations - Students can be encouraged to practise relevant aspects of Tai Chi as relaxation techniques and which can be called upon almost anywhere such as at a bus stop, in a bank queue, waiting at a red light, in a waiting room or in an aircraft, or lying down in bed and so on. In the Tai Chi for Health class we can draw on meditative techniques and music to great advantage.

Language - The teacher needs to be aware of the language used and the concept imagery. Martial or violent imagery is not conducive to relaxation and stress release for many people. Use verbal instructions, which include mixed imagery of sound, colour, smell, texture and light. If verbal instructions are delivered too rapidly, participants will become frustrated (not relaxed!). By expanding the imagery, by recalling all sensations will develop a rich and rewarding experience for everyone. The tone of the voice will also impact on the effectiveness on the Tai Chi task.

Discipline & Concentration - Be aware that some people have great difficulty relaxing and they resist the feeling of "letting go" to a great extent. Be patient. Sometimes it may be appropriate to partly close the eyes either standing or seated (depending on where the students are in the Tai Chi for Health Matrix of Performance) and keep the muscles of the body completely still. This requires considerable discipline in itself. If concentration is disturbed, ask the person to remain still with eyes closed (only if seated) and try to begin the concentration again. Train the class that there will nearly always be sounds in any situation such as coughing, telephones, cars and so forth. The skill is to not be physically distracted and to regain concentration as speedily as possible.

Timing - Remember the teacher is not performing hypnosis when focussing on learning how to relax. The aim is not to put them to sleep. They should be able to hear the teacher's voice clearly at all times. The students should not "drift off" but stay focussed and alert. When approaching the close of a segment with the class involving stillness (seated or standing), the teacher should bring them back gently by asking them to open their eyes, shake their fingers gently and return to normal.

Tension - There appears to be a close relationship between muscle tension and the global feelings people describe as STRESS. Many of us have recognised that exercise, in particular low to moderate rhythmic exercise which is simple enough and uncomplicated enough not to cause us stress itself - contributes to the relief of physical and psychological tension. For this reason, Qigong breathing exercises are best performed for beginners with upper body only standing or seated.

Muscle Activity - After the muscles have finally settled down and when in deep sleep, there is zero muscle activation (unless in REM [8] sleep). Achieving a state of deep relaxation can reduce muscular activity from about 10% to 0% depending on the teacher's skill, technique and the ability to continue to practise and improve.

Activity in Muscle

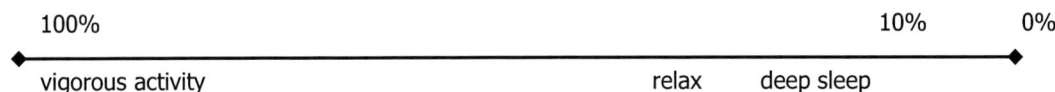

100%		10%	0%
vigorous activity		relax	deep sleep

Relaxation positions of choice:

1. Lying flat supine position, legs apart with hips rotated outwards and arms relaxed turned outwards, palms upwards (see Modifications Unit 1.73).
2. Lying curled in a comfortable foetal position. Underneath arm curled to support head and top arm relaxed onto the floor, with or without a pillow (see Modifications Unit 1.73).
3. Sitting in a straight chair, feet flat on the floor with hands in the lap. Head must be over the spine, neither forward drooping nor extended.
4. Alternative position for those with back problems. Lying supine with knees bent. Feet placed hip width apart on the floor and then knees placed gently leaning together (see Modifications Unit 1.73).

The FOCUS of the relaxation component should be to impart a SKILL that the participants can draw on to relieve their physical and/or emotional stress

Most Common Relaxation Techniques - The only limitation on how any of the following may be included with a Tai Chi for Health program is the "imagination" itself in relation always to the Tai Chi for Health teacher's Duty of Care.

Segmentation - This method divides the body into parts, which are relaxed in sequence. Most common segments are: feet, calves, thighs, buttocks, abdomen, shoulders, arms, hands and fingers, face. Learning to relax the shoulders is perhaps the best approach for the beginner to Tai Chi for Health.

Tuning in to the senses - Students can be introduced through the principles of Tai Chi for Health into connecting mind-body through focussing on one or more of the senses - sight, hearing, smell, taste, touch.

A Special Place - In learning visualisation techniques, there are places common to most people but each person has their own experience: a garden, a room, a rainforest, a beach.

Journey - Visualisation techniques include - travel to distant places such as the mountains of Peru, the Great Plains of Africa, Russia, Australia and the Nullabor - in fact anywhere - documentaries, films, books, life experiences are the resources. The teacher's own imagination is the limiting factor - "*You don't have to go to the Antarctic to know it's cold*"

Recall - This means the teacher researches and resources the "memory", giving the detail with word pictures. This can range from visualisation such as seeing people in national dress, or different types of birds to recalling names of rivers, mountains, cities. This requires a lot of concentration and adequate time for processing to search for answers.

---

[8] REM - Rapid Eye Movement is a phase of sleep patterns

Self-Healing - The teacher leads the student on a journey inside the body to "see" it repairing. This is a most difficult area to engage with and requires knowledge of basic body structure and function and an acute sensitivity to the cultural, historical and medical background of the students. It is very important that the teacher does not use anything that is not understood or potentially harmful. Here the danger is that some word images may trigger a negative response by an association of images with some dramatic event in the life of the student and can cause harm. While this is self-healing using the power of the mind, this is best left to a qualified health professional and should not be part of the standard Tai Chi for Health class.

Breathing – This highly successful method focuses on the air going in and out of the nose or mouth. Counting cycles one through seven with continued focus on the breath is the main aim. If the mind begins to wander on other thoughts, then begin again on number one. This is one of the Tibetan teaching methods and is the method of choice for uncomplicated and unemotional focus and quietness.

Cultivating Better Health with Qigong and Tai Chi - Many people understand that Tai Chi is gentle slow movement patterns involving legs and arms coordinating to make smooth curves and soft changing positions. Some of the main principles are: continuous, flowing movement, differentiating between substantial and insubstantial weight transference, suspending the head from the crown, understanding the intention of the movement, turning the waist, opening the joints, lowering the shoulders and elbows, sinking the body, using the least possible effort to perform the desired movement. Generally, as the movements are performed, the focus is on one thing completely. For example, maintaining posture by keeping the crown and base of the abdomen in line. Learning to focus will gradually assist in "quietening the mind".

The three main aspects of the disciplines of Qigong are:
- Meditation
- Movement
- Breathing

Practice will develop confidence and competence and in turn will facilitate an increased awareness of how the following concepts will give substance and benefit to the Tai Chi form and movements:
- Relaxation
- Concentration
- Meditation
- Harmony
- Breathing

Don't be confused by "meditation". It is merely an ability to visualise, for example, seeing in the mind's eye - the hands brushing over the surface of water, separating the clouds, caressing a tree, looking at the at the Southern Cross pointing the way, the Brolga stretching its wings (see Unit 5.50 - *Australia Dreaming*). We all do it. Sometimes there is no need to visualise anything. Simply focus on the breathing and try not to be distracted. Sometimes the simplest task has the most profound effect. When learning a movement, practise first the legwork, then the arm work, then put them together with the breathing and imagery (see Unit 1.42 for sectional practice). Once the individual parts have been consolidated and put together, practise each movement segment perhaps eight times or until the movement of the body is flowing and coordinated and the mind is focussed and calm.

It is important to not expect perfection or to be an expert. Aim for the following five qualities in practising Qigong and it will be an excellent beginning FOR CALMING AND RELAXING:

Slowness   *Lightness*   *Clarity*   *Balance*   *Calmness*

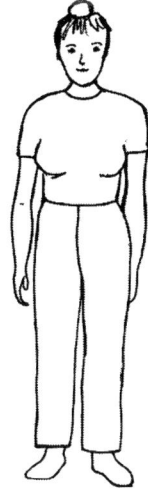

1. The Brain signals the glands and the nervous system to change to a relaxed state including deep, slow brain waves.

2. Slowed in the rate of breathing.

3. Decreased sweating.

4. Decreased muscle tension.

5. Decreased blood pressure and heart rate.

6. Body functions return to normal state.

Preparatory Position - Below is a guideline for the preparatory position and a few hints to get you started. The initial or preparatory position for all the following movements is as follows:

- Stand as if suspended from the crown of the head
- Line up the crown and the middle of the base of the abdomen. This alignment will tilt the pelvis slightly and soften the knees
- Place body weight equally between the ball of the feet and the heel
- Feel a lengthening up the legs and spine
- Slightly depress the sternum
- Allow the dorsal muscles to soften
- Relax the trunk
- Place the head back over the spine
- Tilt the chin down slightly
- Eye line level

This stance has postural benefits as it encourages an upright spine in an ideal and anatomical position and relaxes and exercises muscles. Combined with deep breathing, it also helps to balance the mind- body energy.

Power of the Mind - It is well known that positive mind power can help healing. There are many examples in life demonstrating the amazing power of the mind controlling the body. Tai Chi integrates both body and mind, using the conscious mind to direct the internal force and the internal force directs each movement. When practising Tai Chi one focuses on all movements and the coordination of the body. The mental training in Tai Chi will enhance clarity of the mind, help relaxation and uplift one's mood. A recent review by doctors from Stanford University (Luskin et al, 1998) on complementary and alternative treatments concludes that mind-body techniques (including Tai Chi) were found to be efficacious primarily as complementary and sometimes as stand-alone alternative treatments to medication: "We know many people with arthritis are stressed and depressed. Studies have shown Tai Chi is effective in relieving stress". (see La-Forge, 1997; Jacobson et al 1997; Jin, 1989, 1992; Brown et al, 1995)

Clearly the immense power of the mind has not been fully estimated. As one of the most powerful mind-body exercises, Tai Chi teaches the student to achieve greater self-control and empowerment. Medical studies have found that Tai Chi improves many facets of the mental state for people with arthritis and other conditions. (see Wolfson et al 1996; La-Forge, 1997; Jacobson et al 1997; Kutner et al 1997; Jin, 1989, 1992; Brown et al 1995)

2.40   SAFETY & HEALTH MANAGEMENT
   2.41   Safety
   2.42   Health Management

2.41   Safety - The Matrix of Performance (see Unit 3.40) provides the framework within which the Tai Chi for Health Instructor ensures that the class or activity is not designed as a "one size fits all". The Duty of Care is significantly different for each individual person within the class or activity and the TCH Instructor needs to be able to modify and structure the activities in such a way as to ensure the safety and wellbeing of each student.

The general factors relating to Safety which affect all student of TCH class can be summarised as follows:
- Medical clearance for exercise
- Observation & monitoring
- Illness and injury
- Warm-ups and preparation
- Working comfortably and safely
- Heat and dehydration
- Fatigue
- Exacerbation of existing conditions
- Self–management - taking personal responsibility
- Cool down after exercise
- Identifying tags – name & health history attached

Older adults or people with chronic conditions require:
- Movements where limitations of eyesight can be overcome
- Movements that can be conceptualised as everyday familiar things
- Isolated movements – separate legs and arm moves to reduce frustration if appropriate
- Include some co-ordinated seated moves and some opposite work – "brain gym"
- Short sequences for attention span, fatigue or pain
- Clear, concise instructions
- Time to be unrushed
- Options for rest

2.42 Health Management - This section deals with safety as central to grouping people into different populations as per the Matrix of Performance (see 3.40) that is relevant to the design of an appropriate Tai Chi for Health Exercise program for the individual student and group:

- AGE
- HEALTH
- FITNESS
- SKILLS

A brief profile of each group includes an outline of the most important factors requiring special consideration in the design of a safe program.

The following are **general safety guidelines** for all students regardless of health conditions, age, fitness and skill levels:
- Health screening is essential (see Unit 4.60 – paragraph 4 under Participant Understanding)
- Personal responsibility and consent form (see Unit 4.60 – paragraph 2 under Participant Understanding)
- Every student has a "name badge" (see Unit 4.60 – paragraph 2 under Participant Understanding; and Appendix 6)
- Students informed about dehydration
- Explanation of what is comfortable (see Unit 4.60 – paragraph 2 under Participant Understanding)
- Explanation of legitimate option of breaks and observation (this is not the "soft option")
- Ten minute rule for working with chronic pain
- Reduce possibility of heat stress - loose clothes, fans, drinks
- Observation and monitoring of health condition within class (see Unit 1.43 Mirror Image Teaching)
- Students on antibiotics, colds or flue not to come to class (see Unit 4.60 under paragraph 8 Sickness or Injury)
- Signs of discomfort or ill health
- Three seconds rule – student to take personal responsibility for not holding a posture for more than 3 seconds
- See also Unit 4.60 – paragraph 4 under Health & Safety

AGE - As a general rule, as the body ages, there is a lower rate of adaptation to exercise and recovery from exercise. Older exercisers tend to be weaker, slower, and less powerful. They have reduced balancing skills, are less co-ordinated and less agile than other younger exercisers. The biggest changes are:
- Bone density decreases
- Muscle atrophy
- Tendons and ligaments aren't as strong
- Joint flexibility decreases
- Cartilage becomes less elastic
- Onset of diseases
- Sensory decline
- Postural changes

Older people remain relatively cheerful and mentally sharp. They are adaptable, friendly, sociable and they generally participate in social activities. Older aged people who are in assisted or full time care are often reluctant to participate in social functions outside their immediate environment. They are content to stay in the comfort and safety of familiar surroundings. However, those who enjoy some measure of independent living look forward to learning new skills to enhance and prolong their quality of life and give relief from monotony and loneliness. They have lived a lot, seen a lot, have a lot to offer and are a joy to teach.

Myths about Old Age - Some older people may be committed to an active lifestyle possibly throughout their lives. They may function at a reasonably high physical level and are probably engaged in regular sessions of tennis, walking, golf, dancing, ten-pin, cycling, swimming. Many of them will be still working or may be heavily involved with family responsibilities and aged relatives.

The following myths about old age should be addressed when designing for class needs.
- Old people are much the same
- Old people cannot learn new things, they are set in their ways and cannot change
- Old people have no interest in sexual behaviour
- Old people will have memory loss and dementia
- Old people are ill
- Old people are a drain on society
- Old people should be careful and not take risks
- Old people like to be looked after and spoiled
- Old age is a time of helplessness and hopelessness
- Old people behave like (some) children
- Old people are depressed
- Old people have no sense of humour

Some older people, however, may have restricted mobility and many of them will be having difficulty coming to terms with some of the disabilities and conditions of ageing. Many, if not most, may not have exercised for many years though there has been a recent increase in the encouraging practice of walking among this group, which is an excellent base to complement their Tai Chi.

How does it feel? - In order to have a better understanding of the target population for Tai Chi for Health Exercise programs, think about or try some of the following:

- TRY   smearing your specs with a little egg white to simulate poor sight
- TRY   covering one eye for half an hour or so
- TRY   communicating to all with earplugs or cotton wool in your ears
- TRY   putting a large rubber band around your ankles. Walk for an hour or so
- TRY   sitting in a wheel chair and try doing the shopping
- TRY   getting about in a walking frame. Allow minimal use of hips/knees
- TRY   immobilising a hip, knee, shoulder or even a thumb for one day and night
- TRY   carrying around 10 kgs of potatoes in a baby carrier tied to your waist
- TRY   wearing padded undies for a day. How long could you stand it if they were wet?

Any of the above can lead to: AGGRESSION-FRUSTRATION-DEPRESSION

HEALTH - Health conditions vary considerably but for our purposes, we have devised three broad sub-categories, which are independent of age and different skill levels (see Matrix of Performance Unit 3.40):

- *Excellent Health – A*
- *Average Health -B*
- *Poor Health - C - Chronic - Physical - Psychological*

The following are additional factors for consideration in the Duty of Care for the TCH Instructor for students with Poor Health conditions regardless of age and skills levels:
- Basic knowledge of health conditions by TCH Instructor such as - Osteoporosis, Arthritis, Diabetes, Heart-lung diseases, Cancer
- Modification for special health conditions
- Working closely with health professionals
- Obvious physical/mental impairments include - loss of hearing and vision, slow response times
- Muscle weakness, poor balance and co-ordination
- Reduced temperature control
- Joint stiffness and immobility
- Reduced concentration
- Increased frustration
- Pain
- May not hear, see or understand instructions
- Inappropriate music can be confusing or disturbing
- Too much information for student can be overwhelming
- Cognitive change or decline
- Depression

Design considerations might include:
- Increasing knowledge by TCH Instructor of specialist health conditions through research and formal training such as the Tai Chi for Health programs offered by Dr Paul Lam and Alice Liping Yuan
- Need for trained assistant helpers to provide additional encouragement & support
- Consider seated activities within class
- Consider chair and rail support for standing work
- Class numbers should be limited to 15 for adequate supervision by one qualified Instructor
- Music should be familiar, light and bright. Sometimes background music will suffice
- Keep sequences simple, use repetitions (without overuse). Short-term memory may be limited
- Allow adequate time for change of weight, change of position or direction. Never rush a move or movement
- Extra care in observation of fatigue, sleepiness, lack of balance, pallor and signs of pain
- Minimise correction of detail, only correct for safety

Some who participate at this level may be fragile in body but tough in spirit. Many older students may have lost a spouse, close friends and children and often have serious chronic health problems. Many have financial worries and concerns for their safety in an ever more confusing and ever increasing technological and impatient world. Some people have a learned dependence on help and support. Generally, these people will be considerably restricted in mobility, strength, flexibility, co-ordination and balance. However, with encouragement and praise these folk can improve their quality of life and their independence in every-day tasks. Often times they do not initiate their own participation in an exercise class and are referred by a health professional or carer. For many, "exercise" is just something they do not do and they do not particularly want to do.

People making decisions about their health and welfare usually decide to encourage participation. Sometimes people of an advanced age and disability decide to "shut down" and are not willing to do anything to slow down the process. Difficult as it might seem to understand, this is their choice, their body and their life. Others, sometimes also in chronic pain and disability "wouldn't be dead for quids". They are keen, punctual and eager to learn and try to improve. Be mindful that this group is always your "better", sometimes your "equal" and never EVER less than you physically or mentally. Patronising behaviour is not acceptable in any of its ugly forms. Usually, most people attending regularly make some measure of improvement, which they will enthusiastically report after their first lesson. They will show it in their faces and by their gestures to you. A working frail aged class, for example, is the most rewarding and satisfying class you will ever teach. They are tough, resilient, motivated, dedicated and grateful.

FITNESS - It is important not to categorise people into groups such as age without regard to other factors such as health and fitness. Fitness is defined here as – aerobic, strength and flexibility and is independent of age and health conditions. For example, an older person may have good fitness but may have a health condition, temporary or chronic, that limits the ability to fulfil certain tasks (see Matrix of Performance 3.40).

The following are factors for consideration in the Duty of Care for the TCH Instructor in relation to Fitness levels of all students regardless of age, health and skills levels:
- Working at the students own level is important for fitness
- Dehydration
- Overworking can create additional muscle tension which limits health benefits of Tai Chi
- Overworking can increase the risk of stroke and heart failure regardless of age and health condition
- Cross training with resistance work with weights can significantly detract from learning how to work the energy systems for internal power, but certainly have benefits with specialised teaching

Design considerations for this group might include:
- Ongoing observation and monitoring by TCH Instructor
- Subject to health conditions, for students with average to good levels of fitness to encourage students to induce an aerobic output by working longer segments rather than having as many frequent rests
- Working at about 70% of capacity reduces muscle tension caused by self-imposed stress & will reduce fatigue
- Strength is not based on muscle size alone
- Daily practice with balanced program to maintain & increase fitness levels

SKILLS - Skill levels are defined here as Mobility (A, B, C) - Sightedness (A, B, C) - Hearing (A, B, C) - Cognitive (A, B, C) (see Matrix of Performance 3.40)

Factors for consideration here for different skills levels are:

- Previous experience in different forms of movement such as dance, martial arts, athletics, football can determine capacity to transfer movement skills
- Lifestyle & work – sedentary habits limit functional movement & incidental activities
- Ability to look, process and replicate movement may be limited with poor sightedness
- Ability to hear, process and replicate movement may limit movement outcomes
- Cognitive skills may not be developed to be able to absorb and memorise movement patterns

Having a grading system either for different classes or for different levels of ability from beginners through to advanced is the modern way to take account of your Duty of Care as a Tai Chi for Health Instructor towards different populations and to avoid the mistake of believing that Tai Chi for Health can be "One Size Fits ALL". Ongoing observation within the class by the Tai Chi for Health Instructor is central to a modern Duty of Care to ensure that you "DO NO HARM" and aim to improve the quality of life for your students.

UNIT 300
TAI CHI KNOWLDEGE

Unit Overview
3.10	**Modern Framework for Tai Chi for Health**
3.20	**Warm-Ups, Training Exercises, Cool-Downs**
3.30	**Tai Chi Principles & Concepts**
3.40	**Matrix of Performance Levels**
3.50	**Tai Chi History & Contexts**
3.60	**Martial Concept of Body and Application**

3.10   MODERN FRAMEWORK FOR TAI CHI FOR HEALTH
3.11   Introduction – Safe, Secular and Scientific
3.12   Origins of a Modern Tai Chi for Health
3.13   Paradoxical Logic – The Semiotics of Yin and Yang
3.14   Tai Chi as Qigong for Health
3.15   Tai Chi as Moving Qigong – Technique & Principle

3.11   Introduction - Safe, Secular and Scientific - This Unit introduces the reader into the modern world of Tai Chi and Qigong from a position consistent with the three tenets of Tai Chi for Health – Safe, Secular and Scientific. Safe refers to the overriding responsibility as Tai Chi for Health Instructors of a Duty of Care to "do no harm" to students. Secular means that there is no religious or metaphysical significance in any aspect of the practice and theory of Tai Chi for Health. Scientific involves the understanding and practice of Tai Chi for Health to be based on evidence based research acquired through the biological, physical and social sciences, through reasoned and logical argument capable of being substantiated by empirical evidence as distinct from the authority of myth, metaphysics, superstition, tradition or lineage (see Lam 2006; Ehrlich et al, 2006, and Arthy 2005 & 2006)

In the past decade, new models for the delivery of Tai Chi for Health programs have emerged in Australia and successfully exported into the international arena. These have been pioneered by Dr Paul Lam (Tai Chi Productions, 2009) with the radical extension of Tai Chi practised as a martial art into a science and research based, secular and modern form of exercise. His particular model for delivery of Tai Chi for Health centres on a licensed form of training and accrediting a hierarchy of leaders, instructors and trainers, specifically targeting health and fitness professionals in the safe delivery of a modern Tai Chi for Health. His inspired approach focuses on modern and "effective teaching" techniques (Lam 2006a), applying scientific and modern forms of knowledge about specific health or medical conditions thus extending the benefits of Tai Chi as a secular and modern health art to a much broader range of people. As part of this transformation and modernisation of Tai Chi for Health in Australia, Alice Liping Yuan and Henry Zheng (Exercise Medicine Australia, 2009) have similarly developed a specialised range of Tai Chi for Health programs providing a licensed form of "training the trainer" targeting health and fitness professionals.

We are now moving into the realms of specialised management of medical and health conditions involving mild to chronic forms of disease and pathology. These variables are now being factored into the Tai Chi for Health teaching programs in addition to other variables such as age, general health and fitness levels of the participant. Thus the specially trained Tai Chi for Health Instructor should be in an excellent position to begin to make a significant and measurable difference in the broader community. With the driving force of "making a difference", the training of the Tai Chi for Health Instructor is about creating an awareness of the complexities and responsibilities of a modern Duty of Care which is represented in this course as the Matrix of Performance levels (see Unit 3.40). We are living in a time of corporate and professional responsibility in a society which is considered by some as becoming increasingly "litigious", but which really means people are becoming better educated, they know and understand their legitimate rights of not having harm done to them by anyone providing goods or services in a modern, consumer oriented society.

The role of the consumer is about become better informed and educated about choices available, and this of course includes consumers of Tai Chi for Health (see Consumer Protection Unit 4.48). Duty of Care, specialised training, risk management, safety guidelines and precautions and so on (see Unit 400) are now or should be hallmarks of the expectations of not only in the delivery of health and fitness services, but also in the delivery, the teaching, the instruction of Tai Chi for Health in the community. The consumer of Tai Chi for Health has a legal right to expect the TCH Instructor to be properly trained in all aspects of a modern Duty of Care relevant to the needs of the particular participant as consumer of this valuable community health service.

Tai Chi for Health thus operates within the secular framework of modern science based research informing the Duty of Care responsibilities of competent Tai Chi instruction whereby not only health, fitness and mobility levels of the individual student are paramount but a proper understanding of the range of legal and ethical responsibilities of the TCH Instructor are essential (see Arthy, 2005). Tai Chi for Health as a concept, as a strategy is able to deliver a much broader range of classes, courses, workshops, and activities relevant to a diverse range of people who would benefit from competent and professional instruction. Such a concept includes the ability to teach Tai Chi at various levels of competency from beginners to advanced levels where the central focus is on Tai Chi as a Health Art capable of being delivered with a proper understanding and commitment to safety issues and harm prevention as well as to health enhancement.

Training of the Tai Chi for Health Instructor does not require martial or fighting techniques, which may be found in the traditional training of the martial arts instructor. Nor is it necessary or even desirable for the Tai Chi for Health Instructor to become inculcated into Confucianism or Daoist metaphysics that underpins many of the traditional practices of Tai Chi as a martial art. In the public relations arena, Tai Chi is often portrayed as a Daoist art, which focuses on learning to be in harmony with Nature, where conflict with Nature is characterised as contributing to illness, poverty and disease. This view cannot be justified by evidence based historical research, but represents a pervasive myth founded on mystical and patriarchal origins of Tai Chi for Health emerging from Confucian and Daoist metaphysics and superstitious social practices. Historically, such practices in China have combined to legitimate the feudal social order, including the inferior role of women and grinding poverty for the vast majority, justified by the "Divine Right of Kings" to rule through Nature's way and the Mandate of Heaven. [9]

In the context of a modern Tai Chi as secular health art and exercise science, such atavistic, metaphysical and historically aberrant views of the origins of Tai Chi are anathema to public-policy development of Tai Chi to be accepted, promoted and practised as a secular health art and exercise science which claims to be based on evidence based reasoning and empirical scientific research.

> The way for Tai Chi to be propagated by official bodies is through scientific studies. Governments and large organizations have heard about the benefits of Tai Chi as have many physicians and other scientists. But they need proof, the kind of proof that only scientific studies offer. Currently, the going word for health planners worldwide is "evidence based". To be supported, a program needs to have scientific evidence, just as a doctor is required to practice evidence based medicine. (Lam, 2006)

Central to the strategic public policy direction of Tai Chi for Health is the Sun Style of Tai Chi as an integral feature of a range of courses, and instructor training programs, which can be offered for the beginning student as well as the serious Tai Chi for Martial Arts practitioner who is interested in embracing the philosophy, vision and genius of Sun Lutang. In the words of Sun Lutang, "all people – men, women, the old and the young" - may wish to experience the challenges and opportunities of Tai Chi as a Health Art through the Tai Chi style that was the first to promote Tai Chi for health to the general public and the first to offer Tai Chi for women, and through a teaching, learning and instructor training framework that articulates, understands and embraces modern "Duty of Care" responsibilities and evidence based research as the basis of practising and promoting Tai Chi as a secular Health Art.

Tai Chi for the beginning student can be somewhat overwhelming due to the very different concept of health, fitness and exercise associated with the mystical and oriental art of Tai Chi practised in a modern world. This Unit aims to de-mystify the underlying principles and origins of Tai Chi so that Tai Chi and the abundant associated literature can be more readily accessible thus facilitating the opening up of Tai Chi as a significant vehicle for enhancing global health to all cultures and to all levels of society.

A modern Tai Chi for Health focuses on the health, fitness and well-being of the individual student in the teaching and learning of Tai Chi as a safe and effective form of exercise in accordance with modern ethical and legal Duty of Care requirements which are an essential feature of the training for the modern Tai Chi for Health Instructor. Traditionally, Tai Chi has been practiced as a martial art and as such in Australia formal accreditation as a Tai Chi Instructor has only been available through the Level 1 Coaching course of the National Martial Arts Instructor Accreditation Scheme with the Australian Sports Commission with the peak body for Tai Chi being the Australian Kung Fu Wushu Federation (AKWF):

> It is important to be sure the [Tai Chi] trainer is fully accredited with the Australian Kung Fu (Wushu) Federation Inc, which is the governing body for all martial arts in Australia.... When it comes to practicing Tai Chi safely, Master Jin-Song warns: Make sure your instructor is accredited. The Australian Coaching Council is the accreditation body for instructors. The Australian Kung Fu (Wushu) Federation is the bona fide body for Tai Chi and Kung Fu. There are many instructors who complete weekend workshops in Tai Chi and claim to be instructors. It is best that your instructor is fully insured, and properly accredited and has years of experience in Tai Chi. This way you will be sure to enjoy all the benefits and pleasures that Tai Chi can bring. (Goldenglow, 2008)

Tai Chi for Health on the other hand offers a pathway for Instructor training independent from Kung Fu Tai Chi Chuan practised as a martial art. Accordingly, Tai Chi for Health does not include techniques which involve physically pushing, throwing, grappling or sparring as may be found in the traditional training of the Tai Chi Master

---

[9] Traditional Chinese sovereignty concept of legitimacy used to support the rule of the kings. The parallel in the West is the "Divine Right of Kings", the doctrinal "right to rule" anointed and blessed by Gods or Heaven, which places the monarch, the King or Emperor, above the rule of law. (see Robertson, 2005)

as a martial artist. Tai Chi for Health Advanced Instructor Training provides a comprehensive approach to providing expertise in both the performance and the teaching of Tai Chi for Health from beginners to advanced levels of performance. A modern Tai Chi for Health rejects the "one size fits all approach", it is not a martial art, it is non-contact and a gentle, safe and effective form of exercise for a very wide range of people and situations as outlined in the Tai Chi for Health Matrix of Performance (see Unit 3.40).

In this regard, there is an urgent need for the development of an integrated framework for modern Tai Chi for Health, which not only includes evidence based research and reasoning, but includes a modern approach to teaching within graded levels of standards and performance from beginners to advanced (see Unit 6.20) inclusive of a modern Duty of Care relevant to Tai Chi for Health and not Kung Fu Tai Chi Chuan. In Australia today, the Tai Chi for Health Instructor/Leader programs that are available either do not include a teaching component in the program or contain only a basic introductory teaching method. Our Tai Chi for Health Advanced Instructor Training course is intended to fill this gap for those Tai Chi Instructors/Leaders in our local area, in particular, for those who currently have nowhere to turn to achieve an advanced level of teaching expertise other than through the accreditation of the traditional Kung Fu Tai Chi Chuan martial artist with the AKWF (see Open Letter - Appendix 1).

Our course is also offered as a "Pilot" program, providing a template, a framework, a strategy for other Tai Chi for Health organisations and practitioners to encourage the development of similar courses in Tai Chi for Health Advanced Instructor Training, which may of course include other styles of Tai Chi with advanced level FORMS offered as different modules for the practical, performance and teaching component of a Tai Chi for Health. An integrated framework of graded levels of standards and performance needs to be extended even further into the formal academic and training programs of certain health and fitness professionals who facilitate and offer community based exercise and recreational programs. Standardised curriculum levels would thus need to describe skills and competencies necessary to gain effective teaching expertise as an essential part of the accreditation of the different levels of the Tai Chi for Health Instructor.

Such an approach calling for the development of an integrated framework of a modern Tai Chi for Health is entirely consistent with the pedagogic principles within a modern liberal-democracy which demand open and transparent access to higher levels of education on the basis of graded levels of academic standards, achievement and merit. Access to Tai Chi for Health Advanced Instructor training should be made available to all who qualify, and not be limited to a business model of a licensed franchise or to the rules of patronage within the martial traditions of Kung Fu Tai Chi Chuan.

In the modern context of Tai Chi for Health, it is vital that teaching expertise be considered an equal player and should parallel the development of the practical skills and research focus and outcomes of a modern Tai Chi for Health. Underpinning our argument for the inclusion of teaching expertise at an advanced level as an essential component of a modern Tai Chi for Health, is the concept of "keeping an open mind"[10] for the learning and teaching of "Tai Chi as a Health Art" first radically promulgated by Chinese Kung-fu Master Sun Lutang in the world's first publication of Tai Chi for Health titled *Study of Taijiquan* (Sun 1921).

3.12   Origins of a Modern Tai Chi for Health - So as to better understand Tai Chi for Health as a safe and effective form of exercise, we need to unravel different meanings of the term - "Tai Chi" as it appears in the vast literature of Tai Chi and Qigong translated into English. To do this we need to understand that historically "Tai Chi" has at least two significantly different origins – one is a type of Chinese philosophy and the other is a particular Chinese style of Kung-fu or martial art. On the one hand, the philosophical Tai Chi is based on what is called a form of "paradoxical logic", the dialectic of Yin-Yang theory, and, on the other hand, the martial Kung Fu Tai Chi Chuan is promoted as an "energy efficient" fighting style of the Chinese martial arts which like all forms of martial arts has significant health benefits[11].

The term "Tai Chi" as philosophy emerged between two and three thousand years ago in China and over the millennia became absorbed into metaphysical, religious and superstitious cultural practices such as Daoism and Confucianism. More importantly for our purposes, the philosophical "Tai Chi" can be understood as a dialectical form of language and reasoning translated as the "Grand Ultimate" and is used in analysing, classifying and making order out of the world, the universe, nature, or the cosmos.

The term "Tai Chi" as a short form of Kung Fu Tai Chi Chuan, the Chinese martial art has, contrary to popular myth, only very recent historical beginnings. (see Miller,2000; Wile, 2006; Arthy, 2006) In the mid-nineteenth century, a particular style of Chinese Boxing, taught by Yang Lu Chan at the Manchu Imperial Court, was first linked by the scholar Ong Tong to the philosophical principles of the "Tai Chi". Ong Tong was so impressed by the way Yang Lu Chan performed his techniques, he felt that Yang's movements and techniques expressed the

---

[10] see Fifth Concept of Sun Lutang in Unit 3.31

[11] Empirical scientific research suggests that all forms of martial arts have health benefits and are worthy of promoting as such for people of all ages. (Douris et al, 2004; Brudnek et al, 2002; Swiercz, 2005; Binder, 1999; Weiser et al, 1995) The martial arts are actively promoted as unique among most forms of exercise due to the way they blend strength, endurance, flexibility and balance, and are viewed as a form of self-defence against ageing. (Evenson, 2004)

physical manifestation of the principles of the Chinese philosophy of the "Ta Chi" contained in the *I Ching*, or *Book of Changes* (see Jou,1984) written nearly three thousand years earlier. He wrote for him a matching verse:

Hands Holding Taiji shakes the whole world,
a chest containing ultimate skill defeats a gathering of heroes

Thus was coined the term the "Grand Ultimate" Fist, Kung Fu Tai Chi Chuan, translated as the supreme form of Chinese Boxing and was so described as a result of the effective fighting skills of Yang Lu Chan in being able to defeat his opponents through the particular "rules of engagement" that existed at that time in the Imperial Court of China. Yang Lu Chan's "energy efficient" fighting style was thus perceived to reflect the power of nature itself articulated at that time through the Confucian dialectic based on Yin-Yang theory (see Wile 2006).

The philosophical term "Tai Chi" was thus subsequently borrowed by the Yang family and linked to recently "discovered" and "ancient" texts now called the "Tai Chi Classics", all of which provided a great public relations opportunity to capitalise on the powerful cultural mythology, metaphysics and intellectual prestige surrounding "Tai Chi" philosophy, to promote and differentiate the Chen Style adaptation of "Cotton Fist" boxing from other styles of Chinese boxing that existed at the time. However, contemporary evidence based historical research and scientific reasoning strongly suggests that the "Tai Chi Classics" were in fact written and produced by one of Yang Lu Chan's literate pupils who claimed that the origins of these texts and the origins of Kung Fu Tai Chi Chuan were related to the mythical personage of the Daoist priest - Zhang Sanfeng. (Wile, 1993)

For many contemporary Tai Chi practitioners, the "Tai Chi Classics" represent a canon of texts which function as the "biblical" authority for Kung Fu Tai Chi Chuan in much the same way as the "Bubishi" is suggested to represent the "bible of karate" (see McCarthy, 1995). Like the "Bubishi", the historical origins of "Tai Chi Classics" are shrouded in myth and mystery. Paradoxically, the anonymous authors of the "Bubishi" and of the "Tai Chi Classics" both trace the origins of the "efficiency principle" embedded in the different fighting styles back to a common, mythical ancestor in the thirteenth century China - a reputed Kung Fu Master of Shaolin "Hard and Soft" fighting styles, a Daoist priest called Zhang Sanfeng. (see McCarthy, 1995) Specifically, the Okinawan styles of "Tang Te" (Chinese Hands) and Japanese Karatedo (the "Way" of the Empty Hand) also trace their origins back to this mythical Daoist priest Zhang.

Zhang is reputed to have lived in the thirteenth century in China and to have developed a series of continuous postures based on his knowledge of hard Shaolin and soft Daoist Kung Fu. These mythical origins are based on the premise that Zhang made a study on the principles of vital point theory [12] and were disseminated only to his most trusted disciples:

> *Fascinated by the fighting traditions, and proficient in the Shaolin hard styles, Zhang sought to create the ultimate form of self-defense; one that would allow him to subjugate an opponent with only minimal force by traumatizing weak parts of the human body. To corroborate his hypotheses, it is said that Zhang travelled extensively and experimented on both animals and humans. During his analysis, Zhang and his associates discovered that by striking specific vital points, alternative areas became much more vulnerable to even less powerful attacks; thus by pressing, squeezing, or traumatizing one point, striking other points would have a critical effect. Chinese folklore maintains that Zhang Sanfeng corroborated his lethal suppositions by bribing jailers and experimenting on prisoners in death row.* (McCarthy, 1995, pp108-109)

Placing Chinese mythology to one side, the historical origins of a modern Tai Chi for Health began, however, not with Zhang Sanfeng, not with Yang Lu Chan or even his grandson Yang Cheng Fu, not with the Peoples Republic of China in the early 1950s but, with the genius of the Chinese Kung-fu Master Sun Lutang in the early twentieth century.

Who was Sun Lutang and what did he achieve? Sun Lutang was born in 1861 in northern China and from very humble beginnings, he succeeded not only in creating a powerful, effective and practical fighting style of Kung Fu Tai Chi Chuan (see Cartmell, 2003), not only in becoming a famous Kung-fu Master of three major styles of Chinese boxing but as someone who was well educated and had a deep knowledge of the literary arts including Daoism, Confucianism and the ancient philosophy of the "Tai Chi". More importantly for us, however, the genius of Sun Lutang (see Arthy, 2006) was that in Sun's day in the early twentieth century, there was not yet the idea that Kung Fu Tai Chi Chuan was a Health Art and that Sun recognized the health-building benefits by making the connection between the development of "internal" power through natural exercise and its benefits for the individual's health. (see Miller, 2000)

Sun Lutang was the first Kung Fu Master in China to actively promote to the general public the health giving benefits of martial power and training in a similar way as Professor Jigoro Kano had some years earlier in Japan

---

[12] Sometimes referred to as "Death Touch" or "Dim Mak" (Point Pulse in Cantonese & Dian Xue Shu in Mandarin) and is an ancient martial art that consists of striking certain points on the body to cause illness, serious injury or death. The majority of these points correspond to the same locations as acupuncture points. Dim mak is considered an extremely dangerous martial art, which can cause a great deal of damage to the human body. (Kelly, 2007)

pioneered the transformation of the ancient Japanese martial arts to the modern "Do" or the "Way" [13] incorporating a safe and scientific approach to exercise and health. Sun Lutang also broke with the patriarchal Confucian tradition central to Chinese society by establishing the first female martial arts course in the early 1930s. Previously, Kung Fu Tai Chi Chuan had been viewed and practiced exclusively as a martial art for men. (see Preston, 2002; Wile 2006; Miller, 2000) Specifically, Sun Lutang was the first Tai Chi Master to write and publish books to promote the martial arts for health, and Kung Fu Tai Chi Chuan as having health benefits for "all people":

> All people – men, women, the old, and the young – may practice in order to replace temerity with bravery, and stiffness with pliability. Those of you who are extremely weak, who suffer from fatigue and injury or illness, or who have weakened your Chi from the practice of other martial arts to the point that you no longer have the strength to train, all of you may practice Tai Ji Quan. With practice, the Chi will quickly return to a balanced state and will become strong, while the spirit naturally returns to a state of wholeness. Disease will be eliminated and the length of life increased. (Sun Lutang, 1921, p60)

It was Sun Lutang's publications on the "internal" martial arts identifying health and fitness issues, which represents a pivotal point in Chinese history transforming the way in which educated people began to favourably view the martial arts in China. Instrumental in this development was a pupil of Sun Lutang, Chen Wei Ming, also known as Chen Zeng Ze. From their first meeting in July 1915, Chen Wei Ming was to become a long-standing friend and pupil of Su Lutang in Xing-Yi-Quan and Ba Gua Zhang, and a Tai Chi Master in his own right.

In the "Preface" to Sun Lu Tang's first book, Chen Wei Ming wrote:

> The state of being completely rounded out without any break is in accordance with the principle of the Tai Ji. Styles and methods are but its outer form. There are many Tai Ji boxers who perform the long style [of Tai Ji Boxing] and the Thirteen Postures [Tai Ji Thirteen Styles] without understanding the state of being completely rounded out without any break. They are really not true Tai Ji boxers. Mr Sun Lutang is versed in Xing Yi, Bua Qua, and Tai Ji and thus can merge them together. It will benefit the body and mind deeply for martial artists to make a modest study on this principle. (Sun, 1915, see Third Preface, 1919, by Chen Zeng Ze, p 59)

Some years later, Chen Wei Ming also became a pupil of the famous Kung Fu Master, Yang Cheng Fu. In the late 1920s, as one of Yang's "educated disciples" Chen was instrumental in motivating Yang Cheng Fu into transforming the "external", vigorous and combative movements of Kung Fu Tai Chi Chuan into what is today recognised as the gentle, graceful, flowing and "internal" Yang Style of Kung Fu Tai Chi Chuan:

> ...it was through Che'ng-fu's educated disciples that t'ai-chi was adapted for practice by intellectuals, the sick, the elderly, and women. The Yang family thus became the vehicle by which conservative intellectuals could reconcile both the need for self-strengthening and the preservation of traditional culture and progressive intellectuals could embrace a wholesome legacy from the feudal past. (Wile, 1993, p.iv)

This particular Yang Style of Tai Chi represents the newest major style of Tai Chi that is practised world wide today for health and exercise benefits as well as by some for martial and self-defence purposes. The Chinese boxing style practised by the Yang family up until this point was itself a variation of the vigorous and explosive martial style adapted from the Chen Style by Yang Lu Chang, the grandfather of Yang Cheng Fu:

> Hence, the Yang style of Tai Chi Chuan he [Yang Cheng Fu] developed is sometimes called the Big Form. He did away with jumping, foot-stamping, straight punching and other forceful, aggressive actions, which are more appropriate for combat. He also performed the patterns slowly, gently and gracefully, almost transforming Tai Chi Chuan into an exquisite dance, although he himself was a formidable fighter. (Wong, 1996, p.28)

Chen Wei Ming thus represents a key historical figure linking Sun Lutang's articulation, promotion and pioneering publications of Tai Chi as having "health benefits for all" to the subsequent transformation of the "external" and vigorous combat Yang Style Kung Fu Tai Chi Chuan to a new Yang Style described as a health exercise to make it easier for elderly or less able people who may find the original martial style too vigorous. (Wong 1996, p 28)

Chen Wei Ming also was influential in facilitating the "health giving" essence of "true Tai Chi" boxing as accessible to the general public in a strategic and modern way. This time he collaborated with Yang Cheng Fu in publishing in a quasi-poetic form, what is regarded by many today as the consummate expression of Yang Style Tai Chi Chuan known as Yang Cheng Fu's Ten Principles (see Unit 3.34 and Appendix 7). These Ten Principles were firstly published by Chen Wei Ming in 1925 in Chen's own book *The Art of Tai-chi chu'uan*. (Wile, 1996, pp9-14) The health benefits of this new slow and graceful style created by Yang Cheng Fu and promoted by Chen Wei Ming would be further taken up in 1956 by the government campaign in the People's Republic of China in the promotion of Tai Chi as a method of keeping fit through the creation of the simplified 24 Yang Style form, based on Yang Cheng Fu's thirty four distinct postures. (Wile, 1996, pxiii)

---

[13] Professor Jigoro Kano is a significant historical figure in the Asian Martial Arts due to having pioneered the modern "Do" or "Way" (as in Ju-Do or the Gentle Way) in regard to physical education, health and safety within a government- sponsored approach to the "physical education" curriculum. "Do" is the Japanese word for the Chinese word the "Dao" meaning the "Way". The modernisation process of the Chinese martial arts did not take place in the same way as in Japan until the early 1950s through the health and fitness policy implemented by the government of the People's Republic of China.

3.13   Paradoxical Logic – The Semiotics of Yin and Yang - Within a modern framework for Tai Chi for Health, we firstly need to examine the critical role that "language" itself plays in order to access much of the literature associated with Tai Chi and Qigong. The suggestion is made that the fundamentals of Tai Chi are often poorly understood due to a problem of translation from Chinese into Western languages:

This is mainly because of the parts of the Tai Chi Classics that discuss these topics [such as skeletal posture and muscular function] are rather difficult to translate into English or other Western languages (Jiang, 2006, p.6)

What are the "Tai Chi Classics" and what are the specific language and cultural barriers that seem to frustrate an accurate translation into English resulting in the claim of a poor understanding of the so-called Tai Chi "fundamentals"? What is the significance of the term "dialectic" to understanding the relationship between Tai Chi as a philosophy and Tai Chi as a health and martial art? In order to de-mythologise the so-called "fundamentals" of Tai Chi, we firstly need to unravel and examine the "concept of the dialectic" [14] as a specific style of language, a way of classifying and making sense of the world, the cosmos, the universe, nature, people, substance and nothingness, everything and anything, including emptiness. In addition, we need to have some understanding about the application of the "dialectic" specifically within the cultural context of the Confucian world order that survived virtually intact in China until after the Cultural Revolution in the 1970s and the implementation of the "Four Modernisations" by Deng Xiaoping. In short, we need to understand that the Confucian dialectic has represented an ultra-conservative application of Yin-Yang theory where concepts of "Nature", "The Way", conflict, equilibrium and harmony are fused together within complex cultural and social codes of patriarchal authority and governance, which supported and reinforced a feudal social order in China for over two thousand years (see Wile, 2006)

Thus a large part of any difficulty in understanding the literature and concepts of Tai Chi has much to do with understanding different conventions of language and culture. The Confucian dialectic which underpins much of the myth and literature (such as the "Tai Chi Classics") related to traditional Kung Fu Tai Chi Chuan, confronts the modern reader as a clash of language styles between "poetic" and "prosaic" forms of representation, between the abstract "metaphysics of nature" and the concrete "secularity of modern science", and in broader terms between significant cultural differences of the ancient "East" and the modern "West".

As described by the advocates of the Confucian dialectic, an instrumental feature of Tai Chi lies in poetic, romantic and "ineffable" forms of meaning. Here we are confronted with the "end of words' function but not the end of meaning itself" wherein neither images nor words are deemed capable of conveying the locus of meaning. Within this Confucian dialectic, it is the relationship between "xu" and the "shi" (that is, "un-real/real"), which is deemed to take place outside the language of human beings, where there is "meaning". (see Pan 1996) Specifically, it is claimed that these terms "xu and shi" are not only the most important terms in Kung Fu Tai Chi Chuan, but are poorly understood by Westerners. To remedy this, we are not directed towards science or any evidence based forms of reasoning, but to poetry itself. We are told that we need to understand the poetry of the "Dao De Jing" in order to understand the nuances of the terms "xu" and "shi". Thus, by understanding the cultural and philosophical forces, which shape the respective languages, crystalised in words, then it is suggested they will reveal their treasures grudgingly. (Barrett, 2006)

Being and nonbeing produce each other; difficulty and ease complement each other, long and short shape each other, high and low contrast with each other, voice and echoes conform to each other, before and after go along with each other, So sages manage effortless service and carry out unspoken guidance. (quoted by Barrett 2006, from the "Essential Tao" by Thomas Cleary)

Conversely within contemporary Western and modern culture, practical and everyday language does not embrace the language of poetry to convey meaning but relies on "prosaic", "rational" and "secular" forms of language.

For our purposes of becoming better informed Tai Chi for Health students, the language used to describe and analyse Tai Chi for Health within a modern framework, which embraces a modern legal and ethical framework, will invariably describe activities in the modern, conceptual language registers of exercise, fitness, health, Duty of Care and ethical responsibilities. Such language will be secular, rational, descriptive and practical in order to maximise clarity, precision and to avoid the poetic vagueness of ambiguity resulting in confusion, disengagement and possibly even harm inflicted unintentionally on students by the Tai Chi Instructor. [15]

However, it is important to note that a Confucian dialectic is not one and the same as the paradoxical logic of "yin and yang theory". Central to much of the literature concerning explanations about Tai Chi and Qigong practices is

---

[14] Dialectic: an exchange of   propositions (theses) and counter-propositions (antitheses) resulting in a synthesis of the opposing assertions. The idea of a "universal dialectic" is related to the Daoist and Neo-Confucian concept of the "Tai Chi" or "supreme ultimate". The Western influence of the "universal dialectic" adds a progressive element to the inexorable process of change, a concept which is absent in Daoist thought. (see Wikipedia, 2007b).
[15] For example, a student who reads the "Tai Chi Classics" prescription of "turning the waist" not understanding that the waist and hips within Chinese physiology are one and the same, may indeed cause injury. For information on knee injuries caused by Tai Chi Chuan see also Foster (2006) and Wong (1996, pxvii)

the language of paradoxical logic, a logic which describes "things" as being understood in terms of a relationship with other "things", a logic which functions as a process of understanding the world as "opposites" - as a relationship between "Yin" and "Yang".

Take the Yin-Yang principle, which is probably the most important concept in Tai Chi Chuan. The concept is actually very simple, but it has far-reaching and most profound manifestations. But if one does not understand its basic philosophy and regards Yin-Yang as absolute terms instead of as symbols, this may lead to very complicated and fruitless arguments. For example, if one believes that moving forward is always yang, and as such is always used for attack, he misses the essence of this Yin-Yang philosophy. (Wong, 2006b)

Accordingly, in order to understand the rich history, the traditions and secrets of Tai Chi and Qigong, which emanate from Chinese history and society, we need to take a closer look at this paradoxical logic of Yin-Yang theory.

It is the relational aspect or concept of Yin-Yang theory, which is essential to any understanding of the literature and oral traditions of various Asian forms of martial arts, and most especially – Kung Fu Tai Chi Chuan. In order to understand the power of this "relational" concept, we can begin with the idea of contextualising Yin-Yang theory itself as one of the key ingredients in many of the oral and written traditions within Asian society and in particular Chinese culture. Put simply, the relational concept of "Yin" and "Yang" represents a key communication tool, a system of classifying the world and the universe, an important way of analysing everything in terms of "opposites" – the world, the cosmos, the environment, people, nature, society – literally anything, everything and nothing are all concepts capable of being classified in both relational and absolute terms of "Yin" and "Yang".

It is important to stress that unless we can begin to understand the relational aspect of Yin-Yang theory within a modern framework of Safe, Secular and Scientific, our journey into becoming safer, more effective Tai Chi for Health students and teachers will significantly be inhibited, and possibly even blinded by an obedient silence commanded by a traditional authority based on lineage, metaphysics and superstition – in short, by the Confucian dialectic. In a very real sense, we have already begun our linguistic journey of discovery by examining the familiar antonyms of the "poetic" and "prosaic", the "metaphysical" and the "secular", "ancient" and "modern", and "East" and "West" – these are conventional antonyms.

Where can we find some equivalent to Yin-Yang theory within our own experiences? We are already familiar with the concept of "East and West" as a way of dividing the known world into two parts - Western civilisation and Eastern civilisation. Closer to home and to our own educational experiences, we can ask - what language tools do we use to understand our everyday realities, to help decode meaning about the world around us? We turn to the dictionary and a thesaurus both of which are readily accessible for literate people to de-code the meaning or significance of words in relation to other words, ideas and concepts. In the West, the thesaurus in effect represents the classic dictionary of the "Yin" and the "Yang" of western thought processes. The thesaurus is by definition and practical use, a text of opposites – of both "synonyms and antonyms" – of all things similar and all things opposite.

Where else can we look to see the equivalent power of Yin-Yang theory embedded in Western culture? The modern financial and business word could not survive, it could not cope with the vast amount of information which would be utterly useless were it not for the simple "Yin-Yang" concept of "Debits and Credits" within double entry bookkeeping, the origins of this technology being attributed to Benedetto Cotrugli in the fifteenth century in Italy. Some people even suggest that double-entry bookkeeping is itself derivative of Yin-Yang theory (Yun 1984; and Hyon & Park 1988). But whatever the historical "truth" of this claim might be, what is important for our purposes is to acknowledge the historical fact that the invention of dualistic or binary code of commerce, namely double-entry bookkeeping has been instrumental in revolutionising the Western world of business by adopting a method that recognises the duality of all business transactions – the double-sided aspect of every transaction also demanding a specific context within which the "Yin" and the "Yang" of the business transaction or the "Debit" and "Credit" needs to be located.

Similarly, the modern world of computing could not possibly have come about without the invention or discovery of another "Yin-Yang", or dualistic code called binary mathematics and its application to modern digital technology. The binary code itself was "invented" in the West by Leibniz who is acknowledged as having been motivated by the influence of Chinese cosmology, in particular, by the *I Ching*, the *Book of Changes*. (see Jou, 1984) In the West, it was Leibniz who thus recognised the power of Yin-Yang theory linking this to how the elementary building blocks of "zero and one" could be transformed in principle to build literally everything, and how it contained an efficiency and purpose that is mirrored in today's modern world in the twenty first century in the shift from the technologies of the analogue to the digital age.

Finally, we have in the West a range of formal studies in the Social Sciences, which focus predominantly on the same paradoxical logic of Yin-Yang theory, and one of these studies is called the "Science of Semiotics". This is the scientific study of the relation between "the Signifier and the Signified" (see Barthes, 2001; Eco, 1976). In philosophical terms, Western thinking is mostly based on Aristotilian logic and focuses on theorems of "truth", on notions of objectivity. Semiotics, however, is a relatively new social science concerned about understanding the world as a conceptual relationship between what is "true" and what is "not true" and is sometimes referred to as the "theory of the lie". [16] The reason for this is that if that "something", some "object", cannot be used to signify or represent a "lie", it cannot be used to represent any form of "truth":

> *Semiotics is concerned with everything that can be taken as a sign. A sign is everything which can be taken as significantly substituting for something else... Thus semiotics is in principle the discipline studying everything, which can be used in order to lie. If something cannot be used to tell a lie, conversely it cannot be used to tell the truth: it cannot in fact be used 'to tell' at all.* (Eco, 1976, p.7)

Within this analytical framework then, what is "true" or what is "false" does not stand alone, there always needs to be some context by which to make some judgement based on some criteria through which "true" and "false" propositions can be evaluated, where "facts" do not exist alone but stand in a logical relation to "evidence". Within a semiotic analysis, conceptual objects such as "God", "Nature", "Truth" or "The Way" cease to become transcendental, [17] they can be demonstrated through the signifying relationship as being socially produced constructs.

Within a secular and semiotic analytical framework, the "sign" or "signifier" can be represented as a "word", "image", "concept" or "object" and thus stands in a relationship to something else for there to be meaning and this meaning is the "signified". Thus within Yin-Yang theory, the relationship between the "Yin" and "Yang" in the field of semiotic analysis is simply defined as the relationship between conventional opposites as part of a signifying relationship to derive meaning. Strategically in everyday situations, we often define "something" in relation to the opposite, by what the "something" is not, by a process of elimination. Police investigations and medical diagnoses often use this strategy of "inductive and deductive forms of reasoning", by ruling out what is not the case to arrive at what might be the case, but invariably within a scientific framework of establishing evidence to support a set of facts formulated around a working hypothesis.

In any signifying relationship, as with Yin-Yang theory, there always needs to be some context whether this is historical, legal, cultural, natural, geographical, and so on in order to derive meaning. In the West, semiotics (see also Chang 2003), is a relatively new social science and has become an increasingly important modern educational discipline applied in a range of disciplines from the training of business managers, marketing consultants, advertisers, film makers, public relations experts through to architects and town planners. In the broader field of cultural anthropology, semiotics and related structuralist tools of analysis are deployed in the study of literature, religion, myth, superstition and folk-lore. (see Barthes,2001; Levi-Strauss,1977)

The purpose here, however, is not to suggest that the reader or Tai Chi for Health student or teacher should become an expert in semiotics, accounting, binary mathematics, digital technology, or Yin-Yang theory but to highlight the underlying significance of the cultural classification system of Yin-Yang theory which first emerged in China between two and three thousand years ago, and which is now an intrinsic and analytical feature of Western culture including everyday business and commercial practices. In other words, part of our project is to inform and empower the Tai Chi for Health student to help understand the intellectual and generative power of the ability to "make connections" based on the building blocks of "synonyms and antonyms", of the relational aspects of Yin-Yang theory. It is also important to recognise that this dualistic way of thinking as a social technology in China became absorbed into metaphysical, religious and superstitious practices such as Geomancy, Feng-Shui, Confucianism and Daoism. The appropriation of Yin-Yang theory into cultural and social forms of governance was thus instrumental in justifying the Imperial Mandate of Heaven manifested in the patriarchal, misogynist and ultra conservative social order in China, and legitimised as the "Harmony of Nature". This ultra conservatism based on the cosmology of the "Way of Nature" served to significantly inhibit the modernisation process that began in the West a few centuries ago and in other parts of Asia a hundred or so years earlier. Consistent with the logic of the paradox, both the technology of semiotics and Yin-Yang theory can be used for "good" or "evil", for "democratic" or "fascist", for "progressive" or "regressive" purposes, for the application of "modern" or "primitive" forms of governance.

3.14   Tai Chi as Qigong for Health - There are currently more than 3,300 different styles and schools of Qigong (Wikipedia, 2007a). Do we need to know about all of these before we can understand anything about Tai Chi and Qigong? How can we simplify? How can we begin to make sense of a complex set of possibilities that may be available within the Safe, Secular and Scientific framework of a Tai Chi for Health?

If we are looking for an effective and "energy efficient" "Way" of doing this, the suggestion is to turn immediately to a semiotic approach using the binary code of Yin-Yang theory. For specific guidance on this topic, we can turn to Dr Jwing Ming Yang who has produced a number of texts on this very broad and complex topic, all of which will greatly assist us and serve as an excellent starting point. (see Yang, 1991, 1996, 1997 and 1999) Dr Yang outlines

---

[16] See Karl Popper (1974) whose philosophy of modern science is based on the idea of "falsifiability', if any hypothesis is not capable of being falsified, then it does not have any scientific validity.

[17] Transcendence is a concept central to many religious practices and within Daoism (or Taoism), the textual authority for transcendence is outlined in Verse 1 of the Tao Te Ching: "Transcending - The Tao that can be told is not the universal Tao. The name that can be named is not the universal name (Tzu, 2005, p.7)

a framework upon which we can build and whenever we get lost or confused, we can refer back to the basic building blocks of Yin-Yang theory which he so succinctly outlines in the context of Qigong. A representation of this framework is as follows:

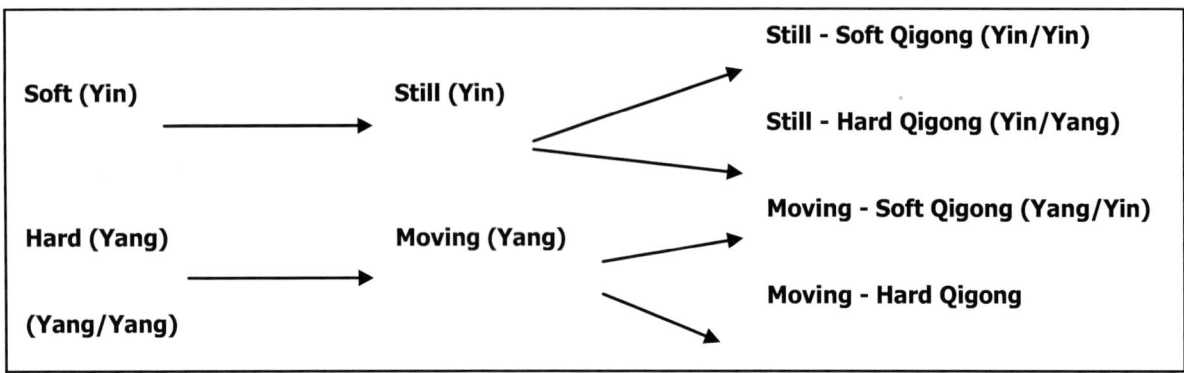

This framework relies on a common understanding of two sets of conventional opposites or antonyms -

- **Soft and Hard**
- **Still and Moving**

In regard to our present topic of Tai Chi and Qigong in the context of Tai Chi for Health, the specific meaning of the terms "soft/hard" and "still/moving" can be usefully classified using Yin-Yang theory as follows:

Still - Soft Qigong
- No movement, everything relaxed
- Breathing – Abdominal
- Body - Calm and relaxed whether lying down or seated
- Overall - Yin – relative to all other categories
- Tai Chi – no posture or form

Still - Hard Qigong
- No movement, some part or all parts of body tense
- Breathing – Abdominal or reverse abdominal
- Body – Some part of upper and/ or lower body in tension
- Overall - Yang relative to still/soft but yin relative to moving soft or hard
- Tai Chi - Wuji position – beginning and end of form or movement

Moving - Soft Qigong
- Movement of part or whole of body – minimum muscular force – relaxed
- Breathing – Abdominal or natural
- Body – Standing or seated with movement and minimum muscular force and relaxed
- Overall – Yin relative to moving/hard but yang relative to still/soft
- Tai Chi – Soft flowing movement through the form and application

Moving – Hard Qigong
- Movement – internal styles of martial arts - minimum use of muscular force – but tensed
- Breathing – Reverse abdominal
- Body – Movement with explosive muscular force and tensed
- Overall – Yang relative to other categories – Yin or Yang relative to style of martial art
- Kung Fu Tai Chi Chuan – Martial applications within form or application – point of contact

As we can see, each broad category can be used as basic building blocks, to begin to construct a more complex set of possibilities by increasing or decreasing the yin or yang relational factor. For example, some martial forms or styles of Kung Fu Tai Chi Chuan, Chinese styles of Kung Fu and Japanese Karate Katas or forms have both soft and hard aspects to movement, slow and fast, high and low positions in attacking and defending. [18]

Most martial artists would claim that their own style of martial arts combines both soft and hard aspects of movement and stillness within the martial applications. Many of the significant differences between martial styles often relate to tradition, ethics and rules of engagement and supposed differences are often over-emphasised and

---

[18] For example, the name of the Japanese style of Goju Ryu karate-do was based on the Eight Poems of the Fist from the Chinese text the Bubishi (see McCarthy, 1995) with the third precept: The way of inhaling and exhaling is hardness and softness'. "Go" means hard and "Ju" meaning soft.

superficial and ignore the commonalities between various styles. (see Liu, 2006) Sumo wrestling for example, has a set of "rules of engagement" which has a great deal more in common with that of Kung Fu Tai Chi Chuan's "rules of engagement" of "Push Hands", than say Judo, Tae Kwon Do or western boxing.

Following Sun Lutang's idea that, whether Tai Chi is practiced for martial and/or for health purposes, there is no need for the development of exceptional physicality, the flexibility of the circus performer or excessive muscular strength [19] in order to be a proficient, and "energy efficient" martial artist or to be fit and healthy.   Thus within this framework, Tai Chi for Health can most effectively be based on "Moving Soft Qigong" and may also include some component of "Still Soft Qigong".   The overall emphasis in Tai Chi for Health is on learning to relax, not to be tense, to learn to use the mind to relax the body and most importantly, and at a more advanced level learning to know how to do all of these things while co-ordinating breathing with movement in a flowing and relaxed way. This does not exclude by any means, the exercise and health enhancing value of tension in the extension and contraction of muscles, ligaments and tendons, in the performance of Tai Chi for Health:

> The best situation is when yin and yang mutually interact with one another at all times. Therefore the emphasis solely on relaxation and softness without any tension is insufficient and misleading. (Chu, 2006)

3.15   Tai Chi as Moving Qigong: Technique & Principle - When we look at the yin and yang of "breathing", we realise that this is something most people take for granted in their every day lives. It is something done automatically without needing to think about it, where there is a balance or equilibrium with the rhythms of the body in relation to the environment. We become aware of breathing when something changes or interferes with this balance. We may become aware of breathing in terms of factors or things both "internal" and "external" to the body.

With the "external" factor, the balance or equilibrium will be compromised by any number of reasons – whether caused by walking up a hill, or if the air is impure, whether too thin with not enough oxygen or filled with smoke or fumes, odours and smells, or smog. With the "internal" factor, the life-giving, fundamental importance of air become paramount when our bodies struggle to get sufficient air in or out of the lungs or the proper quality of air is altered regardless of the cause. Without air, without being able to breathe properly – life itself becomes problematic. Breathing thus concerns the broad spectrum of life from what might be considered normal through to environmental and health "pathology" factors, which affect our capacity to breathe naturally.

Accordingly, the practice of Qigong, which includes a study of breathing, needs to be extremely careful and responsible in order to observe the safety aspects of students. It needs to be comprehensible and based on an informed understanding and scientific basis of the normal to the pathological functioning of the human body. As an absolute minimum for safety issues, the Tai Chi for Health Instructor should be properly trained and certified in Senior First Aid and remain current with that training for Cardio Pulmonary Resuscitation (CPR) by attending a CPR update every year.

In Tai Chi for Health, should students be taught anything specific about "breathing" and "Qigong"?   The conventional wisdom in many Tai Chi schools is to not worry about breathing when performing the Tai Chi form. It is suggested that all that is really needed is to just breathe naturally, relax and not tense up. And after many years of practice, it is also suggested, the co-ordination between breathing and the movements will eventually occur naturally without having to think.   Many Tai Chi schools also teach Qigong as a technique something separate from practicing the Tai Chi form.

Does this conventional wisdom have a place in Tai Chi for Health? Should the relevance of "breathing" techniques and exercises be ignored within an understanding of the broader principles in the performance of the Tai Chi solo form? Should we see Qigong as something fundamentally different from the practice of the Tai Chi solo form? Let us respond to these questions by suggesting that one of the most beneficial health enhancing aspects of practicing Tai Chi is in breathing itself, when we have developed techniques and ways of breathing which enhance our health and feeling of well-being. So, if this is the case, then does it really make sense to quarantine Qigong techniques from the performance of the Tai Chi form? Does it make any sense to delay the development of breathing techniques, to expect the student to wait years and years, through the "discovery" method of teaching and learning? If we are teaching adults, a modern approach to teaching Tai Chi for Health identifies the Discovery learning" method (see Unit 1.42) as being inefficient in the development of skills. It is not focused learning. We need to encourage the adult learner to focus on both "technique" and "principle" and thus tap into the mind-body focus where technique can effectively be used to illustrate the "principle" and the "principle" can be used to facilitate an efficient way of learning the technique. (see Kirschner et al, 2006)

Thus if we are looking to maximise health benefits for our students, then it makes a lot of sense to bring into play, sooner than later, breathing exercises that involve the mind-body focus of the student as an integrated component of Tai Chi for Health. This does not mean that each student in the class is to be straitjacketed with a fixed pattern

---

[19] See also Kano (2005), who makes similar observations in relation to the practice of Judo as an "energy efficient" martial art and physical education.

and prescriptive rhythm of a so-called "correct" way to breathe and move, where the lung-capacities, the health conditions, age or the skill levels of each student are thereby ignored. We need to have an understanding of the need to be flexible in relation to the main variables of the Performance Matrix - age, health, fitness and capability (see Unit 3.40). The idea of referring to these variables of performance means that the Tai Chi for Health Instructor can ensure that the student is not overloaded, does not become stressed and forgets to breathe normally, by tensing and holding or constricting the breath. In addition to other safety requirements, some students need to be reminded not to hold the breath, regardless of challenges in the performance of movements (see Unit 5.20).

In broader terms, the task of the Tai Chi for Health Instructor is to ensure that students are not only encouraged to work within their own individual comfort zones, that students are not only taught how to do just that, but are taught how to learn to take personal responsibility for their own health within the class so that the student learns to know how, why and when to say "no" to doing something that is unsafe, potentially unsafe or uncomfortable for the individual's own situation at any point in time. It is important for the Tai Chi for Health Instructor to not only know how to modify the form, the choreography, the breathing patterns, the physical aspects of learning Tai Chi but also to know how to assist each student to modify his or her own specific set of circumstances in relation variable levels of performance, that is, those related to age, health, fitness, skills and environment (see Matrix of Performance Unit 3.40). The modern Tai Chi for Health Instructor encourages and teaches the student to be able to say "no" to potentially unsafe movements and breathing patterns, without any fear of feeling that saying "NO" is in someway failure to achieve. In short, one of the main tasks of the responsible Tai Chi for Health Instructor is to teach the student in what circumstances and manner it is entirely legitimate to say "NO" to some technique for movement and breathing, and to understand the special needs of the student in being able to modify.

However, In order to be able to modify, we need to have some standard by which to measure and evaluate performance. In setting up standards of breathing for moving soft Qigong, we can begin by making the observations in relation to the following:

- **Practical Language**
- **Relaxation of Body and Mind**
- **Co-ordination of Movements & Breathing**
- **Co-ordinated Breathing Patterns**
- **Breathing Intention or purpose**

1.   Practical Language: Tai Chi for Health requires a language that is comprehensible, logical and makes sense to the group of students in front of the Tai Chi for Health Instructor. In this regard, it is important to use a style of language that communicates clearly and does not mythologise and confuse. Many of the styles of language used by traditional Chinese Kung Fu, including Kung Fu Tai Chi Chuan and Qigong, involve concepts, metaphors and expressions that are unfamiliar to most people in the West. The important thing to bear in mind is to avoid using a language that will confuse and alienate people who are starting a Tai Chi for Health program. The main aim is to assist people with an exercise program in order to improve one's health. [20] Accordingly, communicating with the new-age language and concepts of Traditional Chinese Medicine (TCM), metaphysical journeys of Christianity, Islam, Judaisim and Daoism as the Way of Nature will potentially alienate some, confuse many, and generally be counter-productive. This is not to deny the educational component of introducing students into an informed understanding of the cultural and historical origins of Tai Chi for Health, but the Tai Chi for Health Instructor needs to focus on the objective of Tai Chi for Health and that is not on a metaphysical, mythical and Confucian dialectic searching for the Way of Nature. The Tai Chi for Health Instructor needs to use a language that is consistent with the three basic tenets of a Tai Chi for Health - Safe, Secular and Scientific.

2.   Relaxation of Body and Mind: Moving Soft Qigong strategically involves teaching the student to learn how to relax by using breathing techniques that facilitate this end. Abdominal breathing is the method of breathing which is oriented towards relaxing and is sometimes referred to as "natural" breathing. However, the use of this term is potentially misleading as it is also perfectly "natural" to use reverse abdominal breathing in certain circumstances when exertion and force are required for some specific purpose. Reverse abdominal breathing is a method of breathing related to the application of force in the martial arts used in techniques involved in pushing, striking or throwing an opponent. Within Tai Chi for Health, however, the use of reverse abdominal breathing is not conducive to relaxation but may have validity to improve certain health conditions which would require specialist knowledge on the part of the Tai Chi for Health Instructor in how and under what conditions such training may be responsibly included in the Tai Chi for Health class. Quietening the mind is one of the challenges within Tai Chi for Health. Focused breathing techniques and exercises can greatly assist in the process of learning to relax.

3.   Co-ordination of Movements and Breathing: Co-ordination here simply means to start and finish both the movement and the breath at the same time. This refers to movements and/ or breathing patterns that

---

[20] In some specialised areas of Tai Chi for Health (within the variables of performance levels) such as chronic conditions or palliative care, one of aims of the program may include to help reduce pain and suffering.

may be identified in terms of - Opening/ Closing, In/ Out, Long/ Short, Slow/ Fast, Upper/ Lower, Left/ Right, Up/ Down, Forward/ Backward, Hard/ Soft. What speed should the movement patterns be? Slow or fast? How slow or how fast? When we are not concerned with co-ordinating our breathing, the speed does not seem to really matter all that much as long as we are not holding our breath and we are breathing normally. In general terms, the speed of movement for Tai Chi for Health and Moving Soft Qigong is performed reasonably slowly. But "slow and fast" of course are also relative terms, this being a feature not only of Yin-Yang logic, but also of our everyday understanding that speed is a relative concept. For example, a car travelling at 120kph may be fast but the speed of 120 kph will be very slow indeed relative to the speed of a 747 Jumbo Jet. By definition, the relationship of the "object" to a specific "context" determines the "absolute" meaning where one person's slow performance may be quite fast to someone else. [21]

4.   Co-ordinated Breathing Patterns - We will look at a detailed analysis of how to co-ordinate movement with breathing using "Wave Hands in Cloud" Sun Style and the upper-body only. While there are numerous permutations, we will look at two possible combinations of co-ordinated movement and breathing − 1. Two breaths sequence; and 2. One breath sequence. These sequences should be in multiples of say three to six for the purposes of practice. Once the co-ordinated pattern is established in the class and practiced a few times together as a group, each student in the class can be asked to perform a number of sequences in their own time, thus enabling the teacher to observe, supervise and offer assistance and corrections. Once this type of exercise becomes familiar to the class, the teacher can ask one or two students in the class in rotation each lesson to pick a form any Form from what they know and then set about to firstly ensure that each student in the group knows the form by demonstrating and doing it as a group and then individually. By removing movement of the feet in this exercise, it greatly simplifies the Qigong teaching session and provides the basis for integration with the moving Tai Chi form and sequence that may be being practised at the time. It also provides the opportunity to introduce key Tai Chi principles and concepts along the way with the Qigong exercise.

(a)   Wave Hands in Clouds - Two Breaths

Before you start this exercise with your class, do a "before and after" experiment, asking them this question: What happens with our timing when we use focused breathing patterns? The answers invariably will be - a relaxed, abdominal breathing pattern tends to slow down the actual movements and enhances relaxation. Reflecting on any exercise, and in this case on co-ordinating breathing with movement, this can provide a concrete way of teaching mind-body focus, becoming aware of what happens to focused activity, whether on principles or in this case on breathing patterns.

In this exercise, we will use the relaxed, abdominal breathing method. For positioning of body we will use the clock with 12.00 o'clock to represent facing front position. Positions "A" and "B" represent eye level or "upper" level and positions "D" and "C" represent waist level or "lower" level". All positions "A", "B", "C" and "D" also represent a specific Reference Point (RP) along the trajectory of different movements.

This particular breathing pattern involves four separate body movements while co-ordinating arms with two complete breaths - First breath - IN-breath then OUT-breath; and Second breath - IN-breath, OUT-breath. This TWO breath combination involves a much more relaxed and slower pace of the "Wave Hands" form than is outlined below.

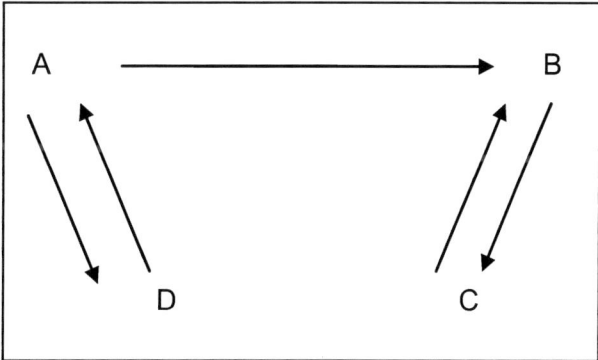

---

[21] See Wong (2006a): "Words are used provisionally, i.e. the meaning is provided for the occasion only. Hence, the meaning of a word used in one occasion may not be applicable in a different occasion. For example, we say that Taijiquan is practiced slowly. Here the word 'slowly' is used provisionally. There are also occasions when Taijiquan is practiced fast. Secondly, the meaning of a word is limited to one's experience and interpretation. The same word 'slowly' may carry different meanings for different people".

FIRST BREATH – starting with expired air in lungs

IN-Breath: The beginning position is the starting RP and in this form we will take this to be - Left Hand (LH) arm showing vertical stop sign at eye level (Upper level at "A") with orientation at 11.00pm, and Right Hand (RH) flat at waist level (Lower level at "D"). LH now exchanges with RH. We can map this exchange movement as LH moves from "A" to "D" and RH moves from "D" to "A". We start the exchange of arms from an expired breath position co-ordinating with this exchange we draw an IN-breath with the two arms exchanging. The RH now is ready to become lead [22]arm for next movement.

OUT-Breath: The starting RP is RH as the lead arm at vertical stop-sign at "A" facing 11.00pm. Lead RH arm now moves across the front of the body to 1.00pm, which is the full length of the lead arm movement. This movement from start to finish is the distance from "A" to "B" and co-ordinates with an OUT-breath. The LH follows consistent with the RH at lower level moves from "D" and finishes at "C".

To map the breathing pattern between "A" and "B" in a bit more detail: the starting point of "A" represents the beginning point of the out breath with lungs and diaphragm beginning as inflated followed by a slow release of air aimed at such speed so as to reach the end point of "B" with no more breath being expired, which is now ready for the in-breath. By definition, co-ordinated breathing happens when the end point "B" the breathing and the movement of the arm finishing at the same time. If we run out of breathe half way between "A" and "B", or if we have lot more breath to breathe out by the time we have arrived at "B", then we have un-co-ordinated breathing. Neither event is bad as what is important is to not breathe too much and thus hyperventilate or to slow down too much so that the intake of air into the lungs is insufficient and thus cause dizziness or even pass out. The aim is to arrive at the same time.

SECOND BREATH - starting with expired air in lungs

IN-Breath: this is the reverse pattern of the First Breath - IN-breath.

OUT-Breath: this is the reverse pattern of the First Breath - OUT-breath.

(b)   Wave Hands in Clouds – One Breath Exercise

The breathing pattern again involves four separate body movements co-ordinating arms with this time only one complete breath - IN-breath and OUT-breath. This variation tends to speed up the body movements and is consistent with a specific martial intention of the OUT-breath involved in the delivery of the force. The breathing technique is thus co-ordinated to maximise the delivery of the force. There are of course other variations or interpretations on the martial intention of this form even within the one breath example given here, but this one here is simpler to perform and compatible with multiple sequences of the same form of Wave Hands in Clouds.

FIRST BREATH - starting with expired air in lungs

IN-Breath: Starting RP is RH at vertical stop-sign at 1.00pm at end of out breath. RH arm now exchanges with the lower LH arm – the exchange is from "B" to "C" for the RH and from C" to "B" for the LH. We continue with the LH arm as the lead arm crossing in front of the body from positions "B" to A". And then the movement of exchanging arms from "D" to "A" and "A" to "D" completes the full movement. This is a long movement sequence which co-ordinates all of these exchanges and movements with an OUT-breath ready for the starting position for the RH arm to be the lead hand to commence again.

OUT-Breath: Starting RP is lead RH arm at vertical stop-sign positioned at 11.00pm at "A" and LH at "D". Lead RH arm now moves across the front of the body to 1.00pm with this movement being mapped from "A" to "B" and co-ordinating with an OUT-breath. In the martial imagery, position "B" represents the point of contact or impact with an imagined opponent.

Variations of Breathing Patterns: Both exercises above can be varied by reversing the movement with the breathing pattern. That is, instead of an IN--breath in the movement, perform an OUT-breath and so-on. Variation means having a choice available to the student in relation to the Matrix of Performance (see Unit 3.40) for the purposes of relaxation, learning to co-ordinate movements, and especially to improve mind-body focus. Some co-ordinated patterns may be easier than others and some may challenge the mind-body focus. These variations can also include a pattern or combination of co-ordinating movements with breathing patterns that may be - Slow/ Fast, Hard/ Soft and then including first the hips, work with that for a while, then feet, body movements and combinations. The permutations are limited by the imagination and knowledge of various Tai Chi forms. For example, with Wave Hands in Clouds, you can use different styles and form – such as Sun Style, Yang Style and Chen Style as variations.

---

[22] We can use the concept of Yin-Yang and call the "lead" hand the "action" hand or the "Yang" hand.

5.   **Breathing Intention or Purpose:** When introducing Qigong breathing patterns into the continuous performance of the Tai Chi form, the rule of thumb is - the First RP is the end point of the previous form and as such, timing for breathing has to co-ordinate and fit in with the rhythm and flow of the form itself.   Different interpretations on the purpose or intention of the form are relevant in deciding which movements might be IN-breaths and OUT-breaths.   If opting for a martial intention in interpreting the form, again there are different interpretations as to what each form and movement might mean in regard to what might be happening in receiving and delivering the force for striking or throwing purposes. "Wave Hands in Clouds" form, for example, has a number of possible variations as to martial intention and application of force.

The art of co-ordinated breathing in the martial arts is considered to be an integral part of enhancing the power of the technique by focussing the internal energy for a specific martial purpose. [23] In the Japanese martial arts this is called "Kiai Jitsu" and in Chinese martial arts is called "Nei Jin". The Japanese term "Kiai" is used to focus internal force when executing a technique and may be expressed audibly in the form of a shout that accompanies some techniques on an opponent or within a solo performance of the "Kata", "Chuan" or form. A relaxed and powerful exhalation can add power to movement where the shout is simply considered to be an audible indication of good Kiai (aligned body structure, focused intent, and good breathing). The sound is not important as the feeling of Kiai can be preserved without making a noise. The Kiai can be silent as it is the coordination of breathing with the physical activity which is important. It is the ability to coordinate breathing with the execution of a Jin movement which is important. The Kiai involves the abdominal muscles and diaphragm and should not be sounded in the throat (see Wikipedia, 2007c).

Within Tai Chi for Health and not for martial arts (Kung Fu Tai Chi Chuan), the focus is on opting for the more health conducing purpose of the Tai Chi forms of exercise. Variations of co-ordinating breathing and movement patterns are thus more extensive and not limited to any specific martial intention. (see Wong, 2001)

3.20   WARM-UPS, TRAINING EXERCISES AND COOL-DOWNS
      3.21   Tai Chi for Health Salute
      3.22   Warm-ups
      3.23   Basic Training Exercises
      3.24   Advanced Training Exercises
      3.25   Cool Downs

3.21   Tai Chi for Health Salute - At the beginning and end of every Tai Chi for Health class or activity, it is important to show the Tai Chi for Health salute. There are strict rules and conventions within the traditional Asian Martial Arts for the salute or greeting. In the Tai Chi for Health class there is no bowing to each other, and the salute is a way of offering greetings and showing respect to each other and to the teacher. The following words may be spoken by the teacher at the beginning and end of each class:

- *Right hand is for Health* (first - show the right hand clenched fist),
- *Left hand is for friendship and humanity* (second – show the left hand flat with fingers stretched), *with*
- *Thumb is tucked in for humility and to keep an open mind* (third – show the thumb pressed against left index finger), *and*
- *Together for Strength and Unity* (fourth – then bring the left open hand and the right fist together)

3.22   Warm-ups - The Warm-up exercises below follow a standard pattern of focussing the mind and warming up the body [24] by loosening the joints and tendons and relaxing the muscles and preparing the student for the training ahead. The pattern here begins with a relaxed and focused posture, followed by – neck, shoulders, spine, hips, knees, ankles, toes and finishes with hands, wrists and elbows.

The following warm-ups are suitable for beginners to advanced students and will need to be modified to suit the specific requirements for the Tai Chi for Health class and students as outlined in the Tai Chi for Health Matrix of Performance (see Unit 3.40). As an essential part of beginning the warm-ups, the Tai Chi for Health Instructor should take the time to "Relax and Focus". For intermediate to advanced students, the Instructor can start bringing into play different Tai Chi principles of movement and mind-body focus (see Unit 3.30) and also combine different movement patterns as part of the Warm-ups. In between each set, or periodically, remind students to be relaxed and maintain upright posture.

First Breath - Relax and Focus
- Standing still – focus, relax and posture check, take one or more deep breaths then
- Tuck the chin in and then slowly look down on out-breath, looking at toes or floor
- Slowly breathing in as arms and palms of hands facing each other gently raise

---

[23] See Toguchi, 1987, pp160-190 for a detailed outline of Zen and Sanchin method of breathing as a system of focussing energy for Goju Ryu karate-do.
[24] For other warm-up exercises used by Alice Liping Yuan in Tai Chi for Health & Falls Prevention program (Exercise Medicine Australia, 2009); and Dr Paul Lam's Tai Chi for Arthritis program see Videos or DVDs (Tai Chi Productions 2009).

- Raise arms outstretched co-ordinating with in-breath to shoulder height tucking chin in
- Slowly lower arms breathing out
- Repeat three times with reminders to relax
- Variations - Slight weight shift from heel to ball in co-ordination with arm movements; different feet positions; different hand shape – palms up and down – rotating at shoulder level; mind-body focus on neck, posture and stretch; for spinal stretch see Cartmell (2006)

Neck – Central Rotation to Both Sides – Playing Lute to Side
- From Open/Close position, both arms move together to left to form "playing lute" position
- Body still, head turns on axis to look at top hand
- Hands and arms move across body to other side
- With head turning on axis to look right at top hand
- Repeat three times
- Variations – Co-ordinated breathing patterns; different feet positions; mind-body focus on neck, posture and stretch

Shoulder Rolls – Relax, Tension, Relax
- Roll shoulders gently forward three times
- Tension is in three places, chest stretch, shoulder crunch, back stretch, relax in between each complete shoulder roll
- Repeat rolling backwards three times
- Variations – Co-ordinated breathing patterns; sequential shoulder rolls; mind-body focus on tension-relax and posture

Shoulders Lift and Press – Relax, Relax, Relax
- Bring arms around from the sides in to cross at front breathing in while lifting
- When hands cross in front, rotate to trace hands in circular fashion over a large beach ball
- Gently trace shape of ball all the way down, breathing out while lowering
- Variations – Different feet positions; raising and lowering body co-ordinating with arms and breathing; reversal of movement; mind-body focus on relaxing and posture, stretching chest, opening joints

Spine – Lady at Shuttle
- From Open/Close position turning left lifting left hand over head and right hand push under elbow
- At same time turning body relaxing trailing leg/knee
- Return to Open/Close position repeat on right
- Repeat exercise three times
- Variations –Co-ordinated breathing; different feet position; mind-body focus on opening joints in backbone, posture and weight shift; top hand under eye level like Chen Style wave hands; Hands in front of chest carrying Tai Chi ruler or balloon extended stretch of "playing the lute" to where it is comfortable

Spine –White Crane Flashing Wings
- Lifting hands to upper chest level then splitting arms continue
- Move left hand upwards and right hand moving downwards
- Stretching both ways
- Exchange and repeat three times each side
- Variations – Co-ordinated breathing; mind-body focus on spinal stretch and posture; Yang Style and Chen Style White Crane stretches

Hip – Foot Forward, Back to Side
- Hands float up front then both arms push back as right heel back feather touch
- Both arms front with right toe back, back to centre then
- Press both arms to left side with toe to right side
- Reverse for each side repeating each left and right movement three times
- Variations – co-ordinated breathing; mind-body focus on, extending the hip joint, maintaining posture, smooth continuous flowing, relaxed and co-ordinated movement of upper and lower body; height differential.

Hip – Step Side, Behind Diagonal
- Hands float up front then right foot to the right side, feather touch, slightly bend supporting leg
- At same time push both arms and hands to left front side on an imaginary wall
- Swap hands & feet with feet stepping behind to cross legged stance
- Ensure body upright and faces front and does not move
- Repeat three times each side
- Variations – co-ordinated breathing; mind-body focus on substantial-insubstantial, posture, relaxed shoulders and elbows; height differential and safety of knees

Knees – Toe Kick Left and Right
- Place hands in Open-Close position
- Bend knee and kick gently front at a comfortable height opening knee
- At the same time place same side arm open palm over kick
- Bring leg and hand back together. Repeat 3 times each side
- Variations – Heel or toe kick; high or low; mind-body focus on posture, relax, stretching, open-close of joints, tension-relax; height differential; co-ordinated breathing

Knees – Brush Knee Push
- From Open/Close position turn body to right side preparing for brush knee push
- Feather touch step with left heel, slowly transfer weight as complete movement
- After completing forward movement, roll back slowly lifting leg to beginning position
- Complete same movement on each side three times
- Variations – One to three punches face and or mid-section levels and varied; co-ordinated breathing; mind-body focus on safety of knee joint, co-ordinated upper and lower body, weight transfer, posture, continuity of movement, relaxed upper body and percentage weight transfer, controlled movement – no jerky movements; safety factor of seeing toes, no "dead" angles.

Ankles – Heel-Toe-Heel Tap
- Lower body, balance and lift right leg forward, feather touch heel, toe, heel
- Bring leg back and repeat on other side
- Lower body, balance and lift right leg 10.30pm forward, feather touch heel, toe, heel
- Bring leg back and repeat on other side 1.30pm forward, feather touch heel, toe, heel
- Variations – Differential stance and direction of tap – front, angle or side; mind-body focus on stretching and contracting ankle, balance and upright posture

Ankles – Rotation – Smiley & Circles
- Full rotation ankles clockwise, then anti-clockwise
- Three times each foot
- Variations – Smiley face with big toe, mind-body focus on ankle rotation with tension and relaxing in between and posture

Hands – Open and Close
- Make a loose fist curling fingers and thumbs
- Open and stretch the fingers and thumbs and separate
- Repeat three times
- Variations – four directions – up/down, in/out; slowly and quickly contract and stretch; curling inwards on contraction and downwards on stretching with palms facing upwards and then other three directions; co-ordinated breathing

Wrists – Clockwise and Anti-Clockwise Rotation
- Slowly rotate both wrists gently from outside to inside then reverse
- Repeat three times
- Variations – co-ordinated breathing; mind-body focus on full rotation and stretch, relaxed shoulders and elbows

Elbows – Clockwise and Anti-Clockwise Rotation
- Slowly rotate both elbows gently from outside to inside then reverse
- Repeat three times
- Variations – Co-ordinated breathing; co-ordinating arms with hips and weight shifting staggering rotations; ying-yang – opposite movements from different positions; mind-body focus relaxing shoulders, smooth continuous movements; different hand shapes – Sun Style, Yang Style and Chen Style

Kicks – Preparation for Sun Style Ballistic Kick
- Left leg forward, right leg backward
- Left hand forward at eye level
- Start gently, swing right leg fairly straight
- Left hand tap either toe or top of thigh, or towards toe
- Upper body to maintain upright posture
- Repeat five times each side
- Variations – sideways straight hip leg lift, turned hip leg lift, rear straight leg lift, rear leg curl kick

3.23 Basic Training Exercises

1. Arms Up And Down
- Stand in a comfortable position.
- Sweep the arms in a curve until just under shoulder height, wrist slightly lifted, fingers pointing downwards.
- Reverse movement in the same curve, wrist slightly down and fingers pointing slightly upwards.
- The trace line made by the fingers forms a quarter of an imaginary circle. The movement is slow and continuous.

2. Stepping Forwards, Stepping Backwards
- Step forward with left foot into parallel by rolling onto the foot heel first.
- The foot, knee and hip should be in approximate alignment with the knee not protruding beyond the foot.
- The natural follow-through movement of the right leg will allow the right foot to be placed gently on the ball of the foot.
- Step backwards on the right foot rolling the foot gently from the ball of the foot until the body weight is balanced, foot, knee and hip in alignment.
- Relax the left leg in a natural way allowing the heel of the left foot to lift gently from the floor.

3. Waving Hands In Cloud
- Prepare: Stand in a comfortable position.
- Turn body slightly to the left.
- Left hand is bent at the elbow, finger tips underneath eye line facing out.
- Right hand angles to left elbow, fingers pointing slightly upwards.
- Leave a small space between the underarm and sides of the body.
- Begin: Arms exchange positions.
- Now rotate hips and shoulders till facing slightly right.
- Exchange arms then rotate body till facing slightly left.
- Movement should be slow and continuous, eye line beyond finger tips.

4. Stepping Sideways
- Stand in a comfortable position.
- Gently transfer body weight to left. Lift the right heel a little, check balance.
- Keeping right foot close to the floor, glide sideways to hip width (or beyond).
- Place toes to floor, check balance.
- Lower heel and transfer body weight to centre as left leg follows
- Rest ball of foot near right foot. Repeat other side stepping to the left.

5. Taking off Gloves
- Prepare: Stand in a comfortable position.
- Place left arm front underneath shoulder line, elbow slightly bent, palm turning in, fingers pointing front.
- Right arm bent at the elbow, forearm angled towards left elbow.
- Begin: Turn left palm down and at the same time turn right hand outwards so that the palm faces up.
- Slide right hand along the underside of the left arm while slowly retracting left arm until hands pass.
- Repeat on other arm commencing at the elbow (as if taking off a long glove.)

6. Out, Out, In Walking
- Prepare: Commencing position feet at "10 o'clock and 2 o'clock" hands resting about the middle of the abdomen.
- Begin: Step forward left heel, foot angled to "10 o'clock". Roll into foot until knee is over the foot. Follow through with right foot, again stepping onto the heel, foot turned out. Third step is directly front, second leg follows through in a natural way resting slightly behind the weight-bearing foot.
- Close to commencement position.
- Repeat all starting with right foot.

3.24 ADVANCED TRAINING EXERCISES

1. Brush, Knee Push
- Turn hips to corner Right. Load arms for preparation for Brush Knee
- Open arms and feather touch to prepare position, Left heel to 12 o'clock
- Transfer weight to L, pass R arm by head and push front
- Transfer weight back to starting position, bringing Right arm back to prepare at Left elbow

2. Waving Hands in Cloud
- Stand with feet open to hip width
- Wave Hands in Cloud first with one hand then the other, then together

- Weight change from one side to the other

3. **Flying Pigeon Spreading Wings**
   - Right foot turned out, place L heel feather touch to front, arms shoulder height, palms facing
   - Transfer weight to front leg right heel anchored, arms sideways, palms front
   - Repeat several times, then on the other leg, and then with reverse arms

4. **Lotus Kick Preparation**
   - Prepare as for Lotus
   - Smack outside of thigh (or leg or foot), hold open leg bent at the knee open position
   - Lower heel to floor, bring arms in from open position to palm up at waist
   - Bring arms back to side, and prepare again for repetitions

5. **Clock Rotation Stepping & Movements**
   - Tai Chi Walking clockwise – two forward, one back
   - Reverse direction
   - Yang Style and Sun Style stepping
   - For added difficulty, add brush knee push with each stepping

6. **Variation on Arm movements – Upper body focus**
   - Starting with one arm raised and the other hand pointing to elbow
   - Perform different patterns involving inward-outward rotation and contra rotations
   - Different patterns will be training movements for Wave hands, Brush Knee push, Parting Wild Horse's Mane and others
   - Variations – different stances, mind-body focus on weight shifting co-ordinating with upper body

3.25   Cool Downs - Cool-down exercises are designed to release tension from the body, to stretch out and relax muscles that have been working and to return the body to its normal functioning.

Lower Body
   - Gently slap or punch each of the thighs, buttocks and legs keeping an upright posture thus relaxing the muscles
   - Gently stretch the hamstring muscles by crossing one leg in front of the other, keeping a straight back and supporting the upper body with one arm resting on the buttocks while gently stretching down with the other hand over the thigh

Upper body
   - Gently and totally relaxed swing both arms around the torso turning the waist allowing each arm to move without any muscular tension allowing the weight transfer from one side to the other in a relaxed way, do this for about thirty seconds
   - Gently move the arms sideways and outward curving above the head breathing in on the way up and then breathing out on the way down. Do this slowly three times using abdominal breathing.

Spinal Stretch – Alexander Technique (see Unit 2.14 (c) Spine)
   - Keep knees soft and arms relaxed throughout the spinal curl
   - From standing upright position, sit on perch, press head to ceiling, tuck chin in
   - Roll neck forward to C7 arms relaxed, and pause
   - Roll down further to end of ribs (T12) arms relaxed and pause
   - Roll down lumbar spine (to L5) – keep knees soft (unlocked)
   - Roll down a little further to a natural pause (Sacrum)
   - See Unit 2.11 for posture and see also Cartmell (2006)

Whole body
   - Tense and relax the whole body by clenching both fists and all the muscles of the body and hold for three seconds while moving your body onto your toes.
   - Then relax dropping the body, unclenching the fists, gently shaking the arms and feet for three seconds.
   - Repeat this three times.
   - Gently shake the relaxed hands and the feet.

Relaxed Breathing
   - Low position – open/close wide to touching; arms-hands trace big round ball to shoulder height and reverse
   - Medium position – open/close wide and crossing with relaxed wrists

3.30   TAI CHI PRINCIPLES & CONCEPTS
   3.31   Sun Lutang's Eight Concepts of Kung Fu Tai Chi Chuan

3.31   Sun Lutang's Eight Concepts Of Tai Chi - Sun Lutang (1921) articulates certain key concepts and principles concerning the practice of Kung Fu Tai Chi Chuan. These were included in a paper presented at the First International Tai Chi for Health Conference in Korea (Arthy, 2006).   The concepts are outlined below using the specific language of Sun Lutang identifying a number of principles categorised as "Sun Lutang's Eight Concepts of Tai Chi", each of which is followed by the author's interpretation using a language accessible to the general reader, thus providing a clear framework within which contemporary health, fitness and martial aspects of Tai Chi can be examined and practised.

1.   Know Your-Self, and Know Others
- Practice the "body" of the art through solo forms
- Practice the "application" of the art with a partner
- Together "body" and "application" represents a complete martial art
- Focus is on beneficial cultivation of one's natural life force as the core of training
- There is great emphasis on the method of cultivating the body

This is the concept of Tai Chi as capable of being practised as a health art, a martial art or both. Practicing forms by oneself promotes health benefits, practicing the applications facilitates an understanding of the intention of the forms, and practising both solo forms and application of the art can lead to health enhancement and proficiency as a martial artist.   One does not need to train vigorously and develop brute strength to become healthy and be competent in the martial arts.

2.   Movement through the Forms is the Kung Fu of Understanding the Self
- Withdrawing is closing, releasing is opening
- When still, all is still, stillness is closing
- In the midst of closing is the desire to open
- When in motion, everything moves, movement is opening
- All movements must be performed in a continuous flow

The concept of strategic movement is on how to practise the solo forms using the conscious mind to focus on all movements as "opening and closing", aiming to practice the solo forms in a relaxed state as continuous flowing movements.   The expression "opening and closing" is the key principle of understanding movement within the concept of "Tai Ji", the principle of mutual interaction of opposites. One needs to use the conscious mind when practicing to understand that strategic movement is based on the balance of opposite movements flowing with some specific intention.

3.   Obtain Opportunity and a Superior Position
- Move the entire body as a co-ordinated unit.
- The whole body must be without misalignment
- Spirit and Qi must be stimulated by raising the spirit
- Do not let your spirit be dispersed externally
- Concentrate your spirit and Qi in your bones
- Front of the hips must have power
- Shoulders must be relaxed
- Qi must be sunk downward
- The head feels as if suspended from above

The concept of strategic posture is on how the biomechanics of the body, co-ordinated movement, posture and body alignments, all combine with the focus of the mind and energy flows in the practice of solo forms and the practical martial applications in order to achieve maximum benefits through minimal force and effort. The position of the head as if suspended by a golden thread from the crown above with shoulders relaxed and pelvis tucked under the hips provide the postural basis of correct alignment which must be maintained throughout the movements of the forms.

4.   The Force is Changed Internally
- The force must come from the heels
- Transformed in the legs
- Be stored in the chest
- Moved in the shoulders
- The leader is the waist, the arms co-ordinate in the attack, the legs follow
- All of these energies are controlled by the intent and not by brute force, use the intent to move the Qi

The concept of strategic force is described as "internal", whereby in practising the solo forms, the conscious mind controls the use of minimal force through the co-ordinated biomechanics of the body, with the waist co-ordinating the movements of the upper and lower body without the need to utilise or develop mindless "external" brute strength. Strategic force is grounded in the feet, progressed through the legs, magnified by the thrust of the hips and waist, carried through the back and transmitted by the hands.

5.   Practising with an Open Mind
- The student can both practice the art and research the extreme depth of the underlying principles, character and teachings of the art with an open mind
- Before moving, check to see if the whole body is conforming to the above principles
- Immediately make corrections if any part of the body is not in alignment with any of the above principles
- This is why the forms must be done slowly and not quickly

The concept of open mind, of the importance of becoming self-regulating is linked to learning how the conscious and open mind needs to constantly focus on how to incorporate the strategic concepts of movement, posture and force into the practice of the forms. It is easy to be hard and fast, it is difficult to be slow and controlled. The student needs to keep an open mind, to develop techniques of consciously observing body posture, alignment and movements, to make adjustments, to reflect on "opening and closing" movements, on "substantial and insubstantial" and on weight shifting, to differentiate between what is "apparent and real", to modify according to conditions "internal and external" at the time of training.

6.   Practising with a Partner is the Kung-Fu of Understanding Others
- Knowing others in movement and stillness
- Give up yourself and follow the opponent
- So as to you may use one ounce to deflect a thousand pounds
- Causing your opponent to fall into emptiness
- All this still involves questioning the self

The concept of yielding to the "other", of feeling the ebb and flow of the "external" force, is facilitated by practising with a partner enhancing an understanding of the principles of deflection and re-direction of force, which is embedded in the martial intention of the solo forms. Practise with a partner may take any form of practice from the minimum of sensitivity training, through to mild or vigorous forms of push hands, through to the ultimate combat form of full contact sparring with a partner where the risk of injury can be high.

7.   Remedy the Problem of "Double Weighting" by Borrowing Your Opponent's Force
- Be positioned correctly
- As soon as the opponent moves do not disturb the actions
- Take advantage of the movements and the opponent throws himself
- The answer is found in yin/yang and opening/closing
- This is what is meant by "Know yourself and know others, and in a hundred battles you will taste victory a hundred times"

The concept of equilibrium is about how to defeat the "other" through strategic force, to remedy the problem of "double weighting" where force meets force, through practising with the conscious mind focussed on how to "borrow the opponent's force" by learning how to follow and stick to the opponent's force. All of this means to understand how weight change in the upper and lower body, whether co-ordinated or not, impacts upon balance and equilibrium. In a martial context, this translates into knowing how to strategically unbalance the opponent or redirect the opponent's force and movement. One of the martial aims of defeating an opponent is to upset the balance or equilibrium of the opponent, and in the internal arts this is achieved not through brute strength as may be the case with the "external" martial arts, but by sticking to, by following and by "borrowing the opponent's force".

8.   Practice Diligently with the Above Principles
- Brute force will naturally dissipate
- You will come to know beforehand the amount of force your opponent exercises
- Over time you will be able to control others without yourself being controlled by others
- Your Qi will quickly return to a balanced state and you will become strong and your spirit will return to a state of wholeness and your length of life will be increased

The concept of diligent practice means practice with focus and purpose incorporating all the principles of Tai Chi. Diligent practice can lead to improvement in health and fitness levels by combining all of the Tai Chi concepts of slow, relaxed, focussed, co-ordinated and controlled movements. Practising Tai Chi for health means that there is no "quick fix" to good health and fitness, but through diligent practice of Tai Chi, it is possible to achieve a "Sound Mind in a Healthy Body" – "Mens Sana in Corpore Sano".

3.32 **Characteristics of the Sun Style Kung Fu Tai Chi Chuan** – extracted & summarised from Cartmell (2003, pp2-3).

1. **Effective Fighting Style** - Most significantly, Sun Tai Chi has immediate practical value as a martial art as the style does not rely on exceptional physicality as a prerequisite for fighting ability. The emphasis is on practicing only and exactly those movements, which can be used in a real martial encounter; form follows the dictates of strategy and technique. The Sun Tai Chi form is exactly as it is to be applied in a fight and is a result of integrated movement under conscious control. This is distinct from other styles of Tai Chi which are designed to train physical attributes primarily through practicing forms which are done in very low and extended stances, where the goal is in improving leg strength, endurance, and flexibility, thus precluding the use of more practical alignments useful in fighting situations. Sun Tai Chi emphasizes the importance of skill, sensitivity, and technique over the development of exceptional strength or speed.

2. **Practical Footwork for Martial Art** - Sun Tai Chi is often referred to as "lively step" Tai Chi whereby the form was designed by Sun Lu Tang to be practiced as it is to be used. The footwork follows the dictates of practicality, with the feet advancing and retreating with the shuffling rhythm common to all combat arts (including Western fencing, boxing, and wrestling). This basic footwork pattern makes it relatively simple for the practitioner to establish the correct whole-body rhythm and alignment that is the signature of all Tai Chi styles. Rather than hiding the method in abnormally wide and deep stances and impractical posturing, Sun Tai Chi basis is in natural movement and rhythm thus providing a method of developing whole-body power almost immediately upon beginning practice.

3. **Health Benefits** - Sun Lu Tang was the first Tai Chi Master to recognise and promote the significant health benefits of practicing Tai Chi. Prior to him, Tai Chi was viewed simply as a martial art, and was practiced as such. Sun Lu Tang made the connection between the development of "internal" power through natural exercise and its benefits for the individual's health and as a method of keeping fit. In addition, it was Sun Lu Tang who was the first to offer a martial arts course to women in the belief that martial arts Tai Chi should be practiced first for health and personal development and not to learn to fight

3.33 **Sun Lu Tang's 3 Stages of Tai Chi** (see Sun, 2006)
- In the initial stages of practice one will feel as if walking on the floor of the ocean. The movements will feel heavy as if all the water was pressing down on the body.
- The second stage feels as if the feet are not touching the floor bottom, but the body is floating within the water. The movements of Tai Chi will feel more natural at this stage.
- The third stage is when the body is light and agile where one will feel as if walking on the oceans surface. At this stage achievement in Tai Chi has been obtained

3.34 **Ten Principles of Tai Chi for Health** - Yang Cheng Fu's Ten Principles were first published by Chen Wei Ming in 1925 in Chen's own book *The Art of Tai-chi chu'uan*. The following is an interpretation of these ten principles included in a paper presented at the First International Tai Chi for Health Conference in Korea (Arthy, 2006). The language used is practical and focussed expressly on the health and fitness aspects of a modern Tai Chi for Health (for a one page poster-size version see Appendix 7)

1. **Posture Head – Golden Thread** – Relax the head, chin tucked in and allow the body to re-align itself vertically, the joints of the spine are relaxed and opened by visualising a golden thread suspending the head with the body underneath completely relaxed with no stress or tension.

2. **Posture Shoulders – Chest and Back** - Relaxed shoulders allowing the chest to sink, with the back slightly rounded in a relaxed state with no tension. This does not mean to allow a stooping forward posture and forgetting the golden thread. Relaxing the shoulders means avoiding the pulled back tensed shoulders of a "soldier" standing to attention.

3. **Posture Waist - Loosen the Waist and Hips** – The capacity for the body to yield and to exert co-ordinated power, while maintaining the posture of head and shoulders, is controlled by the waist and hips. Loosening the waist and hips releases tension in the upper body enabling the lower body to be strong and stable, and re-aligns the natural upright posture governed by the golden thread.

4. **Body Movement – Weight Shifting** - Knowing the difference between "substantial" and "insubstantial" with upper and lower body is the first fundamental principle of Tai Chi related to movement. Differentiating between "opening and closing" movements of the upper body is important to co-ordination and balance. Learning to control weight transference from one leg to the other using a "feather-touch" principle is crucial to maintaining balance, strength training of the legs, and flexibility of the feet.

5. **Posture Arms - Sink Shoulders, Drop Elbows** - Sinking shoulders allows the upper body to relax with arms dropped down naturally. If the elbows are raised, then the shoulders will be tense and the whole body will easily tire and lack strength. Dropping the elbows relaxes the shoulders and allows the body to co-ordinate and flow.

6. **Mind Directing the Body - Use Will, Not Strength** - First quieten the mind, then using the mind to relax the body, opening the joints, stretch and lengthen the tendons and ligaments, relaxing the muscles using minimum force and effort for maximum benefit and effect. Through a relaxed body and a quietened mind, there will be more control of all circular movements.

7. **Whole Body Moving Together - Co-ordination Between Top and Bottom** - The upper and lower body start and arrive together, they move as a co-ordinated whole, maximising leverage through controlled and focussed execution of movements. Direction of eyes, movement and posture of head, hands and arms co-ordinated by the waist, combine with leg and feet movements to become a single unified movement.

8. **Training the Mind - Internal and External Unity -** It is easy to be hard and fast, it is difficult to be soft, slow and controlled. Training the mind is paramount and requires the student to become self-regulating, to develop techniques of consciously using the mind to observe body posture, alignment and movements, to make adjustments, to reflect on "opening and closing" movements and "substantial and insubstantial" weight shifting, to differentiate between what is "apparent and real", to modify according to conditions "internal and external" at the time of training - fitness and health levels, weather and location. To the observer of the performance, the focus of the eyes, the position of the head reveals the intention of the mind.

9. **Continuous Body Movement – Regulated by Controlled Breathing** – Each form is executed as a cycle of "opening and closing" movements in a relaxed and continuous manner connecting with the next cycle of "substantial and insubstantial" weight shifting using the mind co-ordinating the relaxed body and not brute strength. Breathing techniques are used to co-ordinate and focus the appropriate rhythm, speed and intention of the movements.

10. **Mind Enhancing Energy – Relaxed Continuous Movements Through Breathing** – Combining all the other principles of Tai Chi, using slow, relaxed, co-ordinated and controlled movements regulated with appropriate breathing techniques creating the illusion of stillness in motion, a form of moving meditation. The experience is for some a mystical or spiritual perception of being in harmony with the cycles of nature, with the "Tai Ji" as the Grand Ultimate or Cosmos. In practical and secular terms, stillness in motion represents a means of pacing oneself with much practice and more practice, having the attitude, the patience and the desire to achieve a balanced healthy body and mind enjoying the pleasure, beauty and power in the journey of Tai Chi.

3.35   Yin and Yang of Opening-Closing - "Opening and Closing" are concepts which are used frequently in the literature of traditional Kung Fu Tai Chi Chuan and are based on specific applications of Yin and Yang theory. They are primarily aimed at identifying the strategic relationship between movement, breathing and the orientation of force in a martial or fighting context.

> *Therefore, open and close is also known as extension and contraction. Tai Chi Chuan practice is the motion of opening and closing and vice versa. When it is open, it is large and expansive and there is no more space outside. When it is close, it is so compact and tight there is no more space inside. For a beginner, the open motion should be bigger so that there is more stretching on the muscles, ligament and tendons. For an experienced practitioner, the open motion should be smaller and among each open and close motion, there is a subdivision into smaller open and close motions.* (Chu, 2006a)

Within the Kung Fu Tai Chi Chuan literature, however, we find at least two different versions of what is YIN and YANG when related to the concepts of "opening and closing".

The first version involves a practical, concrete and physical context of martial force and application. The "Yin" is deemed to be an "Opening" movement, the IN-breath, the loading up getting ready to deliver the force and the "Yang" is the regarded as the "Closing" movement, with the OUT-breath maximising the impact in the delivery of force at the end point of the movement.

> *Coordinate all closing movements with exhalation and all opening movements with inhalation. During the martial science of inhalation, it is easy to raise the spirit, as well as to circulate the Chi, and to uproot an opponent during exhalation.* (Hwa-Yu T'ai Chi Health and Wellbeing, 2006)

> *Some Yang masters have used the phrase in the classics "Gathering jing is like pulling the bow, exploding it is like releasing the arrow" to explain. There is an opening movement in preparation for a strike (yin) while the actual strike sees the whole body closing up and compressing to deliver the energy (yang).* (Zhang, 2006a)

The second version of what is YIN and what is YANG involves a philosophical, abstract and metaphysical context involving the "nature" of body and mind:

This natural interchange of the inhalation/exhalation, awareness/unawareness, and consciousness/ unconsciousness demonstrates the contrast of "Yin" and "Yang" which is the Chinese philosophy in the Book of Changes (I Ching). When inhaling, the mind is "Yang" active, positive and expansive. When exhaling, the mind is "Yin" inactive, negative and receptive". (Chen, 2006)

Consistent with this abstract notion of the mind, the physical action of extending and contracting the limbs towards a specific RP in the posture and this RP is also contextualised in abstract terms of "stillness" and "movement".

To open is to extend and move. To close is to contract and be still. Opening is yang, and closing is yin. To issue, to extend, or move is yang. To withdraw, contract, or become still is yin. Opening and closing is like the one qi moving through the cycles of yin and yang.... If the student is able to alternate opening and closing as well as stillness and movement, and comes to a deep understanding of their source, the common root of every posture will be clear and one will obtain their mysterious uses. (Sun, 1921, p.57)

It is the RP in the posture which determines the associated movement towards the RP as the key in contextualising YIN and YANG. Opening movement within this abstract classification of "movement/ stillness" is considered as moving towards the OPEN position or RP, which is now like a loaded gun or weapon. This OPEN position or RP thus is deemed to be a loaded explosive force and is classified as YANG, the gun is cocked and ready to fire.

The release of this explosive force in the Closing movement moves towards the CLOSE position or the end RP, which is now empty, now still, and thus YIN. This may appear confusing but in order to unravel any apparent contradiction, it is vital that the "object" in question in any Yin and Yang dichotomy be "relativised" by being placed within a specific context. For example, each version of YIN and YANG in relation to "opening" or "closing" needs to be contextualised within MOVEMENT or static POSTURE, or "movement" and "stillness" and within each context, there needs to be consistency:

In the above examples of "open" and "close", you are right in saying they refer to different matters in different situations. The "opening" in pulling a bow to gather force is different from the second "opening" in extending the limbs. Moreover, there are also different ways of gathering and exploding force. One may gather force by extending the limbs, like pulling a bow, then explode it by compressing the body, like releasing an arrow. On the other hand, one may gather force by compressing the body to focus on the dantian, then explode it by extending the limbs to send the force out. (Wong, 2006a)

In addition, it is important to note that Tai Chi patterns related to breathing should not be prescriptive so as to exclude alternative breathing patterns, but they need to take account of the specific context within which some movement is performed. It has been suggested, for example, that when your hands pull apart or when you are stepping forward, then that is an opening movement and therefore requires an in-breath (see Lam, 2005). Wong (2006a; 2006b), however, suggests that the specific context of "martial intention" is relevant to determine whether a particular movement is either "yin" or "yang" and that stepping forward, for example, can thus be either "opening" or "closing", "defending" or "attacking" and consequently "yin" or yang". In martial terms, there are thus different ways of "gathering and exploding force".

Moreover, within a modern Tai Chi for Health there is no necessary reliance on martial or fighting imagery. Accordingly, the question of "opening" and "closing" does not need to be tied to the martial intention of delivery of force, but can be accommodated within the imagery of choice so long as it does not go beyond the boundaries of the three S's of a modern Tai Chi for Health. For example, the expanding arms involved in the Single Whip Form within Sun Tai Chi does not need to follow the prescriptive OUT-breath demands of a martial imagery in the delivery of force. The expanding arms can be seen to be consistent with an expanding chest, an opening of the lungs and thus much more conducive to relaxing, loosening of the joints and better health through the co-ordinated extension of arms with an IN-breath.

3.36   Other Concepts of Kung Fu Tai Chi Chuan

Double Weighting: This is used in two related martial arts contexts. One is to avoid double-weighting when sparring with an opponent or practising the solo Tai Chi Form, which means the weight distribution should never be static 50/50 or even on two legs. This facilitates the ability to move quicker to respond to the opponent's direction of force. The other meaning relates to avoiding double-weighting with an opponent and that is to avoid meeting force with force, that is, to avoid attempting to challenge the incoming force from that opponent with an equal or even superior force. Both meanings are related to martial application and are part of the "efficiency" principle meaning to avoid placing the body in a disadvantageous position of being more vulnerable to attack, striking and throwing techniques from an opponent. From a Tai Chi for Health perspective, being double weighted may in some situations be beneficial for balance and stability as well as for enhancing relaxation (see Gilman, 1998) for certain people and situations in relation to the Tai Chi for Health variables of performance levels. The value of focussing on "double-weighting" relates to the Yin-Yang aspect of mind-body awareness and enhanced health benefits of balance, co-ordinating and mental alertness (see Ho, 2008, pp6-12).

Relaxed - Sung (or sometimes Song): Sung means relaxed, ready and alert and is achieved by softening the muscles, loosening the tendons and joints of the whole body, releasing tension so that the body will be sensitive and responsive. The "energy efficient" fighting principle means to remove rigidity, to avoid the use of brute force and to allow gentle, relaxed softness within a relaxed body structure, the biomechanical principles of which facilitate efficiency of intention in the delivery of force. This is called "Sung". In order to achieve "'Sung", you must let go of all tension throughout the body, using your focused mind and not brute force to neutralise and defeat the opponent. Sung is also very important for Tai Chi for Health as suggested by Oliver (2007): "One maintains all the body's natural strength, energy and potential and is free and alive. When one is genuinely relaxed, physically, mentally and emotionally one can not only move smoothly, quickly and naturally to deal with an opponent, but one can face life's challenges easily too; which is why Taiji is so highly rated as a system of exercise and meditation which can improve the health and calm the mind." Kung Fu Tai Chi Chuan is considered to be about being the more intelligent fighter arising from the scientific principles, which exploit the deepest and most profound connections between the mind and body. Through returning to a natural state of relaxation, one becomes healthy and strong (Xu, 2007)

Push Hands, Sticking Hands, Sensitivity Training: Two person, push hands training functions to assist the martial arts student into being able to follow the opponent, feel the direction and intensity of force so as to be able to be re-direct that force to neutralise and defeat the opponent. When practising the solo Tai Chi form for martial arts, all movements within the Tai Chi form should be performed in such a way as to be able to move according to the ebb and flow of force with an imagined opponent in mind. This is no different in all martial arts that perform solo katas or forms. In addition, the Japanese Martial Arts call this "Muchimi", meaning giving way, flexibly, "heavy, sticky hands". While pushing hands is not considered a martial art in its own right, it is considered an essential part of the combat training for Kung Fu Tai Chi Chuan:

> *The essential combat theory of Tai Chi Chuan is to use softness or Yin to overcome hardness or Yang and to use hardness or Yang to overcome softness or Yin. So rather than blocking the opponent's attacks we divert or redirect them using evasion and/or footwork at the same time. This is using softness to overcome hardness. The attack has then become 'dead' force and has changed from Yang to Yin. At this point we must also change from Yin to Yang by striking (Yang) the vital points of our opponent (Yin). This is using hardness against softness. In order to train this evasion it is necessary to do a lot of practise on the pushing hands exercises I mentioned earlier.* (Docherty quoted in Davies 2007)

Various approaches to push hands, however, do not involve combat training and are more correctly labelled sensitivity training and thus if properly supervised are suitable for Tai Chi for Health within the limits of the Matrix of Performance (see Unit 3.40)

Yielding, Body Evasion: The yielding techniques in the Chinese martial arts such as Kung Fu Tai Chi Chuan are the same as are found in Japanese Martial arts which is called Tai Sabaki. This concept overlaps with "double-weightedness" where the idea is to evade the force of the attacker by shifting the body, by yielding and sticking, by avoiding the use of brute force and harmonising with the attacker's force. The Japanese word "Ju" involved the yielding principle and relates to "kuzushi", the art of unbalancing an opponent. The so-called Tai Chi Classics refer to the yielding principle as "a force of four taels is able to move a thousand catties", that is, the more familiar expression of "four ounces can move a thousand pounds".

Chi: Chi is considered by some to be the most fundamental and important concepts in all Daoism and relates to all Daoist practices and arts. (Dunn, 1990) It is important to note that this "Chi" as in Qigong (Wades-Giles spelling) is not the same thing as the "Chi" in "Tai Chi". In Pinying spelling they are entirely different – the "Chi" in "Tai Chi" is spelled "Tai Ji" which means the Supreme Ulitmate or Grand Cosmos. The "Chi" as in Qigong is "Qi" in Pinying spelling, but is pronounced the same "Chee" as in "cheese". The concept of Chi (or Qi) means energy. Within traditional Chinese cosmology, it is considered the vital life force, the essence of being, what the French similarly call "elan vitale". It is viewed as the potential energy latent in the body - for which the English language does not have an exact word. (Dunn, 1990) The concept of Chi has application in both TCM as well as many of the Asian Martial Arts, where for example, the Japanese word for "Chi" is "Ki" and features specifically in co-ordinated breathing and movement concepts and practices of Kiai and Aiki. Within TCM, the flow of Chi is considered to follow the meridians and the central storage of Chi is located at the Dan Tien. Western science considers Chi to be energy, meridians to be equivalent of the nervous system throughout the body and the Dan Tien as the centre of gravity within the human body.

Jìn or jìng (勁), or "power," is often confused by Westerners with the related concept of jīng (精), which literally means "semen," and by extension used metaphorically to mean "essence" within the context of Daoist literature and TCM. Jìn or jìng (勁), or "power," also should not be confused with jīng (經; classic/warp), which appears in many early Chinese book titles, such as the Nèi Jīng, yì jīng and Chá Jīng, the fundamental text on all the knowledge associated with tea. (see Wikipedia, 2007d; see also Laronge, 1999)

Thirteen Postures: These represent what are termed the "Eight Gates and Five Steps" of skills training for some martial styles of Kung Fu Tai Chi Chuan and are recorded in the so-called Tai Chi Classics of Yang Lu Chan. The most frequent references to the 13 Postures coming from the writings and teaching of the Yang Style of Kung Fu

Tai Chi Chuan. The Eight Gates are: Wardoff – Peng; Rollback – Lu; Press - Ji, Push – An; Grab – Cai; Split – Lie; Elbow- Zhou; Bump - Kao - all of which represent eight basic movement patterns. The Five Steps are: Stepping Forward- Jin Bu; Stepping Backward - Tui Bu; Look to Left – Zuo Gu; Look to Right - You Pan; Firm the Centre - Zhong Ding. For a detailed explanation of these strategic martial principles and applications see Chapter 3 in Yang (1999).

3.40   MATRIX OF PERFORMANCE LEVELS FOR DUTY OF CARE

Major Variables	Duty of Care Factors	Beginners		Intermediate		Advanced	
		1	2	3	4	5	5+
Age	Children Younger Adults Older Adults Frail Aged						
Health	Excellent - A Average-B Health conditions - C - Chronic - Physical - Psychological						
Fitness - Aerobic	Excellent -A Average-B Poor -C						
Fitness - Strength	Excellent -A Average - B Poor - C						
Fitness - Flexibility	Excellent - A Average - B Poor - C						
Skills - Capacity	Mobility (A, B, C) Sightedness (A, B, C) Hearing (A, B, C) Cognitive (A, B, C)						
Environment	Access Lighting Floor conditions Temperature Humidity Clothing - footwear Position (includes seated, standing etc) Location (includes class, home, park etc)						

3.50   TAI CHI HISTORY AND CONTEXTS – Two Papers
      3.51   Genius of Sun Lutang: Origins and Concepts of Tai Chi for Health
      3.52   Teaching of a Modern Tai Chi for Health

3.51   Genius of Sun Lutang: Origins and Concepts of Tai Chi for Health - The following is the abstract is from a paper (Arthy 2006) presented at the Concurrent Session at The First International Tai Chi for Health Conference held on December 6, Seoul, Korea. The paper presents the argument that a modern Tai Chi for Health has to be entirely consistent in any claims it makes based on scientific and evidence based reasoning so as to maintain intellectual integrity in the public policy arena.   This consistency is significantly compromised if scientific and evidence based reasoning is not equally applied in all areas of research, in particular historical, cultural and pedagogical, and to include both quantitative and qualitative forms of reasoning and research into any contributions made to the practical value of Tai Chi for Health in a modern age.

Abstract - The original motivation for this project was based on a single premise. Over years of researching the histories of the Asian Martial Arts, and in particular, the various myths and histories written about Tai Chi, I came to the conclusion that Sun Lutang has clearly not been given the proper credit for the genius that he was. As recognised by Tim Cartmell (2003), Sun Lutang was the creator of a different style of Tai Chi, which is both, an effective fighting style, and a style very suitable for promoting Tai Chi for Health. Unlike other styles of Tai Chi, Sun Style Tai Chi does not rely on exceptional physicality as a prerequisite for fighting ability and it contains stances and combat techniques that are both practical and highly effective as a Martial Art suitable for people of all ages not just the young. The style also contains a basic footwork pattern, which makes it relatively safe and simple for the beginner to establish the correct whole-body rhythm and alignment that is the signature of all Tai Chi styles and thus is more readily accessible to a broader range of people, men and women, old and young.

This paper has been written to enhance the application of Tai Chi for Health promotion in the twenty-first century through an examination of the radical contribution that Sun Lutang made almost one hundred years ago to the promotion of Tai Chi for Health and to the subsequent transformations of Tai Chi as a Health Art from Tai Chi practised as a vigorous and combative form of Chinese Boxing in the early part of the twentieth century in China (see Wong, 1996; Wile, 1993; Miller, 2000).

This examination outlines a snapshot history of the emergence of Tai Chi for Health based on various facts, evidence and respected published accounts of the historical emergence of Tai Chi for Health and the roles played by Sun Lutang, Chen Wei Ming and Yang Cheng Fu. It is the juxtaposition of facts and evidence, grounded within a consistent and coherent chronology, which questions and challenges the pervasive views that Yang family style of Tai Chi Chuan was the original Tai Chi health art and that Tai Chi is a Daoist art advocating harmony with Nature, and characterising conflict with Nature as contributing to illness, poverty and disease. More significantly for our purposes, is that Sun Lutang was the first Tai Chi Master to break with the patriarchal Confucian tradition by publicly offering Tai Chi to women, and he was the first to write about and publish Tai Chi for Health and personal development and was thus the first Tai Chi Master to promote to the public Tai Chi as a Health Art (see Miller, 2000).

However, the main focus of the paper is on analysing contributions to Tai Chi for Health as specific concepts and principles of Tai Chi which were published by Sun Lutang and by Chen Wei Ming. This examination highlights both the insights and genius of Sun Lutang and the historical significance of Chen Wei Ming in the subsequent motivations to transform the vigorous and combative Yang family style of Tai Chi to the slow and graceful Yang Style Tai Chi as it is practised and recognised today (see Wile, 1993). These contributions are articulated in the paper in a language that is accessible and suitable for the general reader and student interested in Tai Chi as a contemporary secular Health Art.

In regards to research methodology for this paper, an understanding of Tai Chi for Health epistemologically and historically cannot be gained through the academic paradigms of the scientifically controlled experiment, epidemiology or medical research (see Popper, 1974; Kuhn 1970; Lakatos et al 1980). Social and cultural historiography driven by a semiotic analysis (see Barthes, 2001; Eco 1976; Foucault 1977; Hirst et al, 1984; Levi-Strauss, 1977; Rose and Rose 1977; Ryan, 1973; Turner, 1975; Hammersley and Atkinson, 1980) has informed the intellectual engine of the research methodology for this paper in an evaluation of myths of Tai Chi often presented as history and in the presentation of concepts and principles of Tai Chi for Health. Semiotics and Tai Chi philosophy of the Yin and the Yang are tarred to the same East and West brush of paradoxical logic, an unusual but legitimate nexus of intellectual endeavour within a qualitative approach to the social sciences.

In the context of Tai Chi as a contemporary secular Health Art, the paper identifies the radical contribution to Tai Chi for Health made by Dr Paul Lam in the international arena of the latter part of the twentieth century and spearheading the way into the twenty-first century. In addition, the paper outlines the rationale and the necessity for Tai Chi for Health Instructor Training and for public policy development of Tai Chi for Health to be formulated, promoted and practised, not as a metaphysical journey or as a martial art, but as a secular Health Art (see Cheryl, 2001; and Grigg, 1990) which is based on evidence based, scientific research and on the modern Duty of Care principle.

3.52   Teaching of a Modern Tai Chi for Health - The following is an extract from a joint paper (Arthy & Arthy 2006) presented by Elva at the Concurrent Session at "The First International Tai Chi for Health Conference" held on December 6, Seoul, Korea. The stated purpose of the session was to discuss the topic of "How to teach Tai Chi Effectively". In Australia, Tai Chi for Health Instructor Training at an advanced level is locked into a martial arts framework, and limited to the Level 1 Coaching course offered through the Martial Arts Industry Association (MAIA), which includes the Australian Kung Fu & Wushu Federation (AKWF) (for more detail, see Appendix 1 – *Open Letter re TCH Instructor Training*). The extract presented by Elva examines the tensions of the historical and cultural contexts of this topic in the form of a dialectic, between traditional Tai Chi practised as a martial art and the Tai Chi practised under the rubric of health and modern and how this radically impacts on the method and strategy of teaching.

EXTRACT - Introduction - Contexts of Tai Chi - In order to identify possible contexts for our discussion, it is not inappropriate for our purposes, to link our task on "How to Teach Tai Chi Effectively" to the paradoxical logic of Tai Chi philosophy, of the yin and yang. Do we examine the techniques of "effective teaching" of Tai Chi Chuan in the different evolving historical context of "secret transmissions" (see Wile, 1993) through the traditional lineages of particular forms of Chinese Boxing, effective styles of combat first categorised by Sun Lutang as being part of the broader "internal" family style of the martial arts? (see Miller, 2000). Do we evaluate the techniques of "how to teach Tai Chi effectively" through the present-day context of the fighting, combat and martial arts equivalent to those existing in Imperial China at the time of Yang Lu Chan? Specifically in this regard, do we evaluate on an outcomes basis the "effective teaching of Tai Chi" in a martial context where all fighting styles come together under the minimum "rules of engagement" of the modern-day blood-sport "Ultimate Combat" in the Ultimate Fighting Championship (UFC), whereby serious injury or even death is a possible outcome? (see UFC, 2006)

Or do we examine "effective teaching" of Tai Chi in an entirely different context where the aim of Tai Chi teaching is to promote good health and well-being through safe and effective forms of exercise and to do no harm to our students? In an examination of the plethora of radically different contexts of Tai Chi, we will be exploring the question - Is it possible to find a context for evaluating "effective teaching" for Tai Chi for Health that does not demand that martial prowess and a knowledge of fighting and combat techniques are necessary prerequisites?

Within the broader public relations context of Tai Chi being actively promoted as a Health art, it is not uncommon to hear that whatever else Tai Chi has become, "Tai Chi Is a martial art":

> T'ai Chi is fundamentally a close range, counter attacking art. It uses strikes to and from various parts of the body, locks and grips and uprooting techniques in various combinations. These skills are developed through a series of partner work exercises: Sticky Hands develops initial listening skills; Push Hands develops these on both physical and mental (energetic) levels through a wide variety of fixed pattern and free form routines; fighting applications of movements in the forms are developed taking into account skills trained in Push Hands and these can be taken in to more complex patterns and free sparring. (Tabrett, 2005)

The essence of an effective Tai Chi Instructor is claimed to lie in the ability of the teacher to demonstrate the martial ability, power and intention, not only in the solo form, but through Tai Chi's martial "rules of engagement" of "push hands":

> One of the beautiful things about T'ai Chi is the richness of the internal activity, both for health and martial arts…. So you want a teacher with good knowledge, who has received good instruction. Ask them about their training. Ask them what they have learned. Ask them about what goes on inside the Form. They should know push hands – have them push you so they can feel if they have some power. Ask if you can push them so you can feel if they know how to neutralize a push. Giving and receiving pushes should be gentle but something unique and powerful should be happening. (Cobb and Grannis, 2006)

Moreover, it is suggested that if you only learn the movements and not learn push hands, you are denying yourself an incredibly fascinating experience and limiting your knowledge of the art and you are denying yourself the added health benefits that actually come with learning the martial side of Tai Chi. (Mills, 2004) This claim to superior health benefits through the "martial side" traces its lineage of what is "real" or "authentic" Tai Chi back to the time when Tai Chi was practised as a martial art in China before the communist revolution in 1949:

> Schools often started and founded on the reputation and skill of their teacher. If a master was defeated by a challenger, he would often close his school and follow the person with greater skill. If he didn't, then his students certainly did. (Mills, 2004)

This latter comment gives silent witness to the cultural context of a traditional martial form of Tai Chi practised in China when only men were allowed to receive instruction and practice any style of Chinese boxing due to the patriarchal Confucian tradition in Chinese society, which excluded women from government, education and martial activities. Historically, it was Sun Lutang who is stated to be the first Tai Chi Master to publicly break with this tradition by publicly offering Tai Chi to women in the early 1930s, and he was also the first in the early 1920s to write about, to publish and to promote Tai Chi as a Health Art as well as a martial art. (Miller, 2000)

These historical facts about the origins and subsequent transformations of access to Tai Chi for all people, including women, are often ignored or obscured in the historical origins of Tai Chi practiced for health reasons (see Arthy, 2006) and in the claims that "Tai Chi for health" which is practised today is largely the product of the "standardised, and synthesised style" pioneered by the Peoples Republic of China. (Mills, 2004) For some of the adherents to the traditional lineages of "Tai Chi Is a martial art", there is a grudging acceptance that "Tai Chi for Health" actually exists today as "a fait accompli". "It is a great shame," it is suggested, "that the Tai Chi for health players have immense difficulty in recognising there are other levels to Tai Chi. (Mills, 2004) In response to this claim, it is whimsically suggested by one teacher of Tai Chi for Health who alludes to consumer choices made by students:

> I don't emphasise too much martial art to new student, instead endeavouring to promote the health benefits and learning how to relax. As we know, many of our students are middle-aged elderly, so they may not want to enter the martial arena just yet. (Gregson, 2004)

Some contemporary traditional Tai Chi Instructors take an even harder line in their critique of "Tai Chi for health" and include an attack on the belief held by those same traditional "Tai Chi Is a martial art" players who regard push hands as the ultimate martial and combat expression of Tai Chi. It is suggested that Tai Chi which is taught as a slow dance like form and Tai Chi which lauds "push hands" as the crux of the fighting arts are not "real" forms of Tai Chi:

> So what if we are able to uproot! [through push hands training]. He comes back with a blade and cuts us! The push hands was only ever meant as means of learning balance and timing and not for self-defence or tournament There is

push hands and then there is advanced push hands. This is where we learn about the dim-mak strikes and how to use them at close range, this is the real reason for push hands, not for pushing but for striking. ...T'ai chi is dim-mak and to teach it at any other level is to deride this great martial art. I was once asked if T'ai Chi was good for fighting. I told the inquirer that I thought it not! And that idea has not changed much due to the fact that what most people are teaching as being representative of T'ai chi is just a very poor excuse for a fighting art. And so many are teaching at this level that most of T'ai chi nowadays is not good for self-defence. How can someone teach what he or she calls a martial art when they have no idea of how to defend themselves! (Montaigue, 2004)

Another central aspect of the debate on Tai Chi for Health today is in the characterisation of Tai Chi as an "internal" martial art. The focus on the "internal" in Tai Chi is described as being all about the "richness of internal activity", building internal energy or "cultivating the chi" (intrinsic energy), developing an inner force that can somehow be transformed into explosive and powerful ways that do not rely on external or muscular force. It is this so-called "internal energy", which is characterised as contributing significantly to beneficial health and the reason why Tai Chi has been practised historically as an ancient health art. Such a view may in some instances be "involved in some occult practices"[25], but at best is simply misleading, where "internal energy" is represented as some mystical inner force that operates within a vacuum, that has no bearing on physical force, biomechanics, principles of leverage or as part of a range of specific fighting techniques:

The real difference between the internal and external martial arts is not chi, softness/hardness, or which is better for health; rather, it boils down to how specific movements are done in a particular mindset, and how these apply to real fights... For centuries, China has had a great variety of therapeutic Qigong and related health systems that are equally as effective as the internal martial arts for restoring, maintaining and improving one's health, and are far simpler to learn and practice than the internal styles. There was no need to invent complex and often extremely physically demanding martial arts to fulfil the same purpose. Although the internal martial arts may be practiced solely as exercises for physical fitness, they were not created with this goal in mind. The internal martial arts were developed for fighting, with their health benefits more or less side effects of training for martial ability. (Cartmell, 1992)

In addition, the "internal force" in a martial arts context represents a way of applying a range of techniques using the mind-body focus, the "whole-body" principle of attack and defence, the art of giving way, of evasion and yielding, maximising the effect of borrowing the opponent's energy thus minimising the effort or the need for excessive external energy in the application of the martial technique. This principle of "maximum effect through minimum force" and the application of specific techniques utilising so-called "internal energy" are not unique to Tai Chi but are features of other so-called "soft" styles of martial arts, which focus on the "gentle" and "yielding" principle.

The most well-known other "internal style" of the martial arts is Judo which was created by Professor Jigoro Kano in the late nineteenth century in Japan, who pioneered the health and ethical principles "Seirokyo Zenyo" (maximum effect through minimum effort) and "Jita Kyoe" (Mutual benefit) in the promotion and development of a disciplined, relatively safe and educational form of physical exercise, sport and self-defence (see Kano, 1994 and 2005). Judo as an "internal" or "yielding" style martial art, however, does not focus on solo forms, but introduces two person forms (katas) at advanced levels, and thus does not readily lend itself to the type of exercise and health benefits for a broad range of people as do the solo forms of Tai Chi for Health. In addition, the modern combat and competitive "rules of engagement" of Judo and Tai Chi as martial arts are significantly different with the full contact and high impact aspects of Judo being decidedly unsuitable for most older people and people with certain health problems and injuries.

The idea that both "external" and "internal" forces are germane to all martial arts, however, is acknowledged by Cartmell (1992) and is echoed by Zhou Lishang where he states:

The way of Taijiquan is to practice both the internal and external. Not only should we practice tendons, bones and skin on the outside, but also we practice qi inside. So-called qi here includes spirit and will. Only by practising both the inside and the outside can we accomplish health protection and fighting skill.... In the past, there was a term 'internal boxing'. In my opinion, this term is a leftover of discrimination between the schools in the old society. In fact, many schools pay special attention to practise both the internal and external, and hardness and softness in harmony. Their differences are in their methods for exercise and forms. That is, they reach the same goals by different techniques. (Zhou, 2006)

In other words, so-called "internal force" is the application of a range of techniques, which do not rely on exceptional physicality or brute strength in the application of the martial technique, but includes techniques of evasion and re-direction of the opponent's force. Some Tai Chi for martial arts Instructors even suggest that most good martial teachers will point out that to categorise an entire fighting style as being "hard" or "soft" is actually nonsense. Any good martial art will use a mixture of hard and soft physical qualities along with both attacking and defensive strategies, all of which contributes to "real" and not "superficial" health benefits:

From a health perspective, careful practice of martial applications gives the body a much more complete physical workout than exclusively performing slow motion choreography. Furthermore, learning self-defence skills can be of the greatest benefit to those who could be seen as potentially more vulnerable. (Zorya, 2006)

There are thus some who argue based on empirical scientific research that all forms of martial arts have health benefits and are worthy of promoting as such for people of all ages. (Douris et al, 2004; Broudnek et al, 2002; Swiercz 2005; Binder 1999; Weiser et al, 1995) The martial arts are actively promoted as unique among most forms of exercise due to the way they blend strength, endurance, flexibility and balance. (Evenson 2004) They are viewed as a form of self-defence against ageing:

If you want to do something that's fun, different and good for self-defense -- and good for long-term self-defense against disease -- do the martial arts... Dr. Douglas McKeag, a sports medicine expert at Indiana University in Indianapolis,

---

[25] See Yeo (2008, pp19-20) where he cautions about fraudulent Tai Chi teachers and Qigong masters brainwashing their students through psycho-suggestion to believe they have special powers where none existed.

believes the martial arts are a perfectly acceptable way to boost fitness, certainly in middle age it makes a great deal of sense. The sport is capable of delivering the type of stimulus that the body needs to get in shape. But he cautions that, as with any new sport, beginners have to come at it relatively slowly and intelligently. (Medicine on Line, 2004)

Within this broader context of the martial arts having significant health benefits, there are some very hard-line Tai Chi Instructors, however, who are waging verbal war against any notion of a separate category of "Tai Chi for Health" and that Tai Chi should not be practised or promoted as anything other than a martial art and are calling for an end to the "broad church" approach which includes any reference to "Tai Chi for Health":

*The time has come to **completely** (sic) distance ourselves from new-age "Tai Chi" practitioners and reclaim the art for the ordinary martial artist. We also need to destroy the idea of T'ai Chi as a form of "gentle therapeutic exercise" or as some kind of "cure-all". As a martial arts instructor it is **not** (sic) for me to be making claims about healing people. "Tai Chi" is currently marketed as anything and everything from a form of spiritual healing to a method of relationship counselling; as "a path to enlightenment" or even as a beauty treatment. With so much mis-information around, no one needs to feel silly for having been mis-led, but we must now wage war on the charlatans who perpetuate the T'ai Chi mythology and reveal them as the frauds they are. There is nothing magical, mystical or even innately spiritual about T'ai Chi Ch'uan / Taijiquan - it is a fighting art, plain and simple.* (Zorya, 2006)

How then within this confusing array of contexts do we identify the bona fide or effective Tai Chi Instructor capable of teaching "real" or "authentic" Tai Chi with "real" and "non-superficial" health benefits? One way to resolve this issue is to accept the yin and yang of there being two broad poles of Tai Chi in the modern world which involve two distinct and different approaches to teaching Tai Chi – Tai Chi as a Martial Art and Tai Chi for Health (TCH).

Our starting point for TCH is thus to recognise and enthusiastically embrace the idea that TCH Is "a fait accompli" and that no one person or organisation can claim sole ownership of the philosophical term "Tai Chi" which has been utilised over a two and a half thousand year period in China in order to explain the order of the universe, the way of nature, all manner of things related to movement, stillness, time and space, how nature impacts upon and interacts with society, and how culture appropriates nature. The term "Tai Chi" was simply borrowed by the Yang family, thus providing a great public relations opportunity to capitalise on the cultural mythology and metaphysics surrounding "Tai Chi" philosophy, to promote and differentiate the Chen Style adaptation of "Cotton Fist" boxing from other styles of Chinese boxing that existed at the time. We can thank Sun Lutang for being the first to liberate the "Tai Chi" from the exclusive brotherhood of the "boxers" and from the "mandate of heaven" of a Confucian social order by stating that the health giving benefits of martial forms and exercise can be accessed by all people – men, women, the old, and the young which with consistent and focussed practice will restore sound health to a balanced state of strength and flexibility. (see Sun Lutang, 1921, p.60)

The genius of Sun Lutang (see Arthy, 2006) was that in Sun's day there was not yet the idea that "Tai Ji Quan" was a Health Art and that Sun recognized the health-building benefits of practicing "Tai Ji Quan" by making the connection between the development of "internal" power through natural exercise and its benefits for the individual's health. (see Miller, 2000)

3.60   MARTIAL CONCEPT OF BODY AND APPLICATION
   3.61   Solo Form Training
   3.62   Two-person Sparring
   3.63   Push Hands – Sensitivity Training

3.61   Solo Form Training - In many styles of martial arts as exist in contemporary society, training includes the practice of what are termed "solo forms". Solo forms are pre-arranged sequences of various martial manoeuvres which are performed solo and involve movements which are defending and attacking against an imaginary opponent. Kung Fu Tai Chi Chuan (Chinese), Tae Kwon Do (Korean) and Karate (Japanese), for example, are martial arts which all have solo forms as part of the training to be a effective martial artist and all have similarities and differences but in outward appearance resemble each other compared to solo performances of other forms of movement such as dance, Western shadow boxing, acting or mime.   For these martial arts, the "body" represents the accumulated knowledge of the particular style and is represented in the performance of the solo form.   Some styles place a great deal of importance on the "body" of knowledge of the particular style of the martial art, on learning "forms", "patterns" or "katas" while others place more importance on what could be described as a freestyle approach to combat involving two-person forms of sparring.

The solo forms of Kung Fu Tai Chi Chuan include a range of different styles such as the Chen Style, Yang Style, Sun Style, Wu Style and Wu Hao Style - all of which are considered to adhere to a common set of "rules of engagement" deemed to be the concepts and principles peculiar to Kung Fu Tai Chi Chuan. The most popular and well-known of these principles are those were originally written and published by Chen Wei Ming in mid 1920s known as "Yang Cheng Fu's Ten Principles of Tai Chi". The performance of the solo form of Tai Chi practised as a martial art is intended to demonstrate the martial skill and ability of the performer through the Chinese concepts of "Yin-Yang theory", of "defend and attack", "fast and slow", "high and low", "internal and external".

Many styles of martial arts including Kung Fu Tai Chi Chuan encourage the development of martial and fighting skills through continual practice of the solo forms. The levels of skill can be demonstrated at martial arts competitions where a number of judges collectively evaluate the performance of the competitor, not in the specifics of a particular choreography, but in the demonstration of the key principles of combat effectiveness. While different styles may have different emphases on martial ability and strategy, there are common features for all martial styles. For example, regardless of the style, the judge can evaluate the skills of "intention" in the moves by the co-ordination of "upper and lower body", by the efficacy of "body evasion/ yielding" techniques, and importantly, the posture of the head, the body and orientation of the eyes.   However, many martial styles including Kung Fu Tai Chi Chuan prefer not to demonstrate their martial "form" outside the confines of the particular school or style, instead opting for competition within the particular organisational framework. Thus it would be extremely rare to see a Kung Fu Tai Chi Chuan martial arts practitioner entering into a "karate" or even an "all-styles" martial arts tournament even to demonstrate the solo form.

3.62   Two-person Sparring - Not all styles of martial arts however, have solo forms as part of the training but most if not all forms of martial arts would have some form of two person training to represent combat under a set of "rules or engagement" whether for the purposes of competition or specific outcomes such as general "self-defence" or training to kill an opponent as in the military services. For these types of martial arts, the "body" of knowledge of that martial art includes the two-person form or demonstration of the martial ability of the performers.

In regard to the "rules of engagement" as demonstrated in tournaments and competition for two person sparring, we find a considerable divergence within the Kung Fu Tai Chi Chuan martial arts world globally. In the United States and Australia, the rules of engagement are aimed at preventing the use of excessive force where combatants either lose points or are disqualified for what the judges deem to be the use of excessive force. On the other hand, the rules of engagement in China are more similar to a Sumo or Judo competition where the use of external force is not penalised due to the reason that the person on the receiving end of the so-called "excessive force" should have sufficient skills to be able to use proper Tai Chi principles in order to neutralise and deflect the incoming force. In other words, under these "rules of engagement" size (weight and strength) of the participant is important in relation to the skills. Although it is possible for a smaller person to defeat a larger opponent, this will only happen with the superior use of skills. In short, where there are equal skills, size matters and this is the reason in many martial styles such as Western boxing, combatants are matched according to gender and weight divisions.

3.63   Push Hands – Sensitivity Training- Outside the competitive arena of two-person sparring, many modern schools of Tai Ch practise non-competitive and co-operative forms of push hands involving two persons. This is sometimes referred to as sensitivity training and is designed to teach students to relax and become more aware of certain key points of Tai Chi such as yielding where "loose hips" are paramount in deflecting incoming force. The value of this type of drill lies not in demonstrations of ego or in the pursuit of trophies in trying to push the other person off balance but as a co-operative approach were each person helps the other person.

UNIT 400
Legal and Other Responsibilities

Unit Overview
    4.10   Introduction
    4.20   Duty of Care – To Do No Harm
    4.30   Practical Requirements of TCH Instructor
    4.40   Other Legal and Ethical Responsibilities of TCH Instructors
    4.50   Risk Management
    4.60   Code of Practice & Ethics for Tai Chi for Health Instructor

4.10   INTRODUCTION

Information about legal and ethical matters in this course is offered to provide a framework for understanding the legal and ethical obligations which the Tai Chi for Health Instructor has towards to the students, and to the broader community. An important concept to understand about the law is that it can be different between different countries across the world, different within the same country between different States and Local Governments and over time the law can change. Part of the focus of this course is to highlight the complexity of relevant legal matters, in particular Duty of Care, and the need for the Tai Chi teacher not to make assumptions about the law and to always obtain independent professional legal advice.

Another important focus of this course is to provide guidelines for the ethical and professional conduct for the Tai Chi for Health Instructor identified as the *Code of Practice & Ethics* to ensure a positive, safe and harassment-free environment for all participants and teachers. This *Code of Practice & Ethics* is also intended to meet community expectations and justify trust in the integrity of the Tai Chi for Health exercise program, particularly in relation to highest standards of a Duty of Care to do no harm.

4.20   DUTY OF CARE – TO DO NO HARM

Common Law Principle - The "Duty of Care" principle in Australia is based on the British common law and not statute law. The legal precedent of Duty of Care was established in a specific court case where it was found that the manufacturer of bottled soft-drink had a legal responsibility towards all consumers of their products, not just to the woman who had become ill after drinking the contents that contained the sediments of a decomposed snail. The court ruled that it was reasonable for the woman to rely on the manufacturer to supply a product that was not going to make her ill and found that the manufacturer was negligent and was therefore responsible in law for causing injury and harm to her as a consumer. What was significant in this particular case was that, even though there was no direct transaction or relationship existing between the woman and the manufacturer, the manufacturer had a legal Duty of Care responsibility that extended beyond its immediate customer, the retailer who actually sold the soft drink to the woman.

Ethical principle of non-maleficence - Duty of Care is about your legal and ethical responsibility as a Tai Chi for Health (TCH) Instructor for SAFETY with all related aspects of offering your services. It is the common law legal principle, which requires you to provide a responsible and reasonable standard of care to those to whom you provide a service and, in the provision of that service, to protect them from harm. This Duty of Care in common law not only includes the ethical principle of beneficence – "of doing good", but extends to the ethical principle of non-maleficence - "the duty to do no harm". Negligence would be the legal consequence of a breach of the ethical principle of non-maleficence - the duty to do no harm.

Risk Management for TCH Instructor - For the TCH Instructor, Duty of Care carries with it a responsibility to ensure that all aspects of the TCH Instructor's provision of a service are considered, even where certain aspects of providing that service may not be directly under the instructor's control or even related to TCH Instruction. In the first instance, Duty of Care means identifying and minimising not only the potential risk of physical, emotional and financial injury or harm to your students but to non-participants as well. Harm or risk may result out of something you have done or have failed to do for such as persons who are visitors at your class, and persons who use the same facilities at some subsequent time. The wide ranging possibilities related to Duty of Care necessitates the TCH Instructor to have in place a proper "Risk Management" procedure and "Code of Practice & Ethics" for your TCH Class, school or organisation to which you may be operating through or with.

Special "Duty of Care" to Client Group - In establishing the "reasonable" standard of care, one has to keep in mind that not only children under the age of 18 and people with physical or intellectual disabilities, but also aged persons require a greater standard of care. There needs to be an appropriate balance between an individual's right of "informed consent" for personal responsibility to participate in a TCH program and the professional responsibility of the TCH Instructor to ensure a safe program and environment for students and other users of the facilities related to the instruction (see Appendix 2).

Other Legal and Ethical Duties to Client Group and other Teachers – This includes being aware of social justice and equity issues, and other legal requirements and relevant practices to ensure a safe, harassment-free environment for all persons related to or impacted by TCH related activities which may include classes, workshops, demonstrations and social functions.

Non-delegatable Duty of Care - Where a Tai Chi Instructor is operating under license of a TCH program both the course providers of that training program and the TCH Instructor have a non-delegatable Duty of Care in the implementation of the TCH program. (see Romel El-Sheik v Australian Capital Territory Schools, 1999) This is to ensure that the actual delivery of the particular TCH activity by the TCH Instructor has been managed in accordance with "Risk Management" strategies as an integral component of the TCH Instructor training program. The duty is to ensure that such measures are taken as in all the circumstances are reasonable to prevent injury. The duty is not so onerous as to insure no injury occurs at all but to take reasonable care to prevent injury that ought to have been reasonably foreseen.

The central issue here is that the Duty of Care cannot be delegated which means that course providers in the first instance have a legal responsibility to the consumer of the TCH program (see Unit 4.48) to ensure that the TCH Instructor has sufficient knowledge on how to teach students safely, to understand their legal responsibilities and an understanding of the importance to maintain the integrity of the program being delivered to the consumer. This includes ensuring that the TCH Instructor knows how to be sufficiently connected with the individual student in order to provide alternative safe movements for those persons whose health conditions and physical capabilities are restricted and to know how to teach students to take personal responsibility for themselves, to work safely within their own health, fitness and ability levels. The TCH Instructor also needs to ensure that all TCH activities are closely and properly supervised understanding that the traditional "follow me" method alone of teaching Tai Chi is dangerously deficient in regard to a Duty of Care.

In addition, both the course providers of the TCH program and the TCH Instructor have a non-delegatable Duty of Care to ensure the safety of the physical space of the TCH activity for entry, participation and exit for all participants, clients, visitors and other members of the public. There is a legal Duty of Care to ensure that there is a safe environment of facilities and equipment, that there is nothing faulty or potentially unsafe. This includes the need to have a "Risk Management" strategy formulated, for example, to include clearly defined emergency procedures for evacuation. Other legal and ethical responsibilities also need to be included by the course providers in training the TCH Instructor to ensure that the TCH Instructor has a proper understanding of various laws and professional ethical standards. These include - occupational health and safety (OH&S), consumer protection, privacy, discrimination, harassment, copyright, defamation and professionalism of the instructor-client relationship.

The TCH Instructor who operates in the community under the license of the TCH program is therefore legally obliged to operate within all the terms and conditions express or implied of that license, which include teaching within the legal and ethical standards as outlined in the TCH program, not delegating the Duty of Care to anyone, being present at all times and taking responsibility for and being vigilant at all times in the delivery of the TCH program. The terms of the license for some TCH programs may also include the need to update skills and knowledge of TCH on a regular basis. As a specialist TCH instructor for any particular populations, there is a legal Duty of Care on both the course provider of the TCH Instructor Training program and the TCH Instructor to ensure there is a higher skill and diligence than one who is less specialised. In Australia, any injury or harm arising out of a TCH activity which resulted from simply not knowing about the multitude of legal responsibilities for TCH Instruction is not a defence in law – *"ignorantia juris non excutat"*, which as a legal maxim literally means: "ignorance of the law is no excuse". In summary, the course provider of the TCH program has a Duty of Care to the consumer to ensure that the sufficient training in 'Risk Management" strategies covering both professional and public liability have been included in the TCH Instructor training program.

4.30   PRACTICAL REQUIREMENTS OF TAI CHI FOR HEALTH INSTRUCTOR

Provide a safe environment by TCH Instructor
- Facilities and equipment must be safe for users, visitors and others involved
- Liaise with facility providers to ensure that appropriate safety standards are met and monitored
- Safe environment for entry, participation and exit is the responsibility of the TCH Instructor
- The TCH Instructor should have in place clearly defined emergency procedures

Activities must be adequately planned by TCH Instructor
- Use appropriate progressions in the teaching of new skills
- Even for advanced students, new complex skills can be daunting. Ensure that all skills, whether aimed at a beginner or advanced level, are progressed in a safe manner that builds student confidence and competence whilst minimising the risk of injury

Instructor needs to obtain informed consent for participation in the TCH program
- The TCH Instructor needs to ensure that there is "informed consent" by the student as to the guidelines associated with the TCH program (for example see Appendix 6)

95

- Instructor advises the student to obtain clearance from a qualified health professional for participation in TCH program as per a prescribed form (see Appendix 2)
- Instructor needs to teach students how to take personal responsibility for themselves as a TCH student, to work underneath their pain level, to visualize what they are not capable of physically doing, to take frequent rest breaks
- Instructor provides alternative safe movements for persons where relevant
- Instructor needs to be aware that the student may not know whether the planned skill practice or activity will exacerbate his or her incapacity or injury.
- A TCH instructor claiming specialist knowledge for a particular population is bound to a higher degree of skill and diligence

Activities must be closely supervised
- Total adequate supervision by the TCH Instructor is necessary to ensure that training sessions are as safe as possible
- Ensure that any designated assistant has a minimum of TCH Instructor Training and is accredited with the particular TCH program of the target population and are present to supervise training routines
- Ensure the Instructor–Student relationship is safe

TCH Instructors must be able to deal with health emergencies
- Instructors must be able to properly deal with a range of health emergencies
- TCH Instructors must have a nationally accredited Senior First Aid certification, which includes a good understanding of the STOP (Stop, Talk, Observe, Prevent further injury) and RICE (Rest, Ice, Compression, Elevation) routines
- Properly equipped first aid kit, including ice packs available at each training session
- Strategy involving procedures in the event of a medical emergency including student information readily available on the student

TCH Instructors should keep adequate records
- Records should be kept of all students with relevant general information, accurate attendance records, medical clearance and consent forms
- Instructor needs to maintain a database of all students with information from their application forms, including emergency contact persons and attendance records
- Instructor must produce and retain proper documentation of any emergencies

4.40   OTHER LEGAL AND ETHICAL RESPONSIBILITIES OF TCH INSTRUCTORS
TCH Instructors should be familiar with and attend to a range of other legal and ethical issues and requirements including:
  o Occupational Health and Safety (OH&S) requirements in involving other teachers
  o Anti-Discrimination Laws regarding the treatment of students and other teachers
  o Ethical principles and laws on harassment and sexual harassment
  o Legal and ethical principles on intimate relationships between TCH Instructor and student
  o Formulation of Code of Practice & Ethics to ensure a positive, safe and harassment-free environment for all participants and teachers, including information on expected behaviour of teachers and students, and on requirements concerning clothing, hygiene, infectious diseases and policy on health screening
  o Formulation of Risk Management Plan covering all possible activities and consequences of TCH activities

4.50   RISK MANAGEMENT
  4.51   General
  4.52   Insurance
  4.53   Professional Duty of Care
  4.54   General Duty of Care
  4.55   Copyright & Music Licences
  4.56   Ethics & Harassment
  4.57   Occupational Health & Safety
  4.58   Other Areas – Consumer protection, Privacy, Defamation

4.51   General - The key factor in an effective Risk Management plan is based on the common law "Duty of Care" of care principle, which requires the TCH Instructor:
- To do no harm either through commission or omission, that is, through something we do or fail to do, or to avoid being negligent
- To evaluate risks through proper planning, taking account of possible outcomes that to the reasonable person are foreseeable in principle

- To take necessary action based on that plan to ensure reasonable safety for all persons who may be affected by the particular activity or event, including students and visitors and on-lookers to the activity or event.

4.52   Insurance - In today's society, insurance for all manner of things is an everyday occurrence and is an essential part of any Risk Management plan. Being insured does not in any way alter the legal responsibility to exercise the "Duty of Care" and does not prevent anyone from exercising their legal right to seek remedy for injury that may have been caused by negligence of some other person. All insurance policies require a full and proper disclosure by the insured person and failure to do so on the basis of what is relevant or not is not a defense as "ignorance of the law" is never an excuse. If in doubt, the golden rule is to seek proper legal advice to ensure that you have correctly understood your legal responsibilities and liabilities. This advice should be sought prior to and as part of a Risk Management plan.

Negligence - Negligence is the name for a particular civil wrong (TORT) that one person in law has done against another person. Negligence is a failure by the person who has a "Duty of Care" (Instructor) for another person to prevent harm or injury that was or should have been foreseeable by the "reasonable person" test. This other person can be anyone who has come in contact with the TCH activity and may or may not be the student; it could even be a casual passer-by to the activity.

Waiver - The waiver is a document that the TCH Instructor obtains from the student in advance of any activity and should be part of the contract entered into between the TCH Instructor and student. The waiver component is deemed to be part of a Duty of Care that the TCH Instructor has towards the student. It is important to understand that the waiver does not remove the Duty of Care, but provides some evidence that the TCH Instructor has demonstrated a Duty of Care in contractually communicating to the student about the risks involved in undertaking the TCH activities and the contractual expectations that the student also has in regard to taking personal responsibility for participating in those activities. The waiver is a form of evidence that the TCH Instructor has exercised a "professional" Duty of Care in obtaining informed consent by the student (for example see Appendix 6).

Liability Insurance - Various forms of insurance are available to the TCH Instructor. Insurance is an important part of any "Risk Management" plan, so the TCH Instructor needs to be properly informed as to the implications of the function and rationale for insurance. Being insured does not remove the legal responsibility for the Duty of Care towards the student. There are three kinds of liability insurance that the TCH Instructor needs to be familiar with –

(a) Professional Liability: This covers the TCH Instructor in the capacity of giving advice and professional services for any failure on the Duty of Care towards the student, where negligence can be established:

Professional Indemnity insurance protects you from legal action taken for losses incurred as a result of your advice. It provides indemnity cover if your client suffers a loss - either material, financial or physical - directly attributed to negligent acts. (Australian Government, 2009c)

(b) Public Liability: This covers all persons who have a legal interest in the safety of the venue, and may include the owners of the property, any persons (or legal entities such as company or association) involved the activity.

Public Liability Insurance - protects you and your business against the financial risk of being found liable to a third party for death or injury, loss or damage of property or 'pure economic' loss resulting from your negligence. (Australian Government, 2009c)

(c) Product Liability: This covers you for products which you sell and which may cause injury.

Product Liability - If you sell, supply or deliver goods, even in the form of repair or service, you may need cover against claims of goods causing injury or damage. Product liability insurance covers damage or injury caused to another business or person by the failure of your product or the product you are selling. (Australian Government, 2009c)

Insurance Coverage

(a) **Necessity:** Is special insurance necessary for all Tai Chi for Health activities, which includes the giving of advice and services? Should all Tai Chi for Health teachers have special insurance coverage to cover the Tai Chi for Health activity? In some instances, the answer may be no. The full answer to this question is dependent on a number of factors and in particular, the relationship of the teacher with the client and other parties. Is the TCH Instructor and student relationship that of a self-employed professional, of a paid employee, of a volunteer engaged by an organisation, of a volunteer independent from any organisation but offering free TCH activities?

(b) **Existing Insurance for Paid Work:** Is the person offering the Tai Chi for Health activity already covered by insurance as for say - a martial arts instructor, a fitness trainer, diversional therapist, aged-care provider, a health-care provider such as a nurse, physiotherapist, or medical doctor? The short answer must start with examining the existing insurance contract to determine if the activity or giving of advice is included or not. For example, the insurers of fitness trainers accredited with Fitness Australia will only cover TCH programs that have been specially registered with Fitness Australia. If the TCH activity is outside or not included as part of the insurance contract, then the Fitness Trainer will need to obtain special insurance for those other Tai Chi for Health activities.

(c) **No existing Insurance:** If the Tai Chi for Health activity falls outside or is specifically excluded by an existing insurance coverage such as sensitivity training or push hands[26], then what special insurance coverage, if any, should the Tai Chi teacher have? The short answer to this question for all matters to do with Duty of Care responsibilities is that the Tai Chi for Health teacher should obtain proper independent legal advice. Why? The answers will be dependent on the pertinent set of facts and the laws as they exist within the particular jurisdiction where the Tai Chi for Health activity is to be held. In Australia, for example, each State has different laws and there are also other legal variables that govern the teaching a Tai Chi for Health class, many of which are referred to in this course.

(d) **Volunteers with a Community Organisation**: In Queensland, volunteers engaged through a community organisation are covered by the *Civil Liability Act 2003, Qld* (see Queensland Government, 2008). With some important exceptions, this law provides statutory protection for the volunteer from being sued for negligence, but does not remove the Duty of Care that the organisation which engages the voluntary services of the Tai Chi teacher towards the client group and related interested parties. The law governing Duty of Care by an organisation to volunteers is also different from that of self-employed professionals and employees and in most instances in Queensland is covered by the *Workplace Health and Safety Act 1995* (see Queensland Government, 2009a) (see also below under Unit 4.47). Other jurisdictions have separate laws governing volunteers.

(e) **Insurance Contract and Coverage**: The next question arises for the Tai Chi teacher who obtains insurance. If insured, what is actually covered for a possible negligence claim against the Tai Chi for Health teacher? This question can only be answered in regard to the application of the law to the specific set of facts surrounding the case. If the insurer is satisfied that the teacher has made full and proper disclosure in general terms, then the insurer may provide legal representation for any civil action being brought, regardless of the outcome. In other words, the Insurer would stand behind the teacher if the policy actually covers the particular scenario and competencies of the Tai Chi teacher and will guarantee two things – to provide proper legal representation and to settle any successful negligence liability claim whether for "professional", "public" or "product" liability where included in the coverage.

(f) **Duty of Disclosure:** Does being insured of itself protect the TCH Instructor from any claim by others? If insured, can the insurer refuse to accept to represent the Tai Chi for Health teacher and refuse to accept liability in the event of someone bringing a negligence claim? As suggested already, the straight forward broad answer is yes, if there has not been full and proper disclosure made to the insurer. This may be revealed through examination of the factual detail of events leading to injury or if the activity was outside the competencies or expertise of the Tai Chi for Health teacher? This question is vital to the insurers to ensure that they only cover those activities that the teacher is suitably qualified to offer, regardless of the fact that the insurer has accepted the premium for coverage of the teacher's qualified area of expertise and regardless of the good intentions of the teacher.

(g) **Mistaken Intentions – No Coverage:** In regard to good intentions, it may be inconsequential if the Tai Chi for Health teacher mistakenly believes they are covered for certain activities and in reality and in law they are not covered. This may also arise where the TCH Instructor mistakenly believes that the organisation that they are engaged with provided the insurance coverage for the activity. Moreover, where harm results as a consequence of the activity, the teacher may not be covered for any claim for negligence regardless of whether or not there was negligence by the teacher. This means that the insurer may refuse to provide any responsibility of a negligence claim by a third party which would include legal costs associated with any claim being brought, regardless of whether or not negligence could be established against the Tai Chi for Health teacher. In this scenario, the TCH teacher would need to bear the legal and associated costs in a defense against a common-law negligence action, which is indeed very expensive. In short, delivering a Tai Chi for Health activity either in the mistaken belief that the activity was covered by insurance or that the activity was deemed to be outside the level of competence and training will leave the Tai Chi for Health teacher exposed to a common-law action for negligence.

---

[26] AON is an insurer which covers allied health professionals for Tai Chi for Health activities and specifically excludes "combat/physical contact" (see AON, 2009)

(h) **Non-delegatable Duty of Care:** This liability arising out of a negligence claim will also be examined in relation to the upward chain of responsibility which is referred to as the "non-delegatable" Duty of Care (see Unit 4.20) to all organisations and persons who are associated with the delivery of the Tai Chi for Health activity. These include the owners of the venue whether a hall or outdoor area such as a Council park, the owners of the particular Tai Chi for Health program and others who have been party to the certification of the Tai Chi for Health program. The injured person or the family will often bring a blanket action against all persons, or entities associated with the event as part of a negligence claim for the reason that at the outset, the facts and the causality of the injury may not be known (see (see Romel El-Sheik v Australian Capital Territory Schools, 1999).

4.53   Professional Duty of Care – Professional Liability

Screening - Health Information Forms recommended:
- Participant General Information form
- Medical Information form signed by a medical practitioner
- Registration form with disclaimer
- This is an integral part of obtaining informed consent on the part of the student (see Appendix 2)

These forms should be mandatory for every person participating in an exercise class regardless of age, signed and updated annually or before if health circumstances have changed.

Familiarise
- Yourself with the information provided through the health screening process of all people on the floor
- Contact the practitioner if in doubt
- Work with the health care network of the participant where appropriate - e.g. doctor, physiotherapist, acupuncturist, natural therapist, nutritionist, carer

Teach your Class
- Never attend class if unwell, especially if taking antibiotics
- To raise a hand if they become unwell, distressed, dizzy or in pain
- To use their PC - Perceived Capacity for work
- To wear non-slip closed footwear & loose and comfortable clothing
- To bring small pillows for hip/or back support for chair
- To drink water before, during and after the class
- Not to chew gum or other substances in class
- To be able to recognize what is normal for them & report change to their medical advisor
- To wear a name badge for every class with relevant information on the back (see Unit 4.60)

Program
- Should be SAFE and EFFECTIVE and FUN and DO NO HARM
- Technique clear and accurate
- Give rest times when necessary
- Water breaks encouraged
- Acknowledge improvements for effort
- Organize helpers where appropriate

Avoid in General
- Lowering the head
- Using the same muscle groups and weight bearing joints repetitively
- Know the 3 second hold rule
- Any movement that hurts
- Deep knee bends
- Movements that do not flow smoothly
- Locked joints (eg. Straight arms or legs)
- Physical contact with students unless with permission, then only with two fingers (see Unit 4.48 under Assault; and Unit 4.60 under Physical Contact)
- Allowing people into class who are suffering from flu or other viral infection

Specifically Avoid
- Hyperextension of the neck
- Sustained stretching of the neck in any direction
- Excessive circumduction of ball and socket joints
- Standing on one leg for long sequences – three seconds rule
- Anything ballistic except with advanced students and always with safety
- Both arms overhead simultaneously

- Trunk flexion from chair for hip replacements or hip flex greater than 90 degrees from standing position
- Crossing leg over the midline for hip replacements

Take Care
- With body alignment, especially be mindful to press up through the top of the head, lengthen the spine from the waist up and from the waist down. Limbs relax.
- With rotation of the spine. Move hips and shoulders as a unit and avoid twisting
- To keep shoulder-level work just slightly below the joint lengthening and loosening
- To be mindful of seasonal temperature fluctuations and adjust your class design accordingly
- Encourage all students to take personal responsibility, which includes students understanding the three seconds rule and the ten minute rule for chronic pain
- Ensure availability of water
- Supervision at all times of class with qualified TCH Instructor
- No eating or chewing during class

Dr Paul Lam's three Golden Rules (see Lam, 2006a) - These are guidelines when teaching any kind of movement in any class, any sport, any situation involving the delivery of movement practices to other people:

1. **"Pass the Buck" or Refer on** - This rule is a very important principle to work by. There is an old saying "know thyself". People who are teaching exercise are trained to teach exercise not medicine. Even those teachers who are medically trained refer the student on to their own medical adviser and do not practise medicine on the teaching floor. Always refer to the doctor or physiotherapist or health management team when asked questions that refer to the health of the participant. In the modern litigious society make no exceptions.

2. **Listen to your student** - Always take the time to really listen to what they are saying. If you don't understand or are not sure whether how they are expressing themselves is a true picture of what they are verbalising or not, ask them to explain again so that you do understand and accommodate what they are telling you.

3. **Teach your students to listen to themselves** - This means helping them to recognise how the body feels, the level of intensity they are allowing themselves to perform, whether the movement causes pain at the time or after the lesson, whether the exercise is uncomfortable or unpleasant, the sensation of weight-bearing, the ease of breathing and so forth.

Start by teaching the difference between what they can do and what is comfortable, gradually teach the mind-body connection and flow into the Rate of Perceived Exertion. To have control over your body movements and not blindly follow the teacher will benefit the student optimally (and reduce the drop-out rate). The student will stay motivated and will continue to improve performance and achievement.

Remember, your first Duty of Care is to yourself.
Do not teach when you are ill. NOTHING is worth the risk and it is not a good example to set for your students.

Remind yourself that to renew your own energy and creativity, you need to have breaks from teaching – say a week off every term plus extra at Christmas/New Year. To remain teaching over many years, be mindful not to physically overload your weekly teaching program and to plan a fitness challenge for yourself also. Remind yourself also that "nothing changes if nothing changes". If nothing changes, you are stale.

4.54   General Duty of Care – Public Liability

Premises
- Ensure safety of physical space of TCH activity for entry, participation and exit for all participants, clients, visitors and other members of the public
- Ideal situation is a wooden floor
- Cross ventilation and fans
- Excellent lighting
- Clear open layout
- Ensure safe access with stairs, exits, rails, toilets
- Supervise use of kitchen for related social activities
- No hazards including objects and spills
- Do not allow smoking within legal vicinity of training area
- Policy on access to venue and class by visitors, friends, relatives & children

Emergency Procedures
- Risk Management strategy formulated

- Know the exact details of location of your venue for the Emergency Services phone call – (Australia - triple zero)
- Have ready access to mobile telephone or nearby phone
- Senior First Aid in accordance with professional requirements
- Including update with CPR professionally
- Where relevant have a trained first-aider or nurse on standby
- Fully equipped First Aid kit available
- Keep icepacks in refrigerator or carry a cool-pak
- If an incident does occur fill out an incident report
- Keep a large printed emergency procedure plan nearby
- Have a blood spillage/infectious diseases procedure
- Have an evacuation plan in place

4.55   Copyright & Music Licences - Any TCH Instructor, who plays any form of music at a TCH activity in any public forum, needs to understand their legal responsibilities under copyright laws in regard to music and DVD/Videos.

The information sheet (Music G012) of the Australian Copyright Council can be downloaded the web address - http://www.copyright

For specific information concerning public broadcasting of Music licences see web site for

APRA (the Australasian Performing Right Association) http://www.apra.com.au
PPCA (Phonographic Performance Company Of Australia Ltd) http://www.ppca.com.au

In general, if playing any form of music in any public forum, you need to obtain permission from the copyright holders of the music or alternatively obtain an appropriate music license from the authorized body such as APRA and PPCA.

In an open letter to the general public dated April 2005, Dr Paul Lam has given "Free Extra Rights" for his products, his music and Video/ DVDs as follows:

> *Tai Chi Productions and East Acton Videos is granting buyers of our Tai Chi instructional material free extra rights to use them in their classes; to present them in educational meetings and scientific conferences; to show to their patients; to use them during public or private performances for non for profit promotional purpose. Within the confines of your country's legal system, we give you rights to use the following products for the abovementioned purposes without having to pay us or any of our agents any extra fee. We grant you this rights because the purpose of us producing the teaching material is to make Tai Chi accessible to as many people as possible (Tai Chi Productions, 2009)*

However, the ownership of copyright and international copyright law generally in regard to music is very complicated it is best to obtain legal advice where there are any doubts about your rights and responsibilities about playing of music, videos and DVD related to any TCH activity.

4.56   Ethics & Harassment - The Australian Government through the Australian Sports Commission has formulated a comprehensive set of guidelines -

> *Every participant in sport, in whatever role, has a right to be treated with respect, dignity and fairness, and to participate in an environment that is enjoyable and safe. Harassment, abuse and other forms of inappropriate behaviour in sport denies participants these rights. The Harassment-free Sport (HFS) Strategy is the Australian Sports Commission's (ASCs) key initiative to assist in addressing harassment and abuse issues in sport. The overall aim of the HFS Strategy is to create safe, respectful and harassment-free sport environments. (Australian Sports Commission, 2009)*

All TCH Instructors should be familiar with these guidelines which are available on the Australian Sports Commission's website.

4.57   Occupational Health & Safety

OH&S (Occupational Health & Safety) Laws - In Australia, states and territories have responsibility for making laws about occupational health and safety (OH&S) and for enforcing those laws. Each state and territory has a principal OH&S Act, setting out requirements for ensuring that workplaces are safe and healthy. These requirements spell out the duties of different groups of people who play a role in workplace health and safety. (Australian Government, 2009a) In Queensland, the *Workplace Health and Safety Act 1995* (see Queensland Government, 2009a) is the framework within which workplaces and work practices are to be safer for everyone, including volunteer workers. The Act sets out the laws about health and safety requirements affecting most workplaces, work activities and specified high risk plant in Queensland. It seeks to protect your health and safety as a TCH Instructor and the health and safety of everyone at a workplace, while undertaking work activities. Everyone has a personal responsibility to care for their own and others' health and safety at workplaces, while carrying out work activities or using specified high risk plant. The people listed as having responsibilities in their own right, in addition to the TCH Instructor include - visitors, clients or students and volunteers who may be assisting the TCH Instructor. (See Queensland Government, 2009b)

4.58   Other Areas – Consumer protection, Privacy, Defamation and Assault

Consumer Protection: In Australia, there are two levels of jurisdiction: Federal and State governments. Under the Federal umbrella, the *Trade Practices Act 1974* is designed to protect the consumer in their dealings with business, for example by prohibiting conduct which is likely to mislead or deceive the consumer; prohibiting a business from using its superior bargaining power in an unconscionable way and by ensuring businesses comply with product safety and service delivery standards. The government department responsible for the administration of this law in Australia is the Australia Competition and Consumer Commission (see ACCC, 2009). Each State government in Australia is also responsible for compliance with the *Trade Practices Act 1974*. In Queensland, The Department of Employment, Economic Development and Innovation (DEEDI) through the Office of Fair Trading is responsible for administering state legislation – *Fair Trading Act 1989 (Qld).* (see Queensland Government, 2009c)

It is important that all Tai Chi for Health teachers understand that there are implications in the manner and the representations made in offering Tai Chi for Health classes in regard to laws governing consumer protection. For example, persons advertising Tai Chi for Health classes representing themselves as accredited under specific Tai Chi for Health programs such as the Tai Chi for Arthritis or Tai Chi for Health & Falls Injury Prevention programs, could be in breach of the various consumer laws and regulations if there was any misrepresentation about their own qualifications, their performance and teaching abilities, the qualities of particular product or service being offered, or a combination of any of these. Again, the issue of non-delegatable Duty of Care (see Unit 4.20) could come into play moving upwards through the chain of responsibility of parties who are associated with and in some way responsible for the integrity and delivery of the program.

Privacy: The key privacy obligations which apply to the private sector in Australia are the National Privacy Principles (NPPs), which govern the handling of personal information. The NPPs set out a minimum standard for the fair handling of personal information by private sector organisations including individuals. The ten NPPs cover everything from the collection and use of information to data quality and access rights (see Australian Privacy Foundation 2009). The implication for the Tai Chi teacher is that all client/student related information and data must be treated as confidential and in accordance with privacy laws as the very minimum. For example, this will include knowledge of the health conditions and personal details of the client/student such as addresses and phone numbers. It can extend to taking photographs without permission. Or even where there is permission, the use to which the photos may be used will be limited to any expressed or implied understanding as to the particular use of the photograph. It can include having a policy of not allowing anyone other than enrolled students walking in to the class without permission, express or implied.

Defamation: A general definition of defamation is the communication of a statement which claims to be factual (express or implied) and which may damage the reputation or good name of an individual, business, product, and other entities. Slander is defamation made verbally, and libel is defamation made in writing. This is a complex area of the law with different jurisdictions. In Australia, there are two levels of laws – Federal and State with each State having its own defamation laws. The implication for the Tai Chi teacher is to exercise caution when making negative and or potentially damaging statements, about students, other Tai Chi teachers or their products, or health professionals who may be responsible for the health care of the students.

Assault: For the Tai Chi teacher, the civil tort of assault underscores the need to obtain informed consent from – 1. the student or visitor to the class in any First Aid situation; and 2. the student in a class situation for the purposes of physical correction and instruction. In regard to the former this should be covered in an accredited First Aid Course where it would be stated that any physical act of touching someone else without consent or permission can be interpreted as common assault. In all circumstances, you must have permission (express or implied) to touch someone and if this is refused immediately you cannot proceed. Even if there is permission, the "touch" must not be excessive so as to cause injury or harm. For example, if consent was for the "two fingers rule", then the "touch" implies a gentle, responsive and responsible approach to physical correction. (see Unit 4.60 under paragraph 7 Physical Contact)

4.60   CODE OF PRACTICE & ETHICS FOR TAI CHI FOR HEALTH INSTRUCTOR

This provides a professional framework for an independent Tai Chi Health Instructor who operates a Tai Chi for Health school. Also membership of Sakurakan-QUBBA (see Unit 6.50) requires that the applicant agrees to abide by this "Code of Practice & Ethics" as part of conditions of membership.

1   Objectives
  1. Tai Chi for Health & Community Fitness ("TCHCF") has as its key objectives:
       (a) Providing a safe environment for instruction in Tai Chi for Health (TCH).

(b) Providing instruction in the Tai Chi for Health with the focus on health, fitness and well-being in the teaching and learning of Tai Chi within the modern Duty of Care framework.

(c) Promoting a wide range of classes, activities, courses and workshops relevant to performance of Tai Chi for Health at various levels from beginners to advanced levels and for all persons regardless of age, gender, health or levels of physical fitness.

(d) Providing Tai Chi as a Health Art as a gentle, safe, secular and effective form of exercise based on scientific evidence based research.

(e) Supporting research through the social and health sciences for the promotion of a secular and safe approach to Tai Chi for Health.

(f) Promoting and developing mental and physical skills for improving health & well-being

(g) Development of positive self-esteem and self-confidence.

2. All persons participating in a class or course conducted by a TCH Instructor and/or school accredited and/or affiliated with TCHCF must agree to be bound by this Code of Practice and Ethics. The TCHCF reserves the right to make amendments or additions to this Code at any time.

2 Participant Understanding

1. The TCH Instructor accredited with TCHCF may offer –

   (a) Tai Chi for Health class - as a gentle exercise class with the major focus in the class on learning Forms (that is set movements flowing in a sequence). An important aspect in learning Tai Chi in the class from the beginning is to learn to understand and apply the essential principles of Tai Chi which underscore the health and fitness benefits of Tai Chi. The class also includes a focus on Qigong (co-ordinated breathing exercises).

   (b) Tai Chi for Relaxation Class – is a gentle exercise class with also the major focus in the class on learning Forms with learning essential principles of Tai Chi and Qigong or co-ordinated breathing exercises. This class may also contain two-person sensitivity training where the practical focus is to learn to relax the body and mind and to understand the ebb and flow of energy within the performance of the Tai Chi form.

2. The TCH Instructor will identify to all potential students and students which type of class is being offered whether it is a Tai Chi for Health Class or Tai Chi for Relaxation class. While the Tai Chi for Relaxation class may include two-person sensitivity training, both classes are non-combative and do not involve techniques, which involve physically throwing, grappling or sparring with other practitioners.

3. Persons participating in any class conducted by the TCH Instructor accredited with TCHCF agree to do so of their own volition, at their own risk and with an understanding that their health and fitness is sufficient to undertake the TCH class or activity with safety. At all times in both types of classes, participants are encouraged to work at their own levels and to be mindful of safety and health factors.

4. Persons wishing to participate in any TCH class or activity accept that a medical clearance will be required as a condition for participation. The medical clearance should clearly state that the person is able to participate in classes conducted by the TCH Instructor and whether there are any restrictions or conditions applicable. This requirement for a medical clearance is partly to ensure that in regard to health and safety matters, the TCH Instructor has obtained "informed consent" from the student (see Appendix 2).

5. The student agrees to wear in every TCH class and activity, a name badge (see Appendix 6) with details attached behind the badge relating to - in the event of an emergency, contact details, health conditions and medication.

3 Instructor Qualifications

1. All unsupervised TCH Instructors with any TCHCF classes or activities must be a TCH Instructor accredited with TCHCF or other organisation recognized by TCHCF.

2. All unsupervised TCH Instructors are bound by the Code of Practice and Ethics.

3. All unsupervised TCH Instructors must have current Work-cover approved Senior First Aid Certification.

4. All unsupervised TCH Instructors must have in place appropriate public liability and professional indemnity insurance.

5. An accredited TCH Instructor agrees to not provide support, advice, or instruction to any student who offers or intends to offer TCH Instruction, which is not supervised by an accredited TCH Instructor or other Instructor recognised by Tai Chi for Health & Community Fitness.

4 Health and Safety

1. TCH Instructors will ensure that the class area is clear of any dangerous and/or sharp objects that may provide a risk of injury.

2. TCH Instructors will have access at all times to a fully equipped first aid kit.

3. All persons participating in a TCHCF class agree to maintain self-control at all times and maintain all care in the performance of any technique.

4. Any person who, at a TCHCF class or activity, exhibits behaviour that, in the judgment of the Instructor, is a danger to themselves or other participants shall not be allowed to continue training until the TCHCF Instructor determines the danger is no longer present.

5. All persons at any TCHCF class or activity agree to notify the TCH Instructor at any time when something arises which may affect the health and safety of that person or any other person involved in the class or activity at that time.

6. All TCH Instructors accredited with TCHCF must have a Risk Management plan, which includes details of – emergency procedures in regard to health and safety issues related to any class or activity.

5 Training Area Etiquette

1. Upon entering the area, instructors and students will show appropriate respect and follow the etiquette as to the type of class being held.

2. Persons should be punctual, preferably early, so that they are ready to participate when the class commences. If arriving late, a person should wait at the side of the Training Area until the Instructor indicates that a person may join the class.

3. Persons must not eat food or chew gum whilst in class.

4. Food and/or drink (including water) must not be consumed whilst in the training area of the class for health and safety reasons.

5. Mobile phones should be turned off during training. Mobile phones inadvertently left on during training should not be answered. Any person who has special needs in this regard should seek approval from the instructor prior to the commencement of class to leave his or her mobile phone on.

6 Clothing & Class Training Requirements

1. All participants should wear loose fitting clothing. Lycra shorts or tights are not suitable for health and safety reasons.

2. Shoes: Flat, non-slip soft shoes are required for all classes unless otherwise prescribed by a health professional for health and safety reasons.

3. All clothing should be free of inappropriate markings that are inconsistent with community standards.

4. Persons inappropriately attired may not be allowed to participate in class.

5. In addition to the general clothing requirements, persons should bring a towel and filled water bottle to each class for health and safety reasons.

7 Physical Contact

1. In all TCH classes any physical contact by the TCH Instructor is by permission only with individual student and is strictly limited to correction of alignment and posture with the "two fingers" rule. (see Unit 4.48 under Assault)

2. In the Tai Chi for Relaxation class, all physical contact between the TCH Instructor and/ or students is optional and to be clearly explained as to the purpose and limits of the activity.

8 Sickness or Injury

1. Persons must not participate in class if they are suffering from the flu or other viral infection that may be passed on to other persons.

2. Where a student's health on any particular day may be adversely affected by the physical activity of or during the class, the student must inform the Instructor and, if determined by the Instructor, must not participate or must cease to participate in that class. In certain cases, the Instructor may suggest that the student seeks immediate medical attention and/or requests the student to seek medical advice before being permitted to continue with any further classes.

3. At any time when requested by the Instructor to seek medical clearance, the student will secure a medical certificate clearly stating that the student is able to participate in classes conducted by the TCH Instructor and whether there are any restrictions or conditions applicable.

9 Other Health and Safety Issues

1. Persons must not attend classes under the influence of alcohol or illegal drugs.

2. Smoking is not allowed near or in the class area.

3. Persons training must give proper attention to personal hygiene and exhibit clean grooming.

4. Persons with a cut or bleeding injury must cease participating in the class immediately and receive appropriate first aid. Rejoining the class will not be allowed until the instructor has deemed that is safe to do so.

5. Persons administering first aid to a person suffering a cut or bleeding injury must wear protective gloves.

10 Other Legal and Ethical Issues

1. The TCH Instructor and all persons at a TCH class or activity must at all times be courteous, helpful and respectful to each other.

2. Physical contact between persons within any TCH class or activity must be appropriate to the particular class and the situation and necessary for the skill development of those persons.

3. Sexual harassment, defined as being where a person is subjected to un-wanted or uninvited sexual behavior, will not be tolerated.

4. Any form of unfair or improper discrimination based on gender, sexual orientation, ethnic origin, language, colour, or other form of differentiation will not be tolerated.

5. It is unethical for the TCH Instructor to become sexually involved or engage in any intimate relationship with any student of the TCH class or activity in which the student participates.

6. The TCH Instructor should maintain confidentiality on all matters private to each student within the TCH class.

7. The TCH Instructor agrees to formulate and make available a refund policy, which is fair and reasonable and consistent with relevant consumer laws.

8. When advertising the services of the TCH Instructor, such information must be consistent with Consumer Protection laws.

9. The TCH Instructor and/or the student of the TCH Instructor must not engage in any conduct which would bring Tai Chi for Health & Community Fitness and/ or Sakurakan-QUBBA (Queensland United Black Belt Association Inc) into disrepute.

UNIT 500
In-Depth Study of Sun 73

Unit Overview

5.10   INTRODUCTION

The *Australia Dreaming: Tai Chi for Health Advanced Instructor Training course* is a "train-the-trainer" course designed to enhance the teaching expertise of the Tai Chi for Health Instructor. The Sun 73 form has been used as the focus for form and movement but with a view to extrapolate to generic principles and concepts of a Tai Chi for Health which is safe and effective for a wide range of people as reflected in the Matrix of Performance (see Unit 3.40).   What is important to understand is that the course itself outlined in this book, as well as the Guidelines of teaching offered here, include concepts and principles that are transferable to teaching any style and form for teaching Tai Chi for Health. In other words, the task is for the teacher is to be able to make the right connections, to be confident and competent to transfer the knowledge, the ideas, principles and concepts identified in the performance of this Sun 73 Form to the teaching and performance of other forms and styles. Within a modern approach to teaching Tai Chi for Health, we need to understand that a "one-size-fits-all" approach is unsafe and potentially dangerous and that we function within modern Duty of Care where the Matrix of Performance provides the framework and strategies to be able to teach a wide range of people.

5.20   GUIDELINES FOR TEACHING

Modifications – The Sun 73 form is a competition form, specially choreographed with varying levels of difficulty to enable Judges in a panel to be able to differentiate between levels of performance by participants and grade different performances according to standards of excellence. There is of course an elite level where the performance is to be completed within 6 minutes, where it is extremely athletic, vigorous, precise, artistic and would compare with the ability to dazzle the audience to appear as if "floating like a butterfly and stinging like a bee".

Most people who do Tai Chi for Health enhancement, however, do not have the training from childhood, the ambition nor desire to compete at an elite level. For most people, therefore, modification represents an essential ingredient into learning any form. Modification for the teacher, can range from being able to make very minor to quite radical changes in order to suit the attributes of the student as suggested in the Matrix of Performance (see Unit 3.40). The idea generally is that modification should be designed to make the movements more readily accessible for performance by the student without stress or any risk of causing injury. Modifications are especially suggested for postures and movements that are difficult for those students whose physical health is compromised or who lack previous experience in any form of structured physical activity. This means that the student has pain, or that the student is not flexible, strong or robust enough to perform the movement safely in its original form or they simply don't feel comfortable and they don't know the reason. That is enough reason.

Some students will be able to perform a form simply by making the movement smaller – on a smaller frame. By focussing on one principle at a time, the body will improve and the movements will feel easier and more "light". Very gradually, without pressure, the size of the movements will increase. One of the lessons Tai Chi teaches is that of acceptance. Many teachers and some students resist modifying. They feel they should be able to do the form without modification. But why should this be so? Many people try to learn a set choreography, only to discover that they have no choice but to compromise the shape of the movement in some way, but hopefully realise in this process that what is important is the application of the principles of movement through mind-body co-ordination. The principles take precedence over the choreographic form, and SAFETY always takes precedence over all aspects of teaching and performance. The Sun 73 form can be modified safely and in so many different ways, like any other style of Tai Chi, and this includes teaching the form seated with suitably modified movements and strategies to maximise the health benefits for the student.

It should be remembered that with modern teaching techniques, such as visualisation, cuing, and mind-body analysis, and with the persistence of disciplined practice, some students may improve enough to be able to perform the moves without modification and with safety. If they don't, it is a lesson in acceptance of their body as it is, being able to perform the form for *their* body and for *their* health condition safely and in the absence of the guilt of a personal disappointment in their capability. Every person's Tai Chi is truly unique and what is really important is "how is this body working?" When it is moving and relaxed and the movements do not cause frustration and disappointment, the student should be happy and content with their progress. Tai Chi for Health itself is a work in progress for everyone, changing and adjusting as the days turn into months and years. These are some of the ideas and challenges for the Tai Chi for Health Instructor to be creative in being able to modify within a framework of safety.

Modifications of Sun 73 - In addition to the suggested modification to the Sun Style and Yang Style forms (see Unit 1.70), many students will need some caution for the spins and kicks of this set. When about to make a turn consider: maintaining posture and ball of foot and heel small movements to the end position, being mindful of careful transfer of weight. Keeping focus close seems to help some people with balance. Others are more stable with a long distant focus. Three or four step turn, or spin on the heel instead of the ball. This will lower the centre of gravity and be a more stable turn. Instead of turning and spinning in the preparation for the Lotus Kick, simply swap sides by changing to the mirror image of the feet and arms as the transition between Forms 68 and 69, and then adjust the arm at right to be more like the preparation for a Lotus.

Use Tai Chi principles & concepts to enhance teaching expertise of Tai Chi as in Unit 3.30 – Remember that the form is the choreography, it is the approximated shape which needs to be begin the process of learning Tai Chi. Introducing Tai Chi principles too early and without a basic understanding of form and movement may run the risk of overloading or confusing the student. On the other hand, the challenge for the teacher to understand that Tai Chi form and movements that are not aligned with principles and concepts will inhibit the student's understanding of the ebb and flow of movement and thus delay the advancement to higher levels of performance and associated health benefits. It is a balancing act on the part of the teacher to find effective ways of introducing both "Form" and "Principle" to the student in a meaningful, competent and safe way.

Apply concepts, principles and techniques of breathing as outlined in Units 3.14–3.15 – While there are many different approaches to breathing exercises within traditional Qigong and Yoga schools, one of the key messages of Tai Chi for Health that needs to be clearly stated, is that students should NOT hold their breath in any way.[27]

> *Try to avoid adopting a dogmatic interpretation of Qigong and forcing energy circulation, simply use relaxation, concentration and internal feeling to find the most natural pathways. Your body is the most accurate guide and it is important to remain open-minded to the way it feels and reacts … The Qigong exercises utilise deep breathing, although this should never involve holding the breath or forcing the movements. Since inhalation is considered yin and exhalation yang, both should operate together in a fluid circular motion.* (Tai Chi Society of University of Nottingham, 2009)

The overriding factor always with any Tai Chi for Health activity and especially Qigong exercises, is safety. While many approaches to Qigong are quite separate and independent from Tai Chi, it is important to understand that, simply put, movement co-ordinated with breathing represents a dynamic form of moving Qigong, whether hard or soft or a combination of both. It is also important from a teaching perspective to understand that every single form or posture within the Sun 73, or for that matter any Tai Chi form, can be practised as part of smaller sequence, or in isolation or with only the upper body – thus making the task much easier to focus on breathing patterns co-ordinated with movement. It is up to the teacher to find ways to introduce sooner than later and facilitate the enormous health benefits to be derived from focussed breathing exercises into a Tai Chi for Health program or class. The easiest way to begin this process is to break any specific form into short manageable movements using only the upper body, that is, neutralising the lower body with no movement of the feet. Once the student has grasped the concept of Qigong, as co-ordinated breathing patterns, the lower body can be slowly introduced. Firstly, this can be done without actually shifting the feet, but by using the mind-body technique the student can focus on the transfer of weight from one side of the body to the other. Then, short sequences can be introduced, building on what has previously been learned, where the focus now can include other Tai Chi principles and concepts, building towards dynamic breathing patterns that can then be factored into the performance of the Sun 73 form. Adopting the "KISS" principle ("Keep It Simple Sweetie"), it may be better at least for beginners to keep movements simple to be better able to focus on co-ordinated breathing with the movements.

As a motivational activity, the teacher can invite students in the class to choose a specific form (any form of their choice) to practice Qigong at the beginning or towards the end of the class. This presents a creative challenge to the teacher to be able to structure the movement and to co-ordinate the breathing patterns, to allow variations and not to be rigid about the interpretation of the "opening and closing" aspects of co-ordinated patterns of movement with breathing. In this way, the teacher is integrating the Qigong training with the Tai Chi performance and enhancing the health benefits sooner than later to be derived from controlled breathing patterns.

---

[27] Some schools of Qigong regard holding of one's breath as an integral component of their practice and philosophy, and of the martial arts; and advocate holding your breath up to one to two minutes as a legitimate form of exercise (see Lee, 2009). We consider this as potentially dangerous, it is not part of Tai Chi for Health and the suggestion that holding the breath is an essential feature of delivering the force in the martial arts or elsewhere is simply nonsense.

5.30   AN IN-DEPTH STUDY OF SUN 73

Sun 73 is composed of SECTIONS 1-5

Section One – Forms 1 – 22

1 Commencement

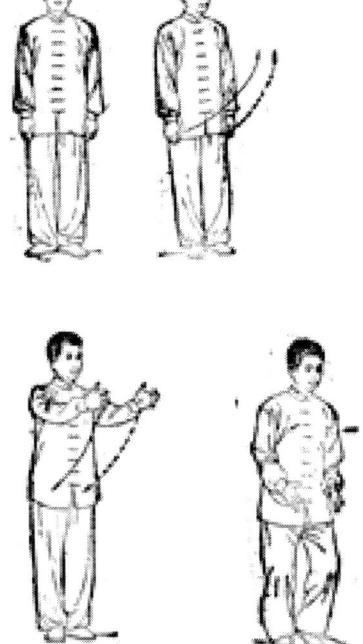

2 Leisurely Tying Coat

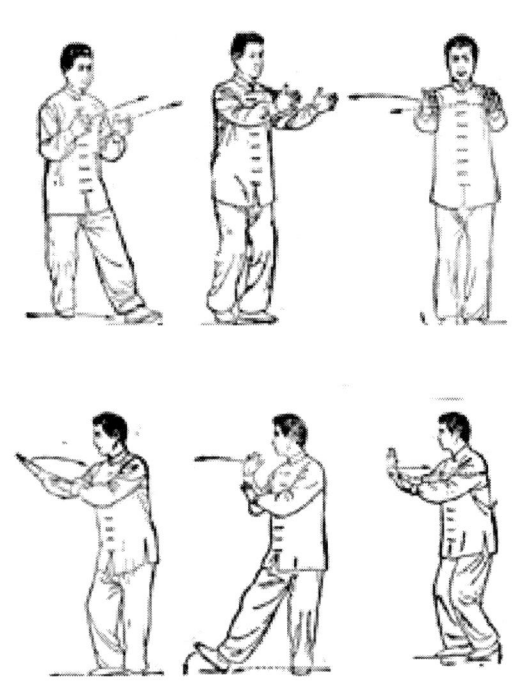

Teaching Hints & Modifications - Starting in Wuji position. Important to focus for at least 3-4 seconds before moving, and run through a posture check, upright posture, tell your body to relax but keep strong through the central core.   Allow time to sink and ground and elevate through the spine before stepping forward.

Teaching Hints & Modifications - Ensure hips and shoulders turn as a unit to stop twisting the spine. Push forward is co-ordinated exactly with the follow step.

3-4 Opening Hands ... Closing Hands

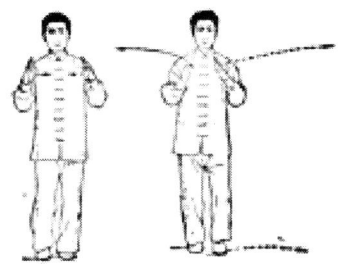

Teaching Hints & Modifications - Keep fingers upright and hands curved. Pull away and press in.

5 Single Whip

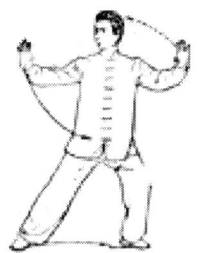

Teaching Hints & Modification - Bring L toes slightly front and orient Dan Tien to diagonal R slightly to assist with the Lifting Hands.

6 Lifting Hands

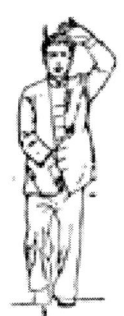

Teaching Hints & Modifications - Sink shoulders and keep lower arm out from body. Light foot in hip line.

7 White Crane Flashing Wings

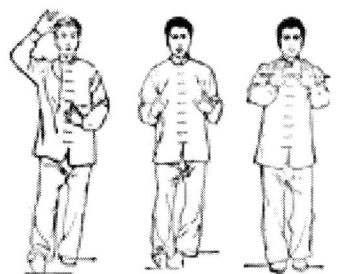

Teaching Hints & Modifications - Heel goes out as hands change passing exactly in the centre. Bring elbows to ribs. Push forward with weight transition.

8-9 Opening Hands ... Closing Hands

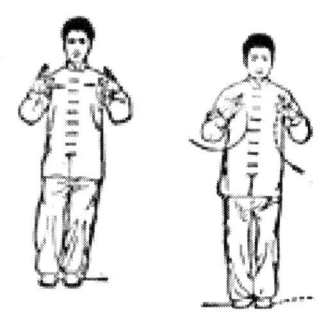

Teaching Hints & Modifications - Feel the energy change through the feet and legs.

10 Brush Knee and Twist Step Left

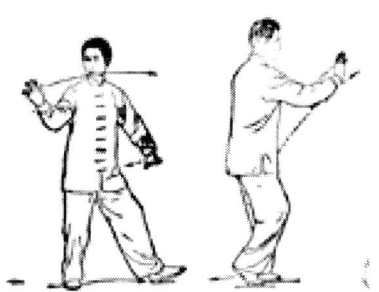

Teaching Hints & Modifications – Encourage student of possible need to modify and to keep off the "tightrope" (wide stance).

11 Playing the Lute

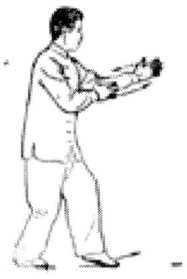

Teaching Hints & Modifications - Pass hands along the arm alignment & co-ordinate follow step with heel of hand pressing to elbow.

13-14 Apparent Closing Up ... Carrying the Tiger and Pushing the Mountain

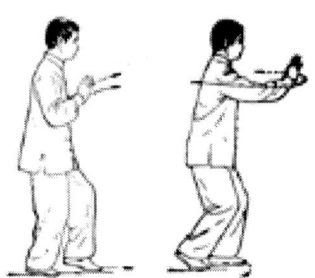

Teaching Hints & Modifications - Keep hands high on chest thumbs facing and shallow curve forward.

12 Step Forward to Deflect Downwards, Parry and Punch

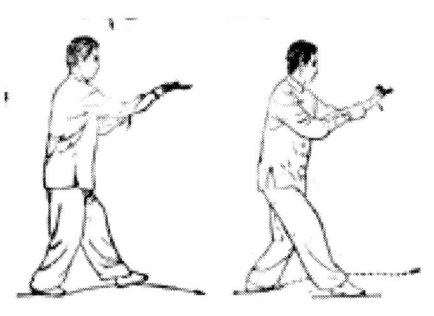

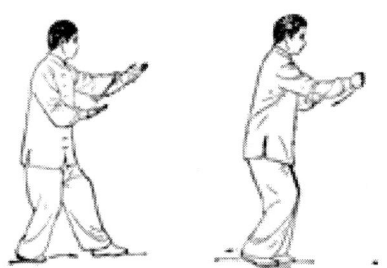

Teaching Hints & Modifications - Turn the waist for the Parry, Parry. Form L fist first then R at R hip for punch. Co-ordinate the punch with the follow step exactly. L fist faces down the R fist punch across wrist through to 9 o'clock, thumb on top pressed down.

15-16 Opening Hands ... Closing Hands

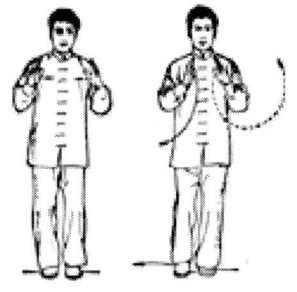

17 Brush Knee and Twist Step Right

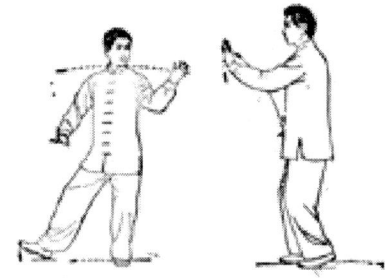

Teaching Hints & Modifications - 1 Look to hand. 2 three stretches. 3 keep hand at the shoulder for transfer and co-ordinate the push forward with the follow step.

18 Leisurely Tying Coat

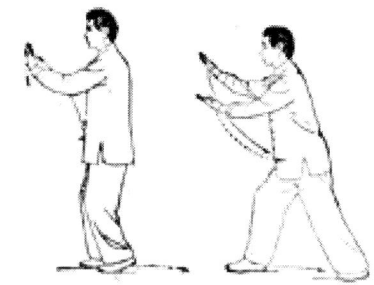

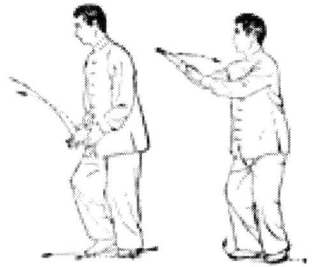

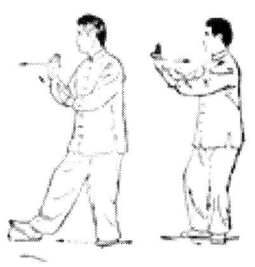

Teaching Hints & Modifications - Sit firmly on step 5 for empty stance with L foot on diagonal. This will minimise spinal twist for the swirl and give good energy. Bring into chest for transfer and follow step and push together.

19 – 21   Opening Hands ... Closing Hands ... Single Whip

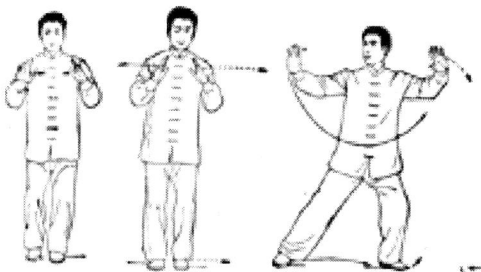

22 Punch under Elbow

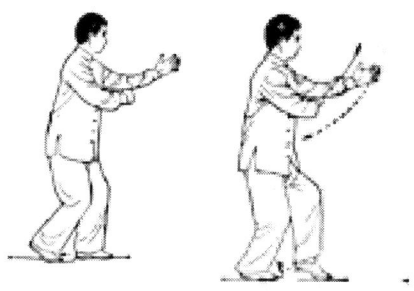

Teaching Hints & Modifications - Prepare punch from chest wall and deliver punch from mid chest to arm pit. Back of hand faces 9 o'clock. To reduce strain on R knee take the half step back to back diagonal. This will be an ideal position for the Brush Knee Push and will be good training for falls prevention.

Section Two – Forms 23 - 33

23 Repulse Monkey Left

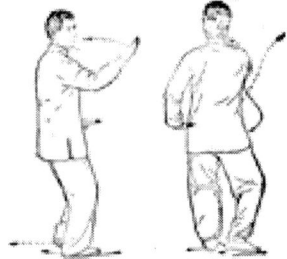

Teaching Hints & Modifications - First Repulse Monkey is to 6 o'clock. Ensure follow step is not too close to heel to allow for transition into Repulse Monkey R.

24 Repulse Monkey Right

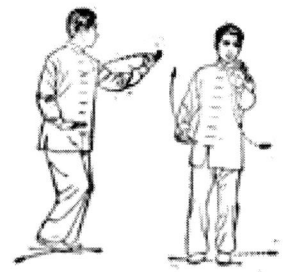

Teaching Hints & Modifications - Unmodified - lifts L toes only and swivels on R toes to face new direction. Modified – steps back R &angles foot to 9'c'clock then lifts L foot to orient body to diagonal for Repulse Monkey R

25 Brush Knee and Twist Step Left

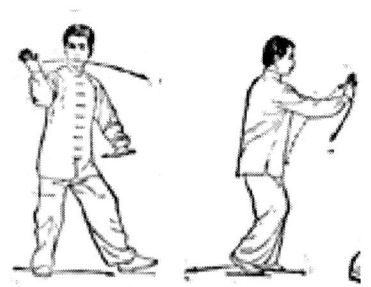

26 Leisurely Tying Coat Left

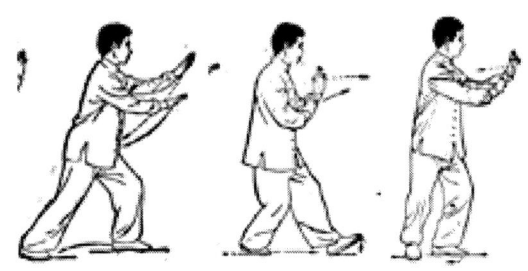

Teaching Hints & Modifications - When pulling back with the arms try to sink the shoulders, and turn the waist slightly so that the low arm is away from the other hand. Co-ordinate the L arm with the L leg.

27-29 Opening Hands ... Closing Hands ... Single Whip Right

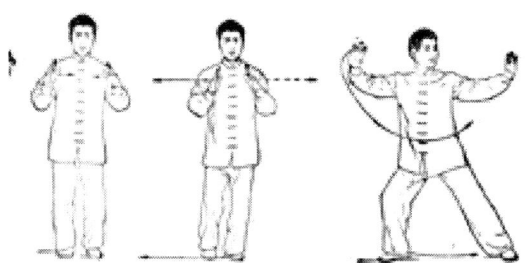

30 Waving Hands Like Clouds Right

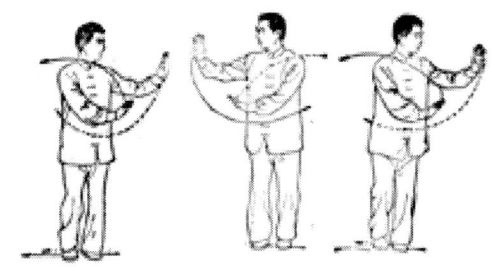

Teaching Hints and Modifications - The placement of the arms should be in front of the body with the turning waist not at the side of the body. For transfer, stretch out leg before the swap.

112

31 Higher Horse

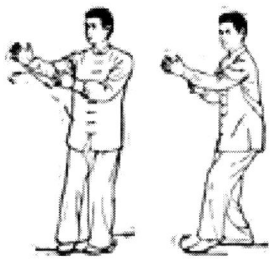

Teaching Hints & Modifications – Place the last Wave Hands follow step slightly behind and on the diagonal. Take time to sink at the end of the final posture before the transition.

32 Toe Kick Left

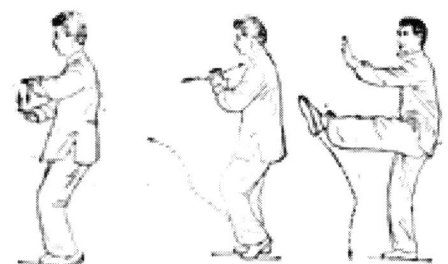

Teaching Hints & Modifications – Hand and leg are in same alignment. Be aware of the placement of the other arm.

33 Toe Kick Right

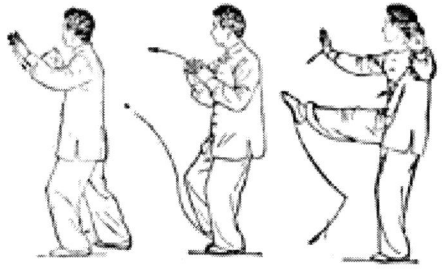

Teaching Hints & Modifications – Gently lower toes to floor to re-align spine until balance is achieved without lowering the foot at all.

Section Three – Forms 32 - 41

34 Step On Firmly to Punch Downwards

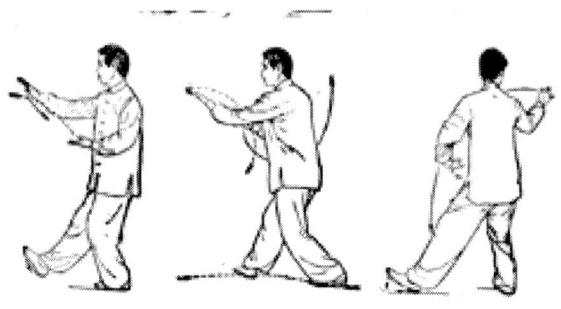

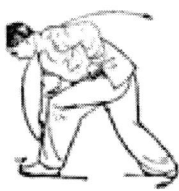

Teaching Hints & Modifications - Keep back upright, weighted mainly on front (70/30), glance down to where the punch is directed. Avoid locking in back leg. L fist is flexed at wrist and horizontal to floor.

35 Turn Body and Jump Up With Both Feet

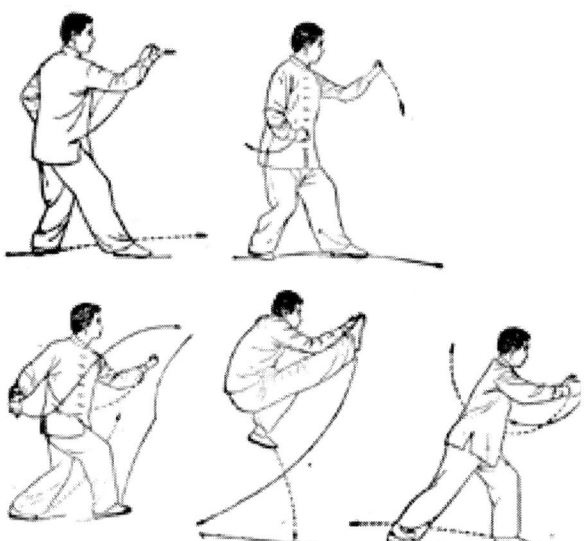

Teaching Hints & Modifications - Turn Body Double Kicks - Legs: Turn to 9 o'clock, step R, step L – same as DVD. Step R again, lift L knee, place L foot straight down, brush R leg fwd straight to pat toe or foot (or bring R leg through bent at knee, pat R thigh), place R leg behind, foot 45 degrees, heel anchored, weight 70/30 to front leg. Arms: same as DVD up to L step. Use L arm to assist lift, open the fist and lower to both hands in front position, width of head, fingers up.

36 Subdue the Tiger

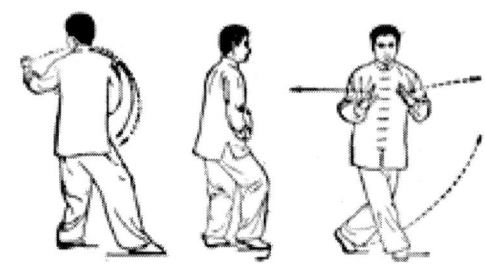

Teaching Hints & Modifications – Transfer weight first. With the step back to diagonal turn the waist and allow R heel to come off the floor. Arms sweep in an oval curve. To train R knee, angle body slightly to corner.

37 Toe Kick Left

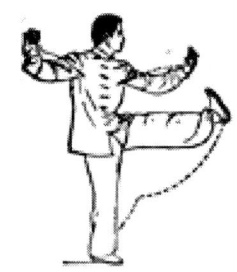

Teaching Hints & Modifications – This kick is a toe kick, not a heel kick as in diagram. Lower the heel to push through for the straight leg kick.

38 Turning Body and Kicking With Heel

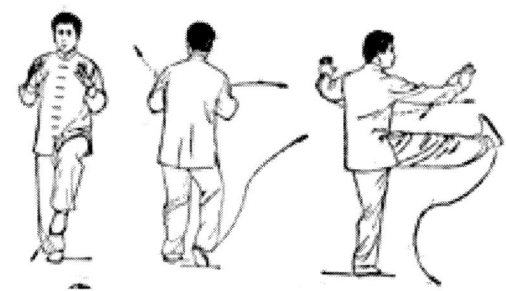

Teaching Hints & Modifications – This can be walked around in 3 small steps to finish at diagonal back. If turning, step close to the other leg and minimize force to control lowering. Heel kick is directed to 9 o'clock. Keep L arm slightly in front of the body.

**39 Step Forward to Deflect
Downwards, Parry and Punch**

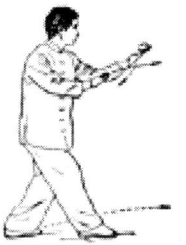

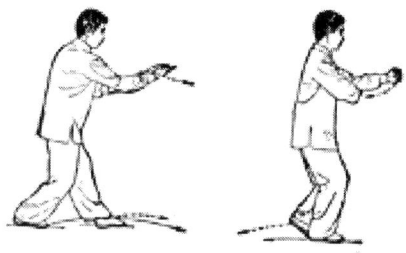

Teaching Hints & Modifications – Keep the
body weight on the back leg to place the heel.

**40-41 Apparent Closing Up .... Carrying the
Tiger and Pushing the Mountain**

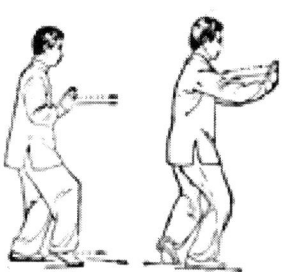

115

Section Four – Forms 42 - 53

42-43 Opening Hands ... Closing Hands

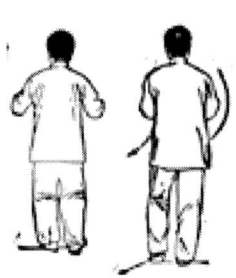

44-48 Brush Knee and Twist Step Left ...
Leisurely Tying Coat...Opening Hands ...
Closing Hands ... Diagonal Single Whip

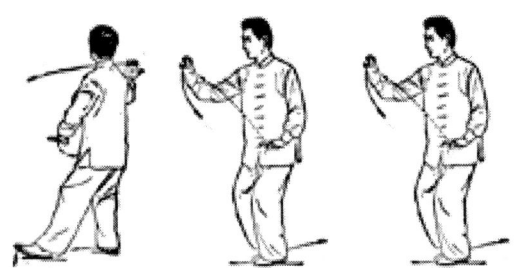

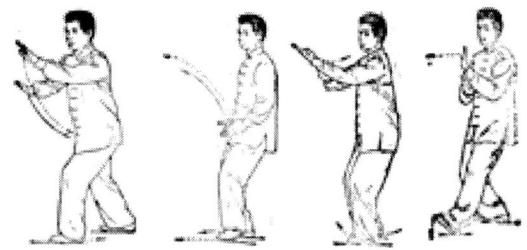

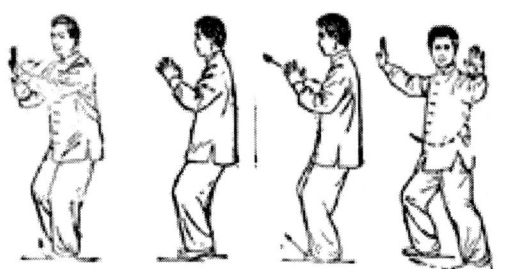

49 Parting Wild Horse's Mane

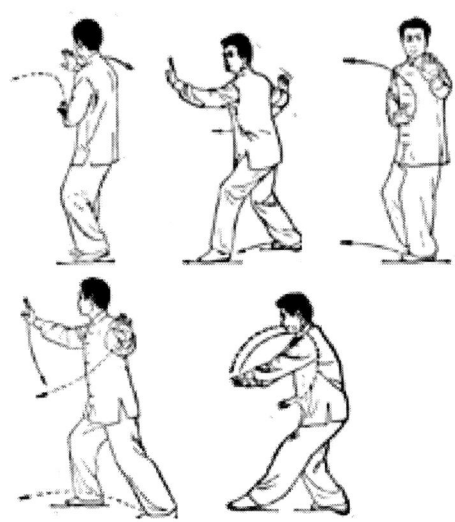

Teaching Hints & Modifications – Allow the moving arm to lower and co-ordinate with the moving empty leg. Follow upper arm with eyes. L leg comes across with arm to step through on heel L. Hands cross R hand aligned with L foot. Circle arms with transfer of weight.

50-53 Leisurely Tying Coat ... Opening Hands ... Closing Hands   ... Single Whip Left

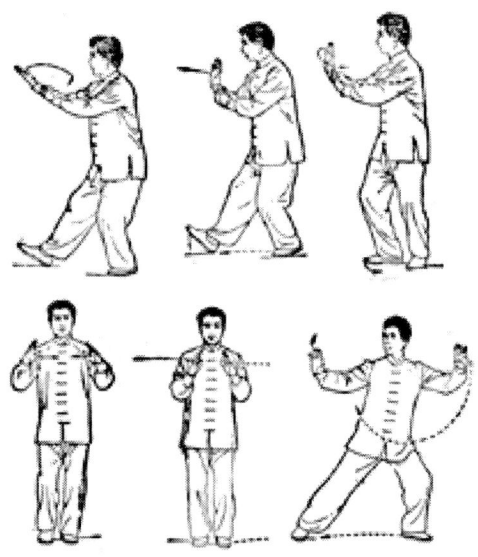

Teaching Hints & Modifications – When changing direction for Open Close, transfer weight cleanly on first leg leaving the other foot clear for toe clearance.

Section five – Forms 54 to 73

54 Waving Hands Like Clouds Left

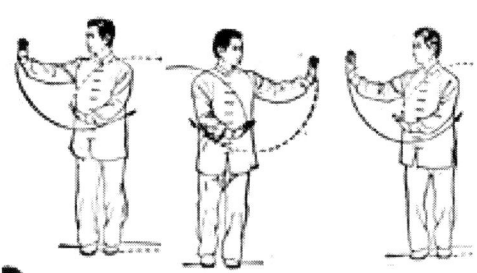

55 Waving Hands Like Clouds and Lowering Movement

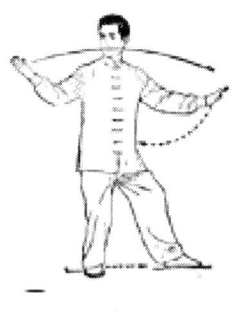

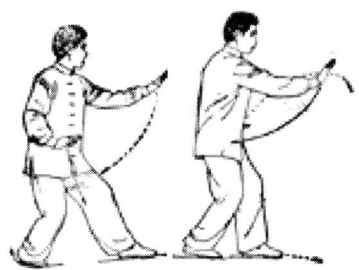

Teaching Hints & Modifications – On 3rd Wave Hands roll the foot toe first on the diagonal to L corner to change weight. Separate arms wide to prepare for the Lowering Movement.

56 Golden Cock Standing on One Leg

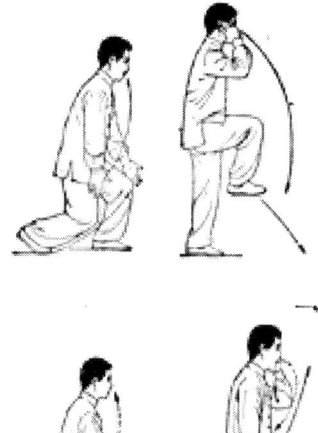

Teaching Hints & Modifications – Turn foot out if turning the waist or leave straight if stepping straight ahead.

57 Fan Back

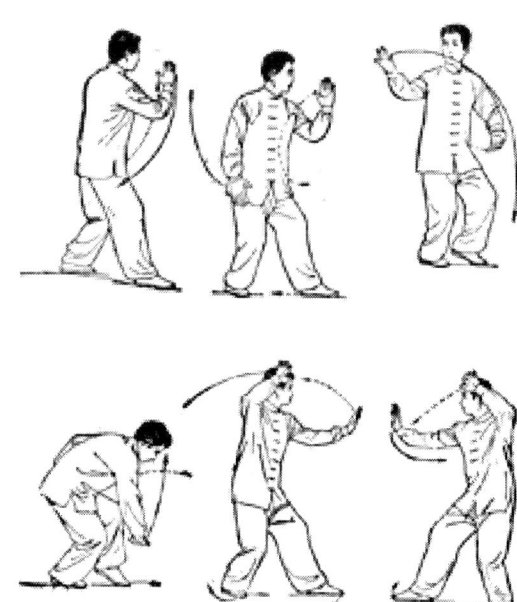

Teaching Hints & Modifications – Remain upright for the pat down. Sink shoulders for the high fan and keep a little weight on the front foot for the delivery of the force.

58 Fair Lady Working At the Shuttles

59 Higher Horse

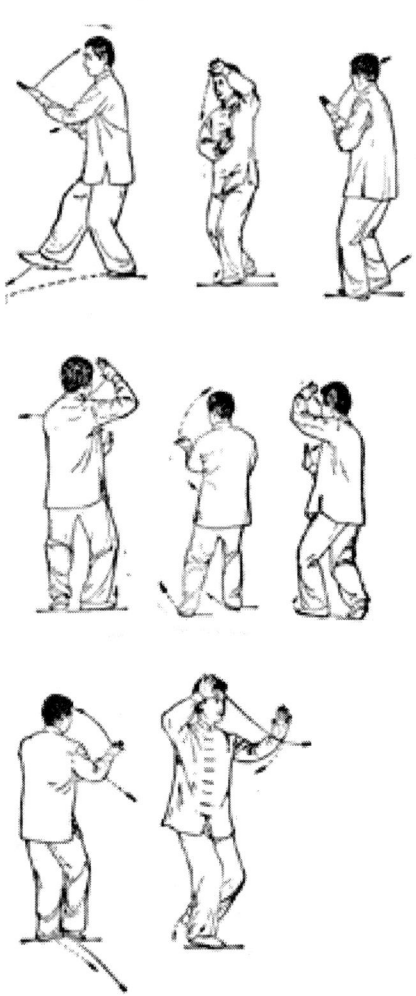

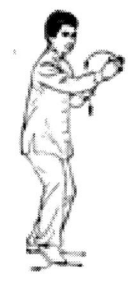

60   Cross Hands and Patting Foot

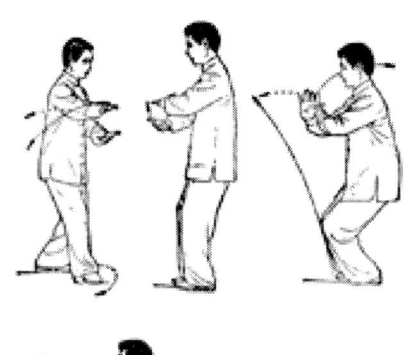

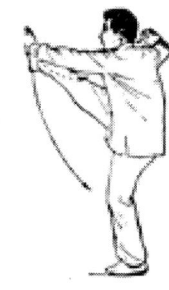

Teaching Hints & Modifications - Really, there is no reasonable modification for Lady except to perform legs concentrating on weight change and direction until legs are consolidated and balance is stable. Practise arms as a separate exercise taking care to press the hand from the mid chest to armpit only and co-ordinate with the spiral movement and push out of the other hand. Practise co-ordinated as a drill before trying the directional change.

Teaching Hints & Modifications – Bend the knees to gather the momentum for the kick. If posture is compromised because of the straight kick or lotus kick, substitute with bent knee patting thigh while maintaining posture.

61 Forward Step to Punch Crouch

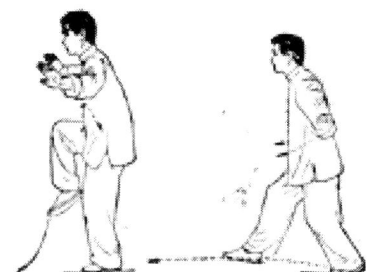

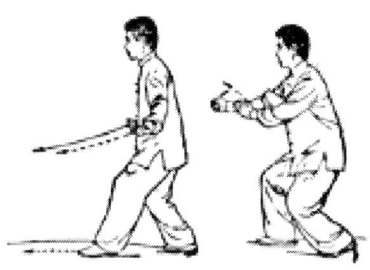

Teaching Hints & Modifications – After the Kick, step down gently onto heel to roll Forward for the 3steps forward.

62   Lively Step and Leisurely Tying Coat

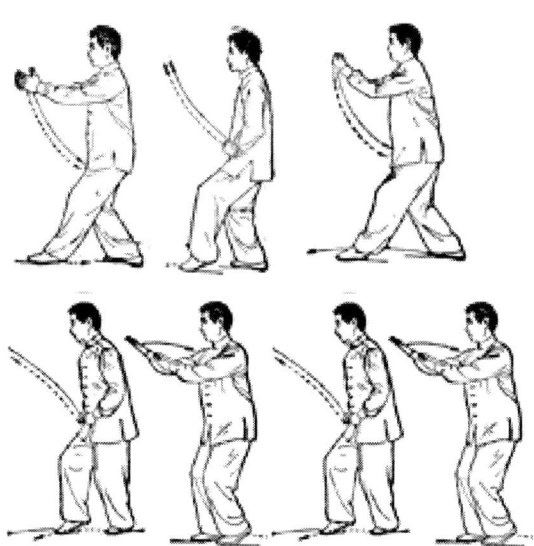

Teaching Hints & Modifications – After the punch, roll the back foot back to step onto R foot for the double punch forward. Keep fists apart.

63-65 Opening Hands … Closing Hands … Single Whip Left

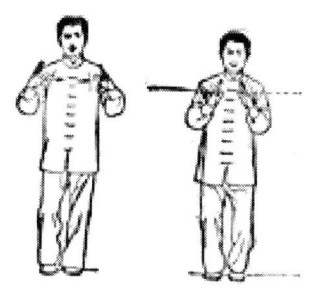

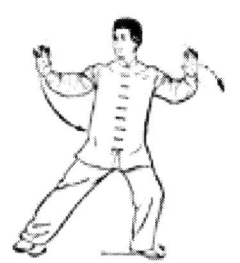

66 Single Whip and Lowering Movement

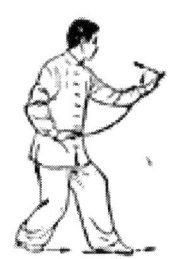

67 Forward Step Seven Stars

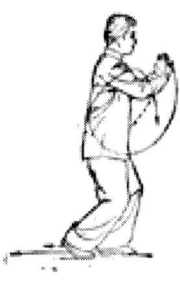

119

68 Backward Step Riding Tiger

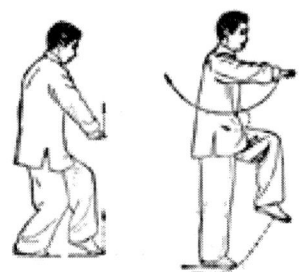

Teaching Hints & Modifications – Maintain upright position before sinking and lifting leg and upper arm together.

69 Turn Body, Lotus Kick

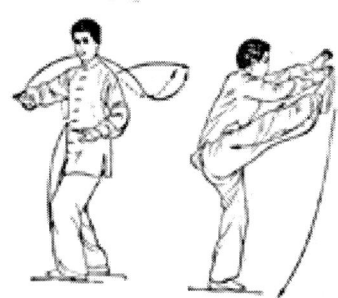

Teaching Hints & Modifications - After the pat down for the preparation for the turn maintain posture and change weight (swap feet position) and adjust arms to opposite side. This will be in the preparation position for the Lotus kick. The weight will be on the L, empty on the R and both arms to the side R (i.e. 12 o'clock).

70 Drawing Bow to Shoot Tiger

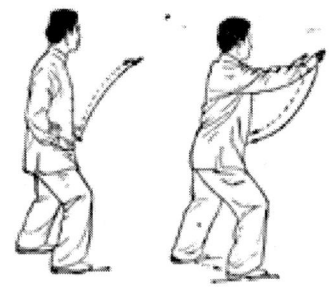

Teaching Hints & Modifications – Lower the foot as if stepping to R diagonal but orient torso to L as weight change.

71 Double Forward Punch

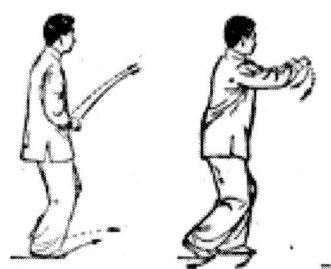

Teaching Hints & Modifications – Begin to turn the waist with the delivery of the double punch dropping the level of the right fist to near the L wrist before the transition to the front.

72 Yin and Yang Merging into One

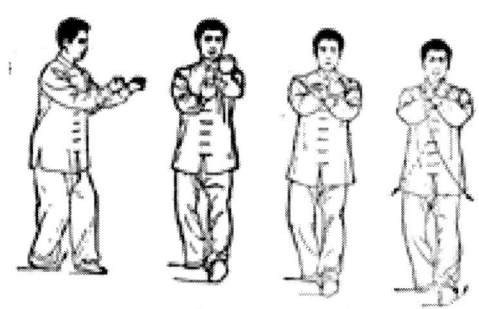

73 Closing

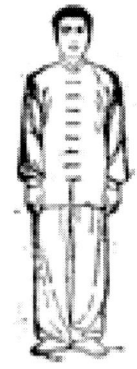

Teaching Hints & Modifications – Remind the student of the importance of the Wuji position and hold for at least 3-4 seconds focussing the mind on breathing and posture.

5.40   Introduction to AUSTRALIA DREAMING by Elva Arthy [28]

A wonderful way to improve Tai Chi is learning how to visualise the form and reproduce it in movement as accurately as possible. Teaching the brain to perceive a posture or the several postures that make up a form is not always easily accomplished. Some people have great difficulty in visualising an image of themselves or of the teacher performing the move.

One very successful method of enhancing the ability to create self-images of body positions and movement patterns is to improve the thought processes that connect an image of the movement to actually executing the movement. Thinking about an image can be vague or clear, easy or difficult. Some images have pieces missing (eg. one arm or the feet – the image is missing) or can be complete in much detail. In Tai Chi such terms as *White Crane Stretches Its Wings* or *Playing the Lute* link an image (crane or lute) with a movement that may bear some recognisable connection to that image – for example, the shape of the arms resemble the wings of the white crane stretching and the movement of the hand mimics the strumming of the lute. Being able to visualise the form as they see it or would like to do it enhances and improves the efficiency of not only learning the forms but the efficiency of the body working technically balanced and well positioned.

Australia Dreaming has been developed with Australian images linked to Tai Chi movements and postures in the Sun Style. My intention was to give students the freedom to focus on colours and images of Australia with the familiar movements they are learning with the Sun Style. The forms or parts of the forms were taken from the 73 Competition Forms composed by Professor Men Hui Feng and taught to me by my teacher Dr Paul Lam. Although we often perform this set in a circle, it can also be practised with the class facing the teacher. Most importantly, the movements should be continuous and flowing with the weight constantly changing. The movements are slow enough and smooth enough to co-ordinate with slow and relaxed breathing.

My driving motivation in thinking about *Australia Dreaming* was to find a special sequence using the Sun Style with images that were uniquely Australian, a special set of forms that would have some familiarity and deep attachment for indigenous Australians. The colours of the sun, the images of birds and animals are meant to evoke easily recognisable pictures of the Australian environment. Tai Chi is now a global experience touching the lives and health for many people of diverse cultures. I have a deep hope that our indigenous Australian family would enjoy practising this short tribute to the land they have lovingly cared for over thousands of generations.

I also especially hoped that children and older people would want to learn more about Tai Chi and in so doing would help to improve their health and give their day-to-day activities strength and calmness as it has done for so many people across the world. There is absolutely no doubt that Tai Chi's gentle, non-threatening, continuous, flowing, weight-bearing, balanced movements practised daily would have a dramatic effect on health and that the deep breathing and focus would unquestionably help to reduce stress, calm and relax and improve the quality of life of many.

I wish to acknowledge the art-work for *Australia Dreaming* to my sister Gail Higgins who is an award winning, international wildlife artist. Her watercolours give the suggestion of the images so that the student can enhance and expand in full bright colour and definition and thus create their own images of their experience or imagination.

---

[28] This is the Introduction written by Elva in the publication titled *Australia Dreaming Tribute to the Ancestors Sun Style Tai Chi* (Arthy and Arthy 2008) which was taken to Tai Chi for Health workshop at South Hadley in Massachusetts held in June 2008. Apart from minor, but important, changes having been made in the imagery, the Qigong set in this book is the same. The first performance of this Qigong set by Elva was at the Tai Chi for Health workshop at Connecticut in 2003.

5.50   Australia Dreaming Qigong 15 Forms

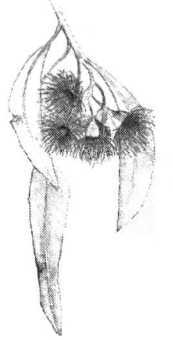

AUSTRALIA DREAMING: Tribute to our ancestors

1   FIRST LIGHT
Silent and cool
Babies cry
Kookaburras begin to laugh

2   FIRST BREATH
Gentle rush of air
Before the dawn
Welcomes the sun

3   SUN RISE
Beautiful colours
Reds and yellows
Break of day

4   BRAND NEW DAY
The day opens
To a bright light beautiful day
A brand new day has begun

5   DESERT WIND SWEEPS THE NULLARBOR
Blowing constantly
Sweeping
The great Nullarbor smooth and flat

6   BLUE SKY, WHITE CLOUDS
Sail across the sky
The sky bright and blue
The clouds large and white

7   GOANNA HIDES FROM THE SUN
In the shade of a large rock
Protected
From the scorching desert sun

8   PERENTIE WAITS
Most feared predator
Its massive legs and body
Fearsome eyes mean danger

9   BROLGA FLASHES ITS WINGS
Stretching
Its beautiful long feathered wings
Revealing its long sleek back

10 JABIRU TAKES FLIGHT
Showing
Its elegant black and white plumage
Before taking flight across the billabong

11 RAIN FALLS ON KAKADU
Large heavy raindrops
Fall on the water lilies' rainbow petals
Amongst the grasses and trees of Kakadu

12 RAINBOW SERPENT GUARDIAN SPIRIT
Totem of life
Of mother earth
Of water and mythical beginnings

13 SUNSET, END OF DAY
Brilliant reflections on the clouds
Warm colours of the setting sun
As far as you can see

14 SOUTHERN CROSS
Pointing the way
Among millions of stars filling the night sky
Shining and twinkling in the moonlight

15 DREAMTIME
Time to rest   Time to sleep
Time to remember the past
To light the way to a better future
A tribute to all our ancestors

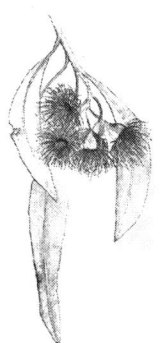

Teaching Hint: *When teaching Australia Dreaming, it may be necessary to repeat individual forms three or more times to develop the imagery and colours. When an image is formed, move onto the next image. Teaching the set is a gradual process. It may take several months to teach the movements, develop the imagery, keep up the flow, relax and breathe comfortably.*

1 – FIRST LIGHT

Silent and cool
Babies cry
Kookaburras begin to laugh

Starting Position - Sun Wuji and Opening Movement- Form 1

1   Sun Wuji is starting Position: arms by side, heels together, toes turned out slightly, focus on relaxing shoulders and upright posture

2   Stepping out to comfortable stance approx wide as hips/shoulders and prepare – *Imagery words start*

3   Lifting arms front to shoulder height and level, palms facing each other, fingers pointing slightly down, relax shoulders, lift to shoulder height and width

4   Keeping shoulders relaxed and sinking elbows, raise fingers – Remember "Toby Tall"

5   Move arms to "open-close" position ready for next movement

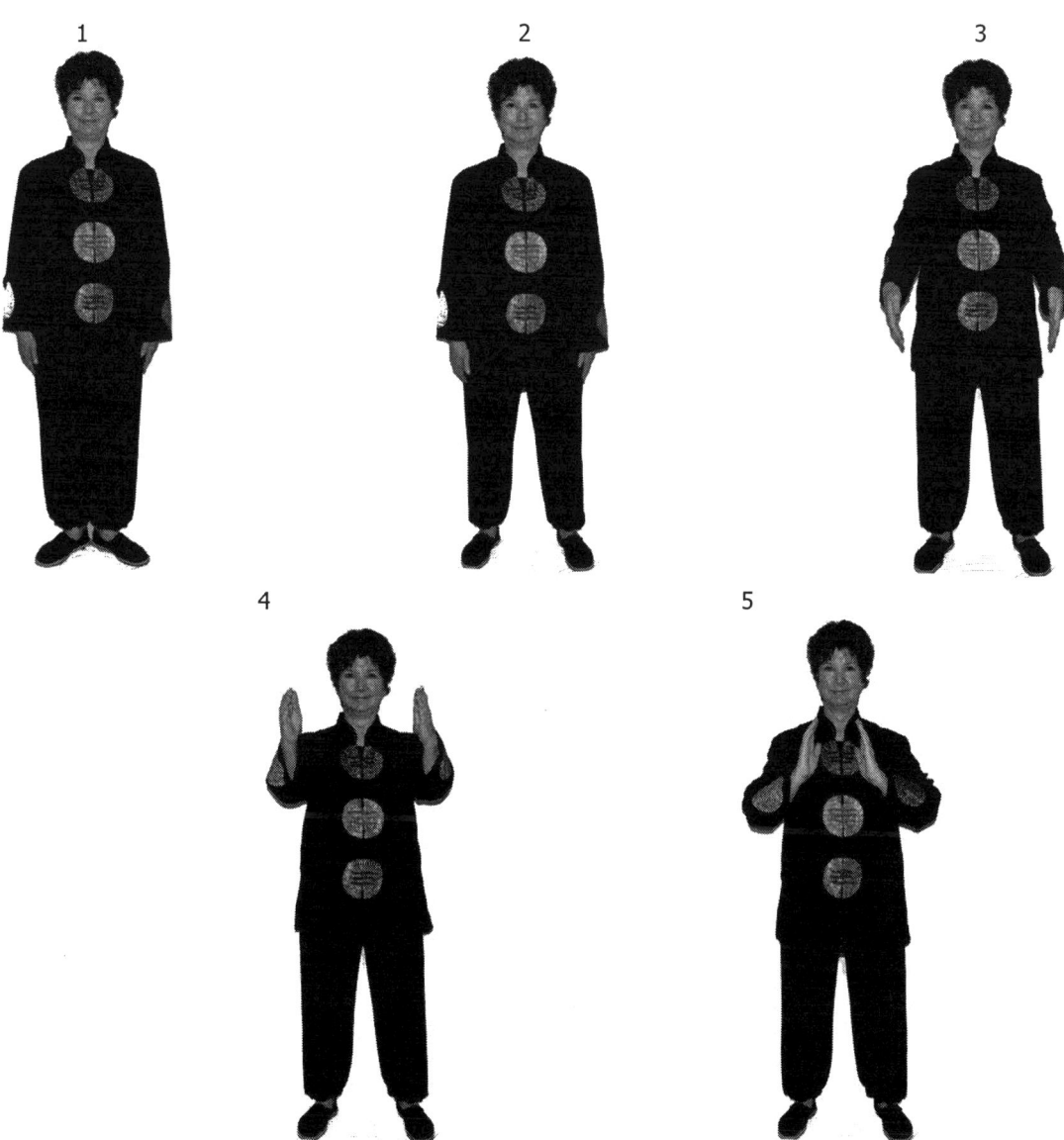

Teaching Tips & Hints – A chance to relax, focus on good posture, imagery and breathing throughout

2 – FIRST BREATH

Gentle rush of air
Before the dawn,
Welcomes the sun

Open and Close Movement- Forms 3 and 4

1   Hands facing each other in front, a face-width distance apart, relaxing shoulders, elbows pointing down

2   Moving hands apart breathing slowly, abdominal breath in, thumbs pointing to shoulders, feeling slight change from one leg to the other with gentle rocking motion

3   Moving hands back together, using mind to feel resistance of air pushing inwards, exhale, back to same as in 1 above

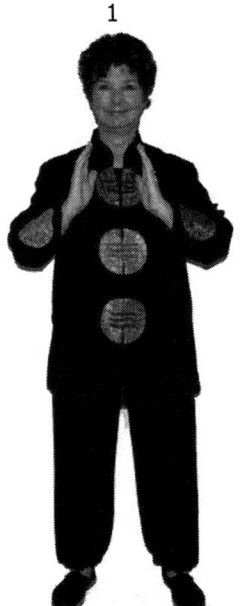
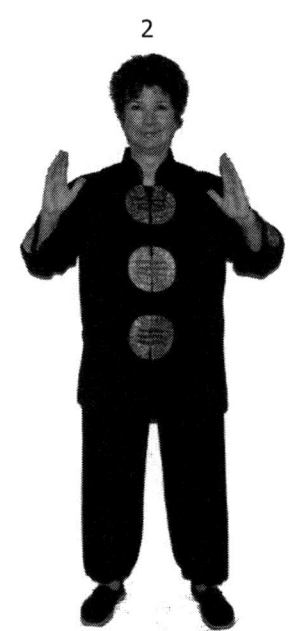
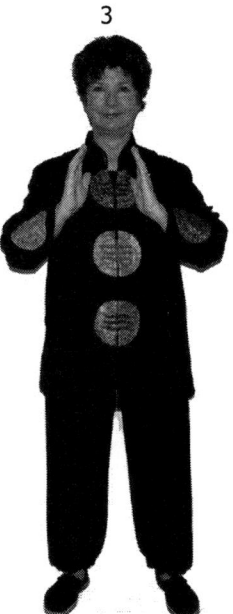

1   2   3

Teaching Tips & Hints - Chance to relax focus on breathing and visualising - choice to repeat once or twice with or without words - keep the knees soft and with the open and close movements - feel the resistance between the palms, pulling away and gently pressing in - imagine you are pressing a balloon

3 - SUNRISE

Beautiful colours
Reds and yellows
Break of day

Single Whip - Form 5

1   Weight to the L and feather touch R heel to the side, push forward with hands slightly fingers staying upright

2   Turn palms to the front - at the same time lower the toes and transfer some of the body weight onto the right leg keeping the knee over the toes - make sure that the base of the body is over the floor slightly more than half way to the weight bearing leg

3   Open the arms wide, palms facing front

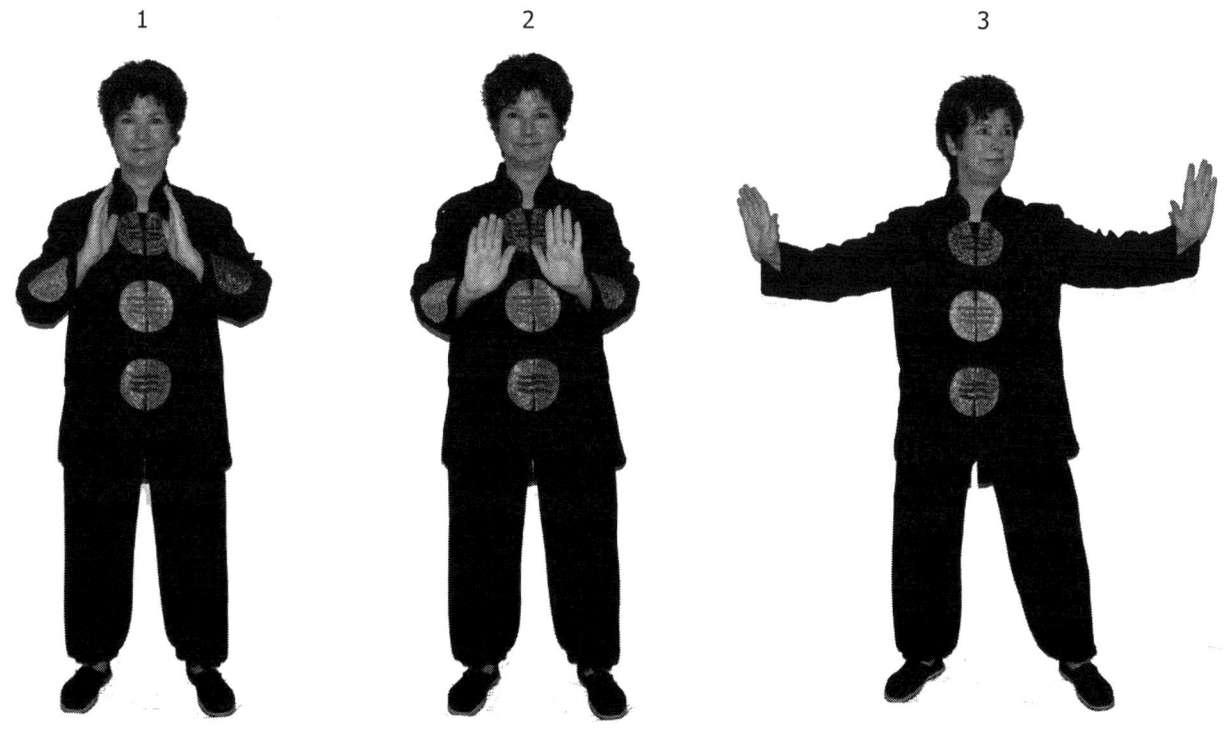

| 1 | 2 | 3 |

Teaching Tips & Hints - Keep the shoulders relaxed - hands should be curved from the heel of the hand to the finger tips and the fingers should be upright – caution- do not force the hands or wrists - use hands in a comfortable way-   at end of form 3 look to the L

4 – BRAND NEW DAY

The day opens,
To a light bright beautiful day,
A brand new day has begun

Parting Wild Horses Mane - Form 49

1   Starting position

2   Curve arms down towards the centre

3   Cross wrists

4   Begin to lift in a circle

5   Open the circle

6   Finish arms to side hands up

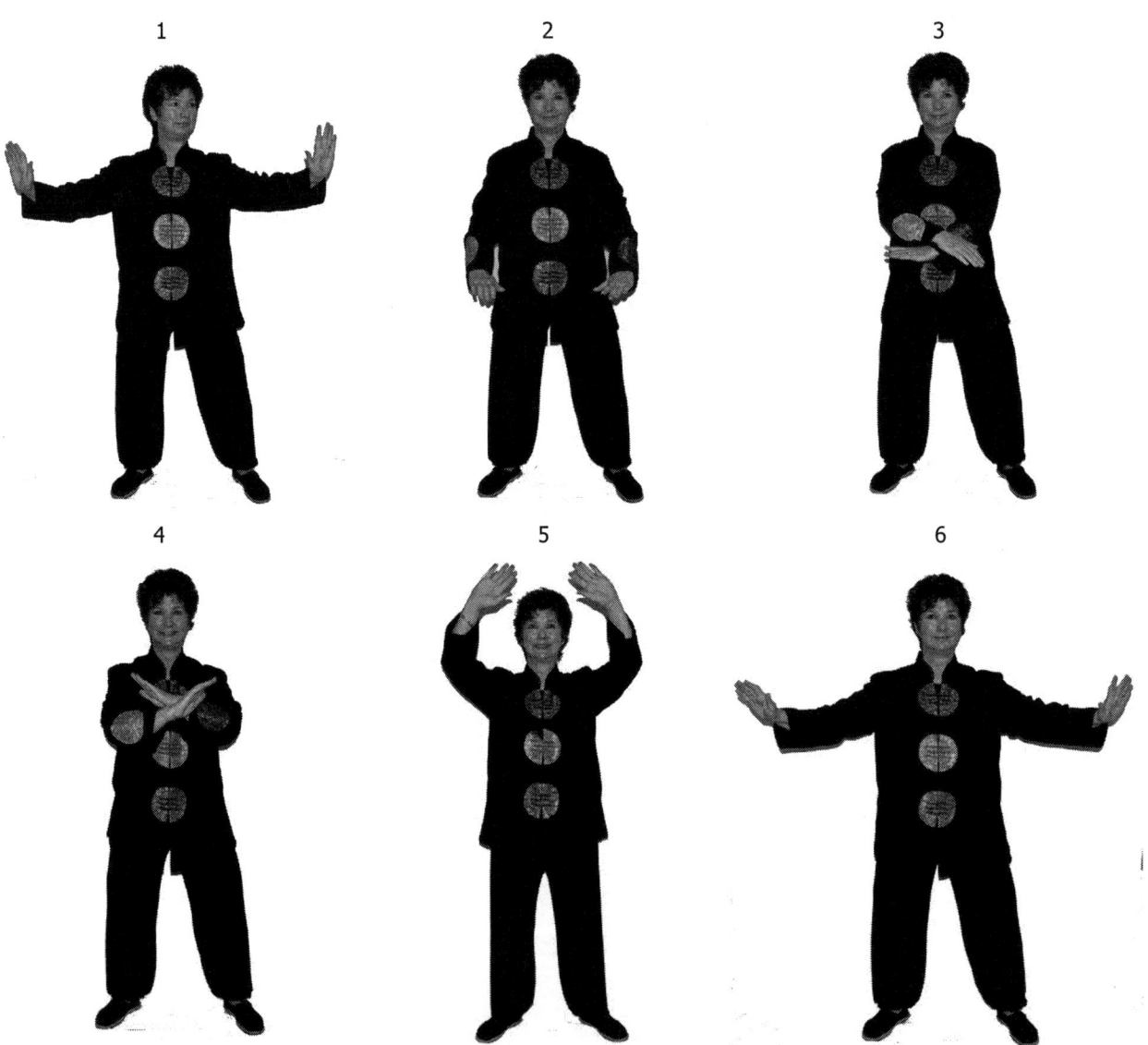

5 - DESERT WIND
SWEEPS THE NULLABOR

Blowing constantly
Sweeping the great Nullarbor
Smooth and flat

Subdue the Tiger - Form 36

1   Starting Position

2   Transfer weight to R, L hand curves low to R side

3   Transferring weight to L, point fingers R and begin to curve back in the same curve

4   Complete transfer to L arms sweeping to L

5–6   Lift and complete the circle, changing weight back to R

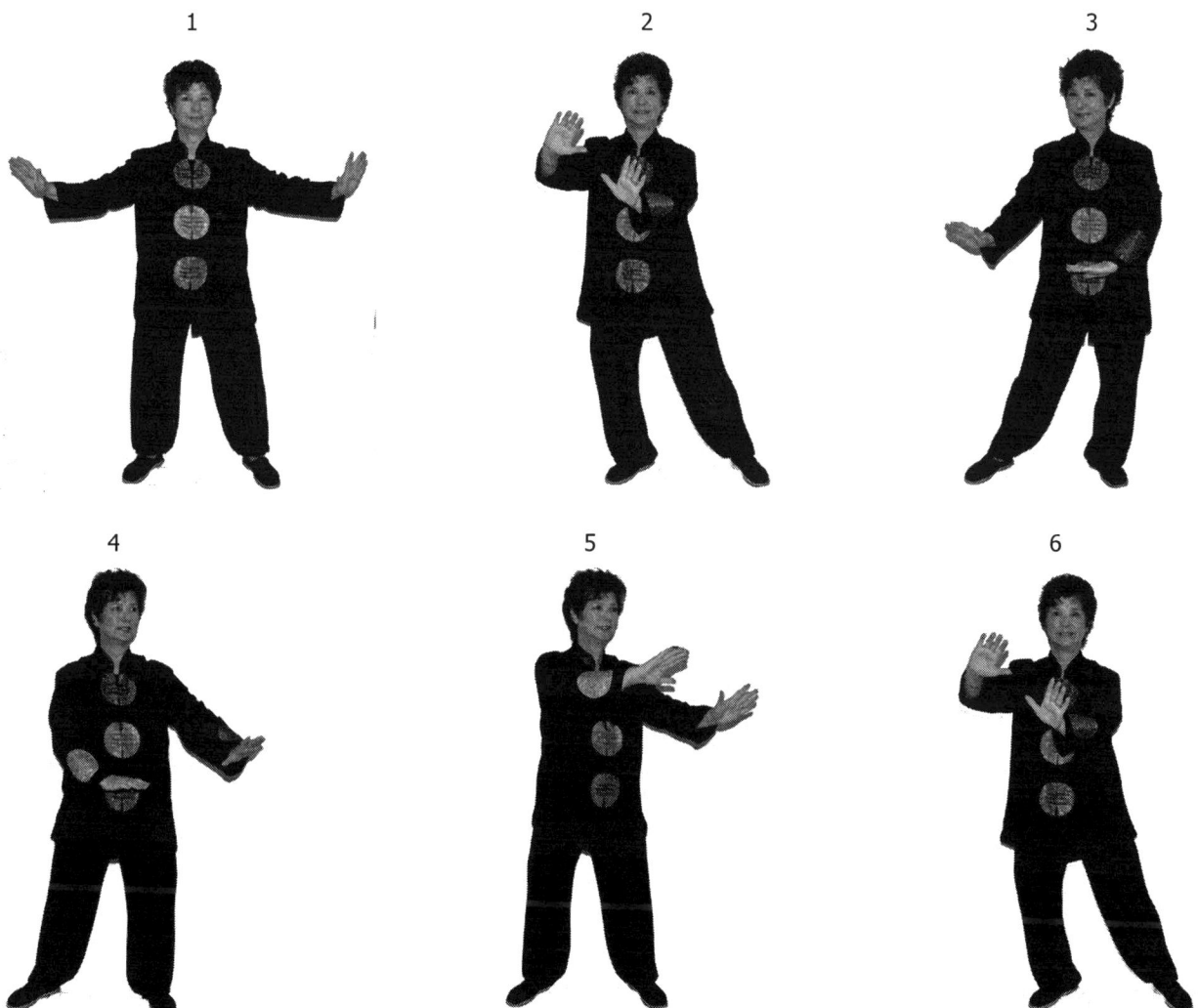

Teaching Tips and Hints

Allow waist to turn with the flow of the curve and slightly anticipate the arms on the return curve

127

6 - BLUE SKY, WHITE CLOUDS

Sail across the sky
The sky bright and blue
The clouds large and white

Waving Hands Like Clouds – Form 30

1   Starting position

2-3   Prepare for wave hands - R hand orients vertical, L hand comes up towards elbow - R hand comes down - step to L and keep arms in front of body as the weight begins to transfer

4-5   Complete the transfer, swap arms and begin to transfer weight back to R

6   Finish to R corner

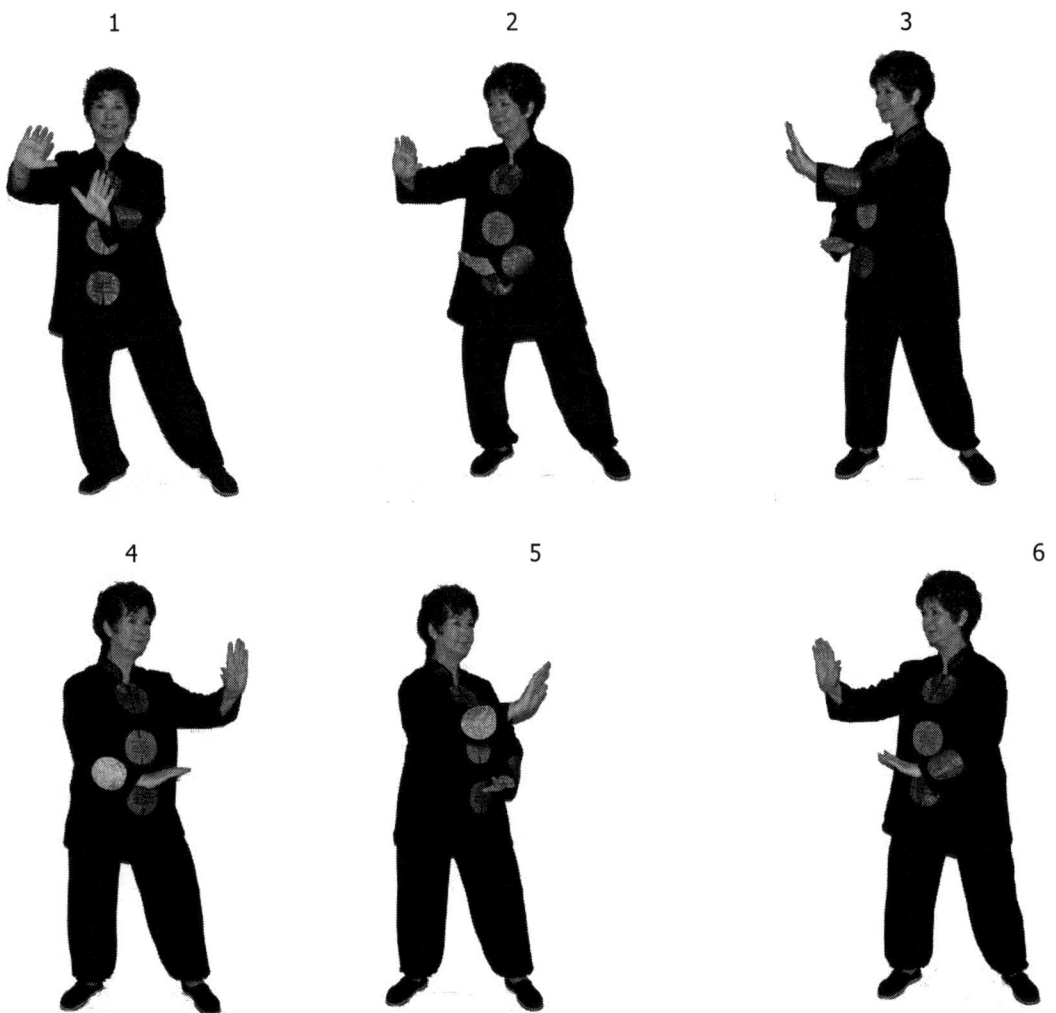

Teaching Tips and Hints

Soften the knees, keep open at the groin and allow to change weight in a natural rhythmical way

7 - GOANNA HIDES FROM THE SUN

In the shade of a large rock
Protected
From the hot desert sun

Fair Lady Working at the Shuttles - Form 58

1   Starting Position

2   Turn L palm up and hug the R forearm sweeping the full length of the arm, R hand finishes at L elbow

3   Point R thumb to centre of chest, R hand lifts above forehead as body turns to the front

4   Spiral the L hand as R hand pushes across the chest, stop as the thumb comes near the arm pit - turn body

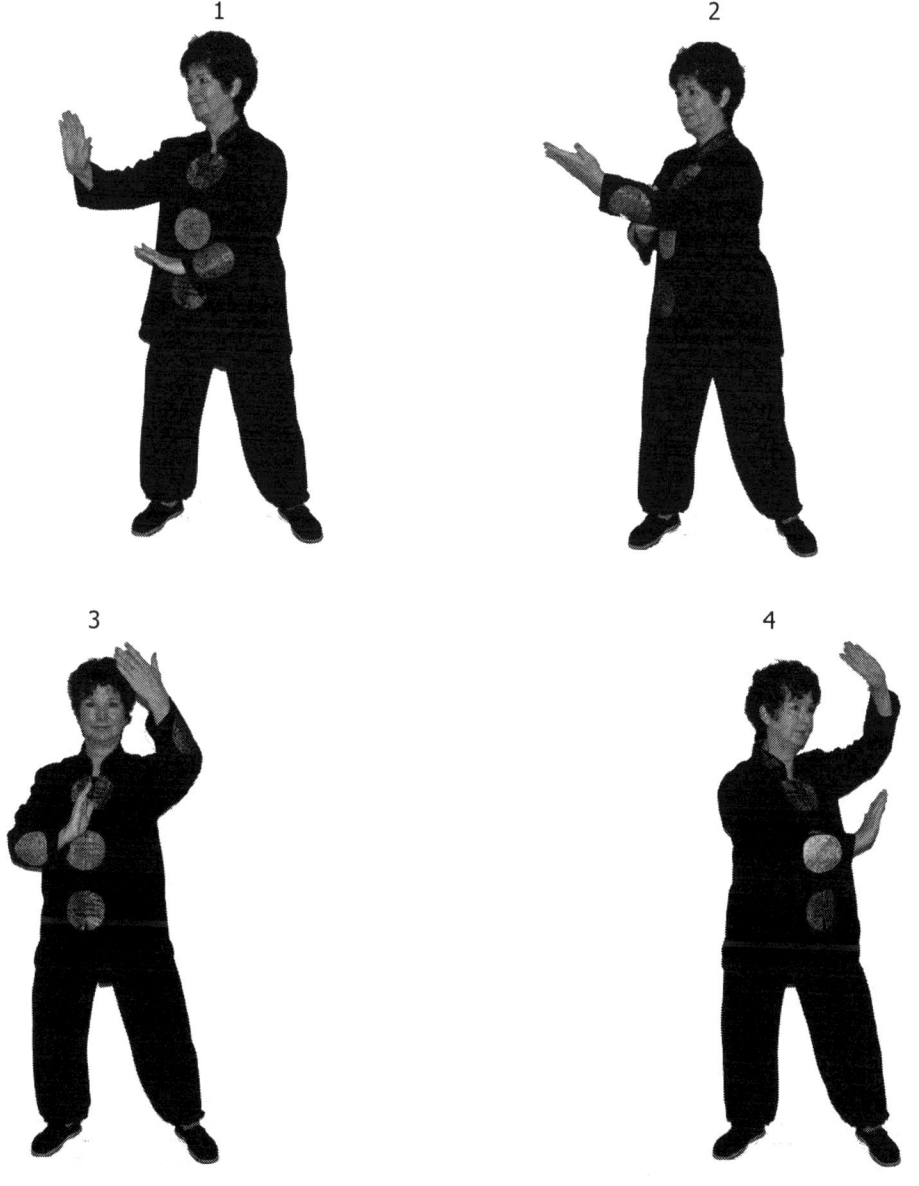

Teaching Tips and Hints - The spiral and push from the mid line with the turn of the body to the L are co-ordinated together exactly

8 - PERENTIE WAITS

Most feared predator
Its massive legs and body
Fearsome eyes mean danger

Step on Firmly to Punch – Form 34

1   Starting Position

2   Lowering Movement – separation of arms begin together - cross wrists and start to transfer weight

3   Open the arms and continue to transfer weight

4   Complete the arms and weight transference, look towards low arm

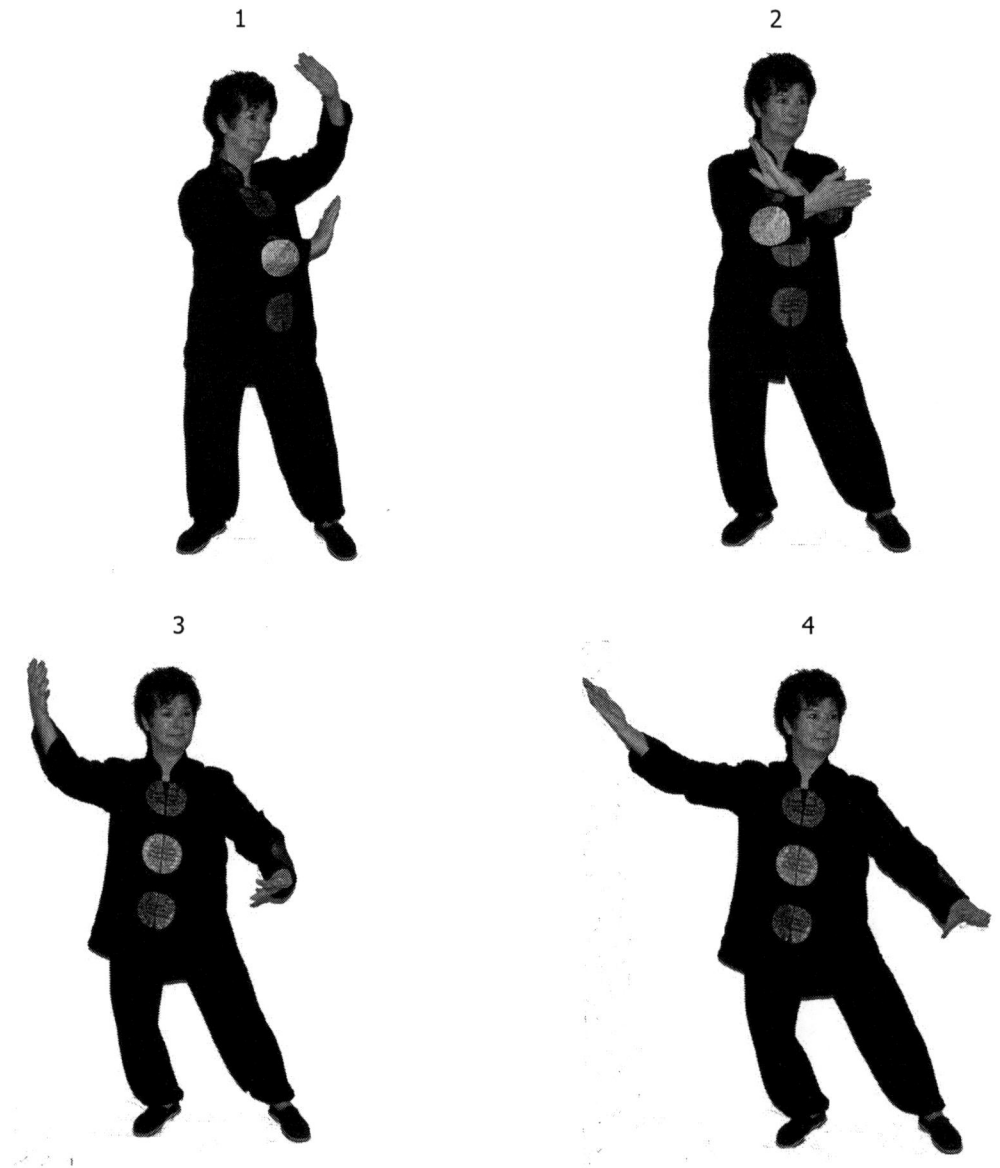

Teaching Tips and Hints - Turn the waist

9 - BROLGA FLASHES ITS WINGS

Stretching
Its beautiful long feathered wings
Revealing its long sleek back

Lifting Hands and White Crane Flashing Wings – Right – Forms 6 & 7

1   Starting Position

2   R arm lifts sideways overhead, palm turned front - at same time L arm sweeps down, palm turned out, weight comes back towards the centre

3   Arms swap with the L hand forming a dropped wrist and R palm front, passing simultaneously at midline

4   Elbows into ribs and push gently front

5   Open arms as in Single Whip

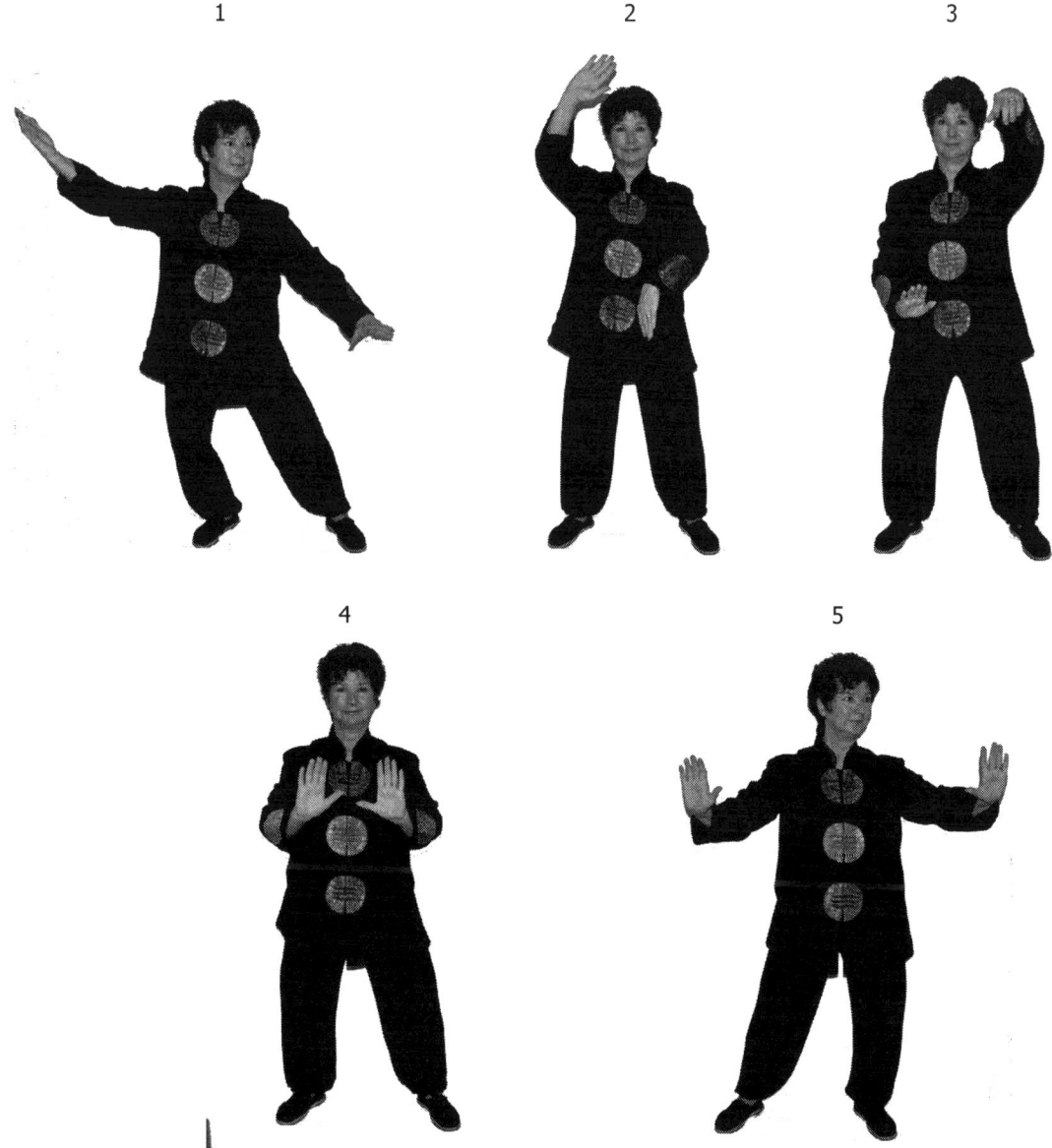

Teaching Tips and Hints - Keep shoulders lowered when lifting arms – the low arm in 2 should be away from the body in the midline

131

10 - JABIRU TAKES FLIGHT   *Showing*
Its elegant black and white plumage
Before taking flight across the billabong

Lifting Hands and White Crane Flashing Wings – Left – Forms 6 & 7

1   Starting Position

2   R arm lifts sideways overhead, palm turned front. At the same time L arm sweeps down, palm turned out, weight comes back to the centre

3   Swap arms drooping the R wrist and raising L palm front, passing in the midline

4   Push elbows into ribs and gently push forward, thumbs facing

5   Open as in Single Whip looking R

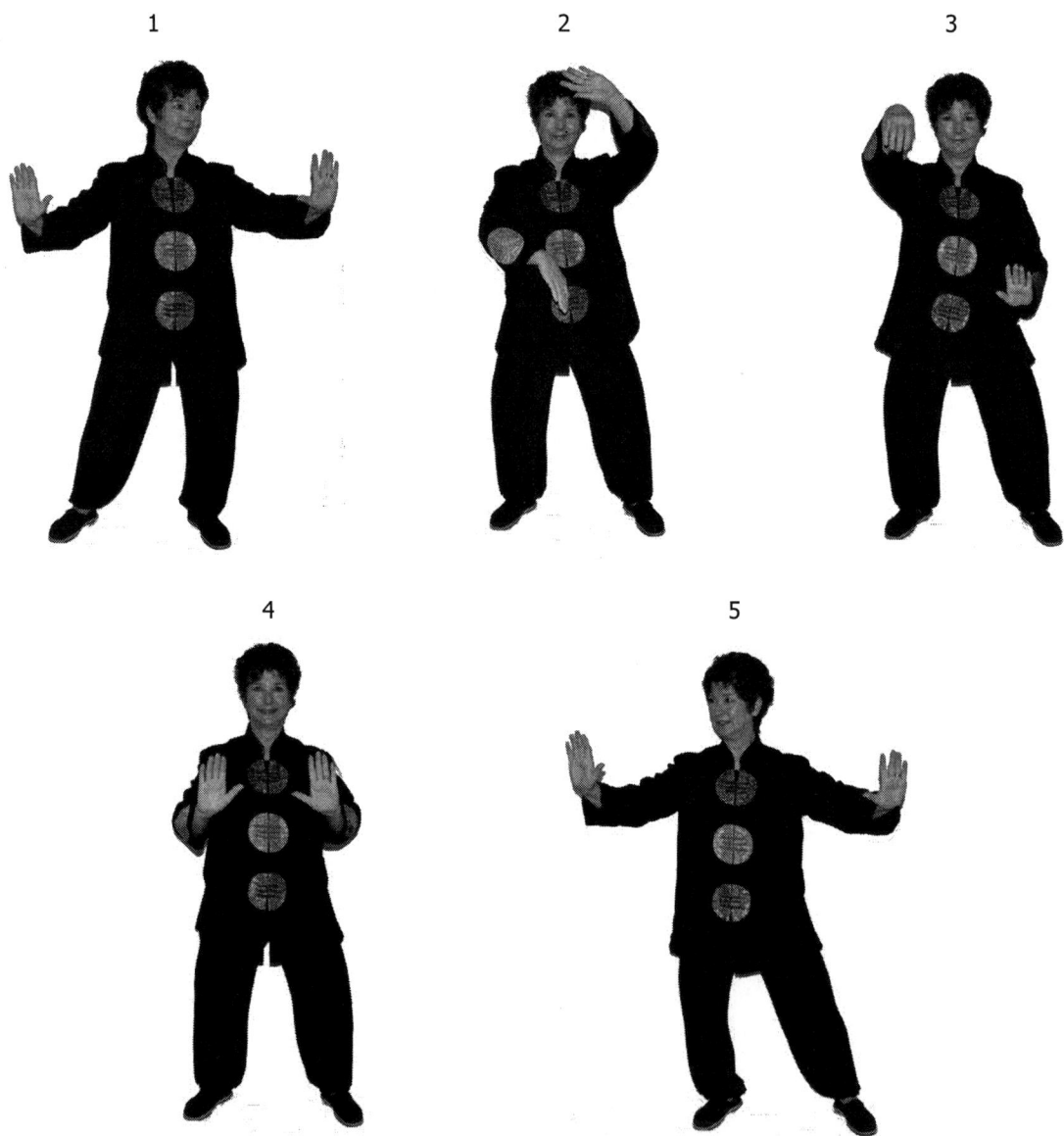

11- RAIN FALLS ON KAKADU

Large heavy raindrops
Fall on the water lilies' rainbow petals
Amongst the grasses and trees of Kakadu

Fan Back – Form 57

1   Starting position

2   L hand comes to centre, palm facing down and R hand sweeps to centre till it is above L hand - R hand then pats down, palm facing down - continue patting down movement with R hand as body turns slightly L

3   Turn underneath hand up as R hand continues to pat - lift L hand until it is over R and body has turned

4   Pat down L hand and lowering movement

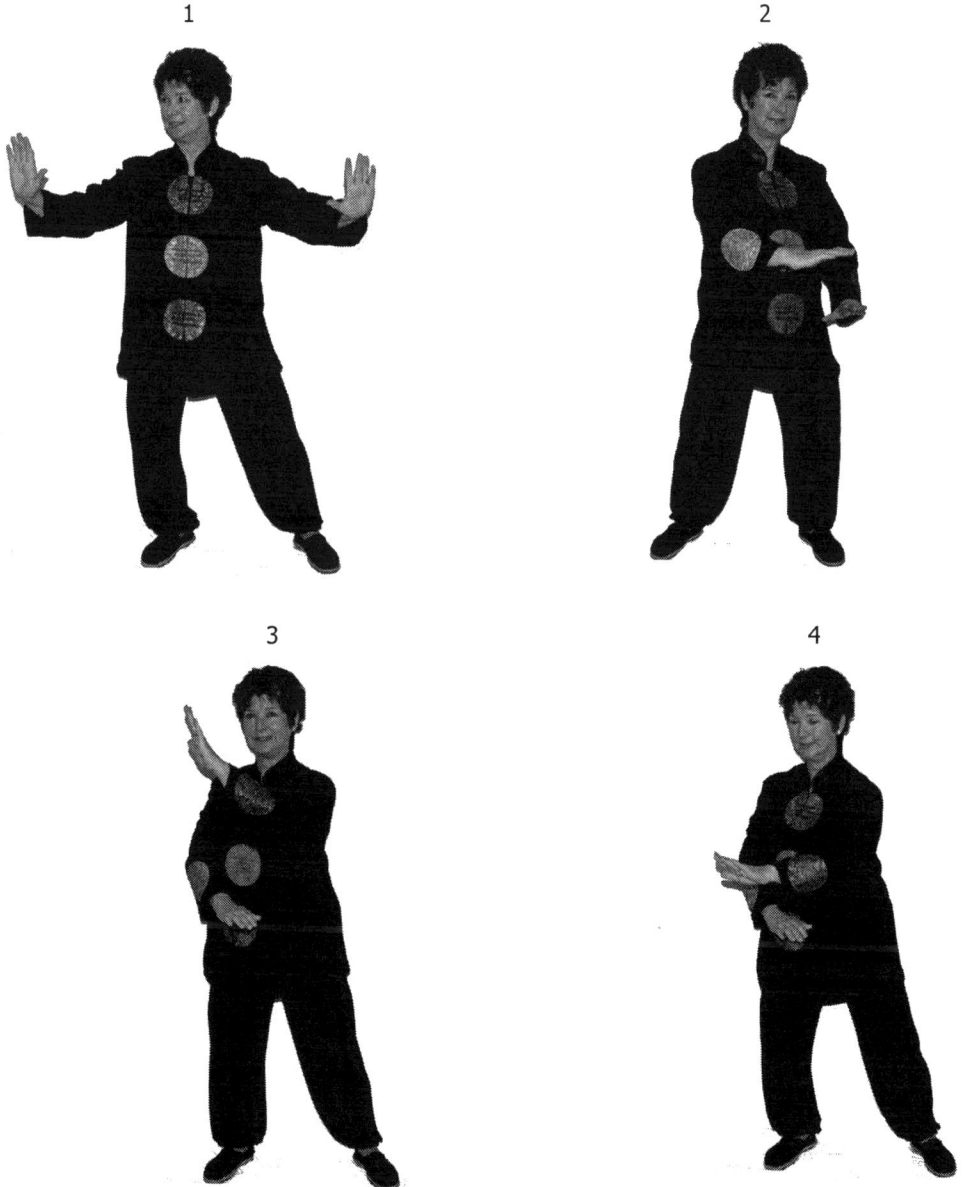

Teaching Tips and Hints - It is important to turn the waist but not lose the upright posture of the spine

133

12- RAINBOW SERPENT
GUARDIAN SPIRIT

Totem of life
Of mother earth
Of water and mythical beginnings

Step Forward to Deflect – Form 12

1   Starting Position

2   Step Forward to Deflect Downwards to Parry - R palm turns over as L hip prepares

3   Slide fingers along forearm until fingers extend to the midline, parry complete weight on L

4   Turn hands together and begin to change weight

5   Slide L hand to front, R hand finishing at elbow, weight to R

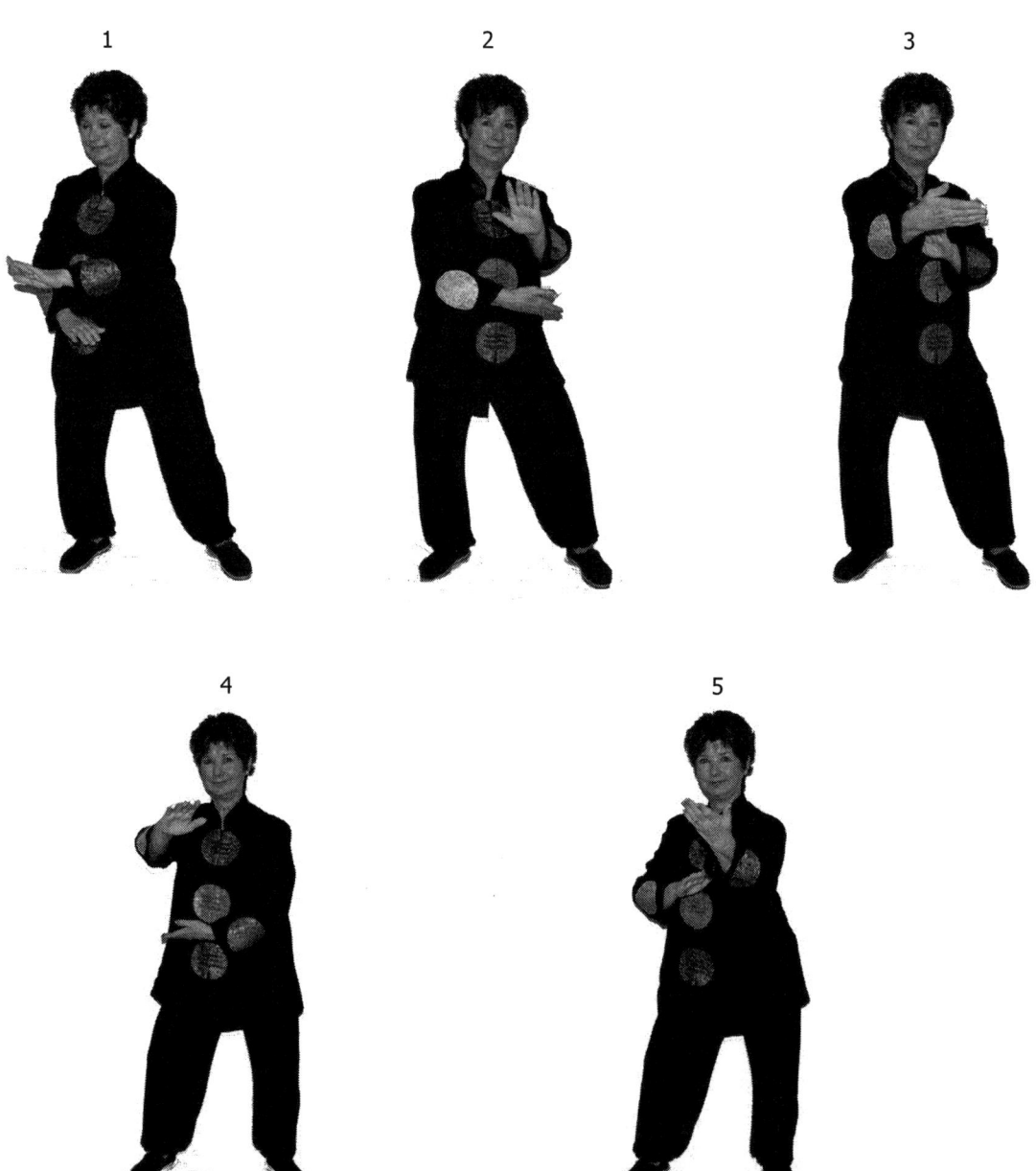

Teaching Tips and Hints - Keep arms close for transition of movement - orient the leading arm directly front while turning the waist to give flow

13 – SUNSET, END OF DAY

Brilliant reflections on the clouds
Warm colours of the setting sun
As far as you can see

Cross Hands and Patting Foot – Form 60

1   Starting Position

2   Preparing to Close - Cross the wrist, pams down

3   Separate both arms in a curve, weight slightly L

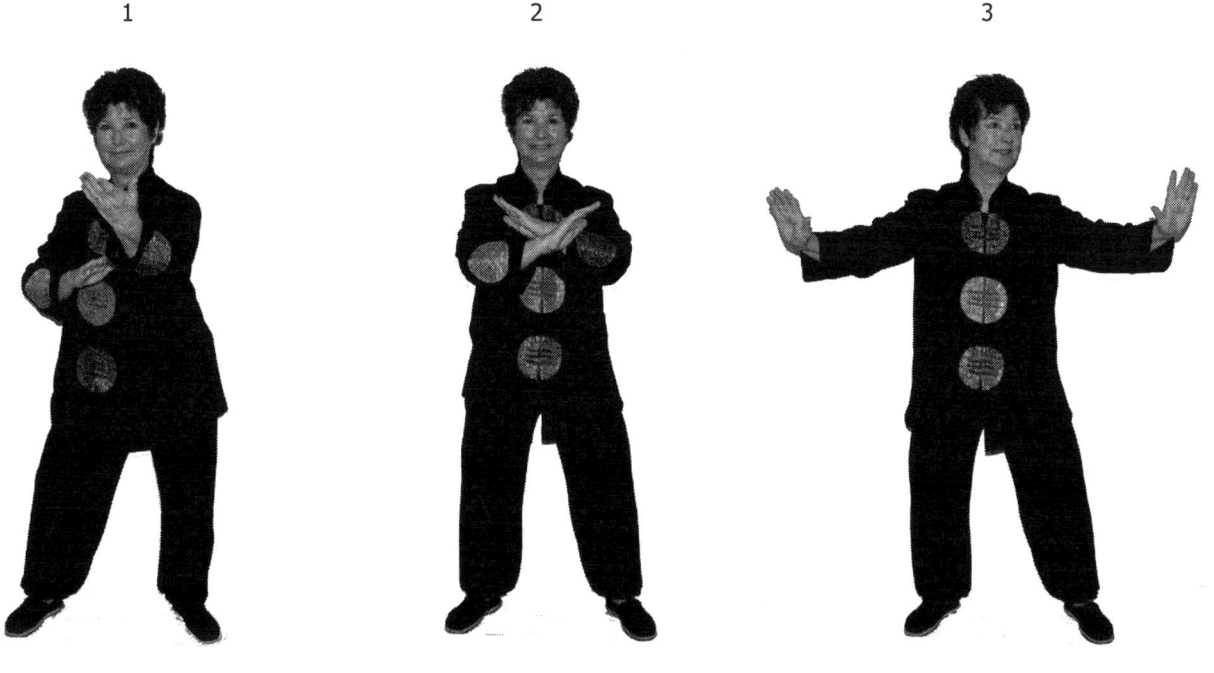

1   2   3

Teaching Tips and Hints - Time to take a deep breath for the opening movement

14 - SOUTHERN CROSS

Pointing the way
Among millions of stars filling the night sky
Shining and twinkling in the moonlight

Single Whip and Lowering Movement and Forward Step Seven Stars – Forms 66 & 67

1   Starting Position

2   Glide the arms down in a curve towards the midline

3   Line up the L arm at shoulder height, R arm is low and close to the body

4   Take the shortest distance to cross hands position or Seven Stars

1

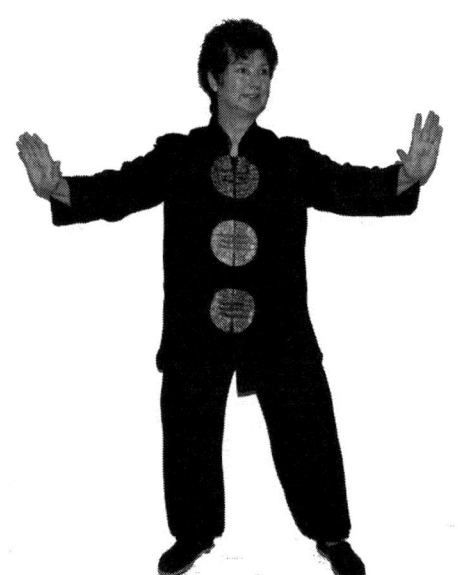

2

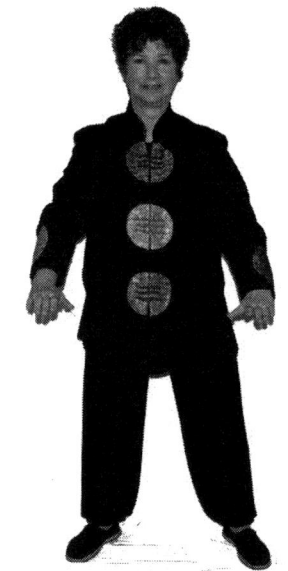

3

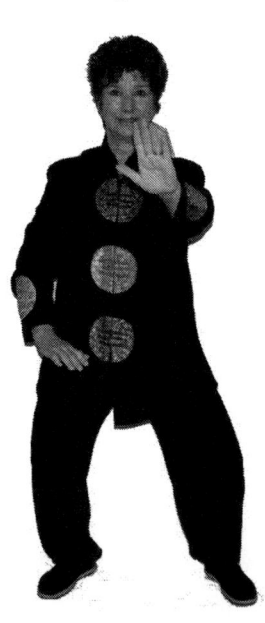

4

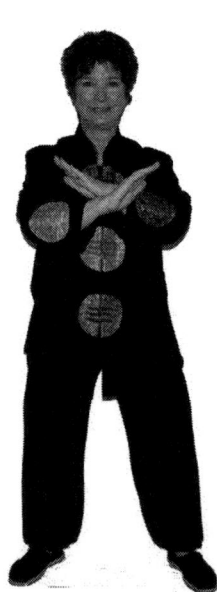

15 - DREAMTIME

Time to rest. Time to sleep
Time to remember the past
To light our way to a better future
A tribute to all our ancestors

Closing Form

1-3   Curve slightly down and out to the side continuing circle to up position

4-6   Curve down and press gently close to the body -close form and return to Wuji

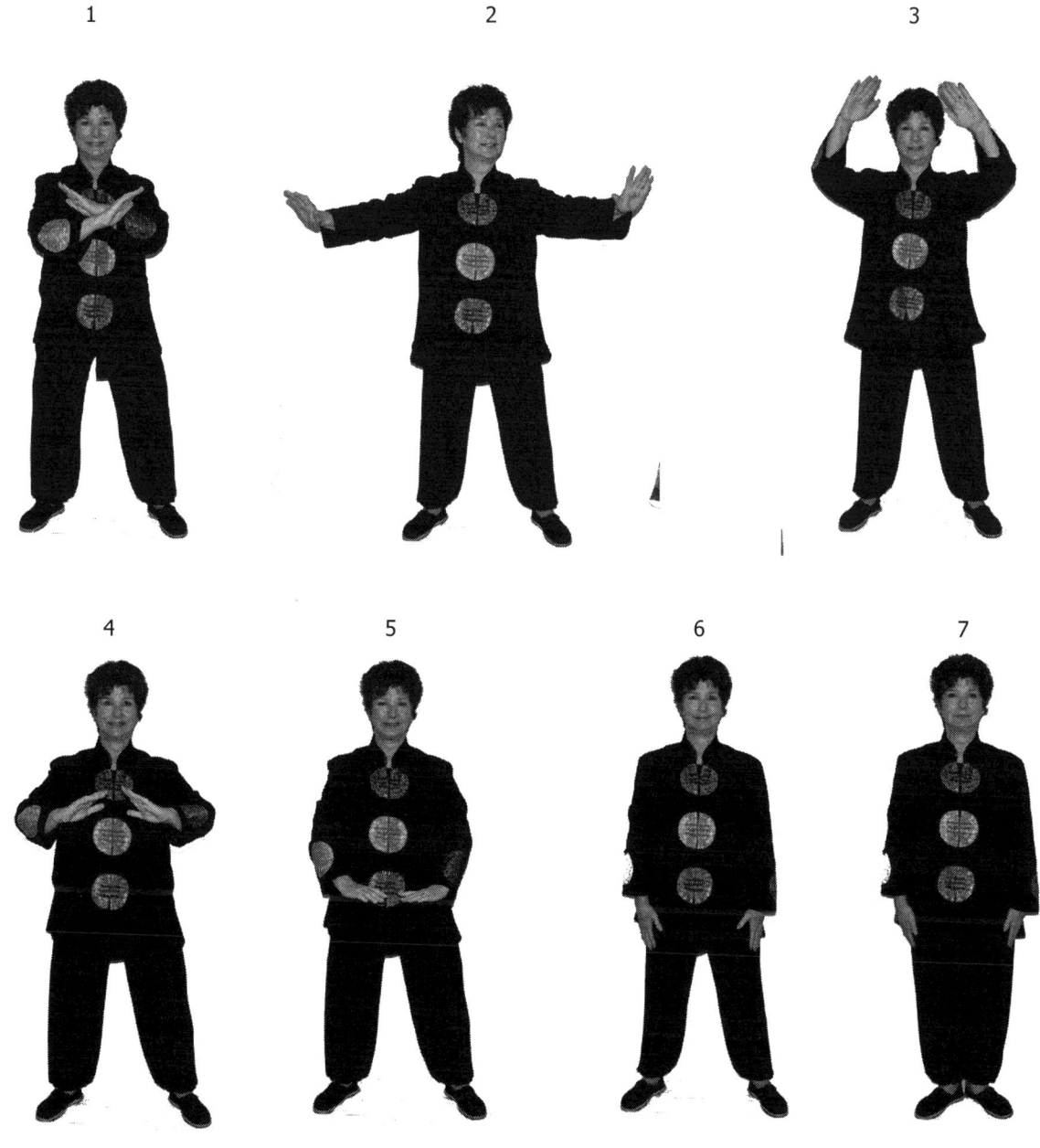

UNIT 600
Advanced Instructor Training

Unit 600	6.10	Introduction
	6.20	Five Levels of Tai Chi for Health Leader/Instructor Training
	6.30	Advanced Instructor Training Course
	6.40	Performance and Teaching Competencies
	6.50	Certification and Accreditation
	6.60	Membership & Accreditation as Tai Chi for Health Instructor

6.10 INTRODUCTION

Tai Chi for Health focuses on health, fitness and well-being in the teaching and learning of Tai Chi within the modern Duty of Care framework whereby a proper understanding of the health and fitness levels of the student has been an essential feature of the training of the Tai Chi for Health Leader/Instructor. Tai Chi for Health as a concept, as a strategy is able to deliver a much broader range of classes, courses, workshops, and activities relevant to a diverse range of people who would benefit from competent and professional instruction. Such a concept includes the ability to teach Tai Chi at various levels of competency from beginners to advanced levels where the central focus is on Tai Chi as a Health Art which is capable of being delivered with a proper understanding and commitment to safety issues and harm prevention as well as to health enhancement.

Thus having some form of a grading system for different classes and/or for different levels of ability from beginners through to advanced is the modern way to take account of the Duty of Care the teacher has towards different populations and to avoid the mistake in believing that Tai Chi for Health can be "One Size Fits All".   The five levels of Tai Chi for Health outlined within this course represent a conceptual framework that is entirely consistent with a modern approach to teaching and learning and in represented by the Matrix of Performance (see Unit 3.40).

At present in Australia, levels one and two have excellent training programs for the Tai Chi for Heath Leader/Instructor which are unmistakeably independent from Tai Chi practised as a martial art. But where does the Tai Chi for Health Leader/Instructor trained at this basic level go for further training in Tai Chi for Health, not simply from a performance level, but from an advanced level of Instructor training? Traditionally, Tai Chi has been practiced as a Martial Art and as such accreditation as a Tai Chi Instructor in Australia at an advanced level has only been available through the Level 1 Coaching course of the National Martial Arts Instructor Accreditation Scheme with the Australian Sports Commission.

However, Tai Chi for Health is not a martial art, it is NON-CONTACT as it does not include techniques which involve physically pushing, throwing, grappling, sparring or combat training as found in the training of the Kung Fu Tai Chi Master as a martial artist. Tai Chi for Health already has a beginning and independent pathway for Instructor training at a basic level and which has now been extended to include advanced levels of training of the Tai Chi for Health Instructor. The Advanced Instructor Training course is aimed at providing a commitment towards Tai Chi for Health Instructor training and in particular to provide intensive training in Tai Chi for Health as safe and effective forms of exercise at all levels as conceptually embodied in the Matrix of Performance (see Unit 3.40).

6.20   FIVE LEVELS OF TAI CHI FOR HEALTH LEADER/INSTRUCTOR TRAINING

Level 1 Leader/Instructor Training - Prior Tai Chi experience is not a prerequisite for participating at this level nor is it necessary for accreditation with the specific Tai Chi for Health Instructor/Leader Training programs. These programs include Dr Paul Lam's Tai Chi for Arthritis (TCA) Instructor/Leader training program and Alice Liping Yuan's Tai Chi for Health & Falls Injury Prevention Instructor training program. Workshops offered are two days for each program and include competency requirements.

Level 2 Leader/Instructor Training - Pre-requisite is Level 1 accreditation with the Tai Chi for Health program. This is the next stage of a beginners' level for persons wishing to update their Level 1 accreditation. The update component for accreditation for Dr Lam's program is a one day workshop and for Alice Liping Yuan's program is a two day workshop, where both workshops need to be completed within two years from the date of accreditation. Level 2 of the TCA program includes training to learn the new 9 Forms of Sun style, to explore tai chi principles and to enhance the performance of the TCA 31 form.

Level 3 Advanced Instructor Training Tai Chi for Health - Prerequisite includes a minimum of a basic proficiency of Sun 31 Form, prior knowledge of Sun 73 form desirable and a minimum of three years teaching experience of a Tai Chi for Health program. The two day workshop involves competency requirements for performance and teaching.

Level 4 Advanced Instructor Training Tai Chi for Health - Prerequisite is satisfactory completion of level 3 and assignment preparation for Practice Teaching at a two day workshop. The two-day workshop involves competency requirements for performance and teaching.

Level 5 Advanced Instructor Training Tai Chi for Health – Prerequisite is satisfactory completion of level 4 and assignment preparation for Practice Teaching. This involves a one-day workshop with competency requirements for performance and teaching, plus a three part Final Assessment – (a) Workbook (b) DVD solo presentation of Sun 73 (b) DVD presentation of Teaching performance. The student has up to twelve months after the workshop to complete this Final Assessment.

6.30 ADVANCED INSTRUCTOR TRAINING COURSE

Overview - the course includes the following:

- In-depth study of Sun 73 Form for Tai Chi for Health (TCH)
- How to be an independent and competent TCH Instructor using Sun Style Tai Chi
- Understanding and application of Sun Style, Yang Style concepts and principles and Tai Chi Classics
- Learning how to modify any Tai Chi form for different levels of ability, age and health conditions and how to adapt a TCH class for different populations
- Various teaching methods and strategies suitable for TCH including - step progression, copy and follow, mirror teaching, concept imagery, motivation, touching, verbal & visual communications – cueing, enunciation, clarity, sign language, eye contact
- Understanding and knowledge of important TCH contexts as they relate to a professional approach to teaching including – "Duty of Care" principles, functional anatomy, history of Tai Chi, social/cultural factors, music, use of language, business-legal, marketing, risk management, occupational health and safety (OH&S), consumer protection, and other ethical and legal matters including privacy, copyright, defamation, discrimination, harassment, and professionalism of the instructor-client relationship

Structure & Focus - The essence of a valued Tai Chi for Health Instructor is not that their performance of Tai Chi at an elite level nor that they can answer every question put to them by their students. It is that they can look at their class and (1) identify what needs to be done and assess whether it is the right time to make or suggest a change and (2) have a broad enough knowledge and skill base to address those needs.

Integral to this objective is the focus throughout the workshops on linking performance of the form with strategies of teaching using the Matrix of Performance (see Unit 3.40). This workshop activity is also linked to assessments at three levels through an extensive set of questions and scenarios that are challenging and thought provoking and to be able to decide strategies and outcomes they could use and develop as a teacher. Students in this course who have successfully completed these assessments all report a heightened sense of teaching confidence and a confirmation that they could answer or research and find the answer to any questions with ability and competence.

Making a detailed study of the different performances of the Sun 73 form on the DVD by Dr Lam, Prof Meng and other demonstrators is a valuable lesson in analysing exercise, comparing and learning critical appraisal and not criticism, training the search for principles and detail so necessary for recognition of all aspects of performance and teaching. It is an exercise in seeing and not merely "watching", it is an exercise in developing the necessary skills of mind-body connections to enhance competent and informed teaching expertise.

Filming their own performance of Sun 73 Competition Form was not about them achieving "perfection" but that they had an opportunity to look at themselves, that they were able to notice their posture and alignments, their consolidation of the principles, the shapes of their postures and so forth. Very often how we imagine our form to be and what we actually do are often very different. Filming their performances can be confronting, but it is an exercise that can be very helpful for the conscientious teacher. There is a lesson to be learned about patience and seeing and accepting then making changes.

The course is structured into three parts with each part representing three separate levels of progression. Workshops are organised as summarised as follows:

Level 3 - Two day workshop
See Appendix 3 for detail on Student Timetable and Assessment
(a) Practical Performance of Sun 73 Form – At workshop
(b) Teaching Performance of Sun 73 Form – At workshop
(c) Written Assignment – Tai Chi Performance - Mind-Body Analysis - Review Sun 73 Sections 1 to 4, and TCA1 & 2. Analyse two forms or groups of forms. Identify differences and similarities between different performances describing movement in terms specified.
(d) Written Assignment – Teaching Tai Chi - Prepare Written Lesson Plan for teaching one form (or group). Identify your target student whether group with ages, levels, health conditions, beginners or advanced or mixture. Based on Lecture and outline include in lesson plan factors specified.

Level 4 - Two day workshop
See Appendix 4 for detail on Trainer Timetable and Student Timetable and Assessment
(a) Practical Performance of Sun 73 Form – At workshop
(b) Teaching Performance of Sun 73 Form – At workshop
(c) Written Assignment: Tai Chi Performance - Mind-Body Analysis - Analyse form from provided lists by reviewing Sun 73 and three separate performances.
(d) Written Assignment: Teaching Tai Chi - Prepare written Lesson Plan for teaching form from list provided with the given scenario. Your lesson plan should address a number of identified factors.

Level 5 - One day workshop
See Appendix 5 for detail on Student Timetable and Assessment
(a) Practical Performance of Sun 73 Form – At workshop
(b) Teaching Performance of Sun 73 Form – At workshop
(c) Workbook – Written Assignment – 73 Questions – 6-12 months to complete covering Units 100 to 500.
(d) Solo Performance of Sun 73 Form – Demonstrate solo performance of Sun 73 Form at a competent standard
(e) Teaching performance – presentation of no more than fifteen minutes of a segment of a Tai Chi for Health class, which demonstrates competent teaching to a student or group of students containing some specific aspect of the Sun Style Tai Chi form. A brief written outline of the Teaching Plan for this performance is required.

6.40   PERFORMANCE & TEACHING COMPETENCIES

All graduates of the course receive certification as to having successfully completed the Tai Chi for Health Advanced Instructor Training Course and that they have demonstrated the necessary competencies as a Tai Chi for Health Instructor as follows:

- To perform and teach Sun Style Tai Chi from beginners to advanced levels to a wide range of people in accordance with the "Matrix of Performance Levels for Duty of Care", that is, with performance variables of the individual student related to – age; health; fitness; skills; and environment in consultation with other Health and Fitness professionals where appropriate

- To analyse Tai Chi form and function using scientific "mind-body" recognition techniques and to have an understanding of movement analysis, scientific knowledge of human anatomy, posture, muscles, biomechanics, ageing, breathing, and the Alexander Technique

- To understand that a modern Tai Chi for Health focuses on the health, fitness and well-being of the individual student as a safe and effective form of exercise in accordance with modern ethical and legal Duty of Care requirements and functions through the social, cultural framework of evidence based reasoning and scientific research through the health and social sciences

- To teach and modify other styles and forms of Tai Chi from beginners to advanced levels in accordance with the "Matrix of Performance levels of Duty of Care" subject to having developed competency in performance of those other styles and forms in consultation with other Tai Chi for Health, Health and Fitness professionals where appropriate

- To teach Qigong, including the Sun Style *Australia Dreaming*, as a safe and effective form of exercise in accordance with the "Matrix of Performance levels of Duty of Care"

- To develop and teach safe and effective exercise programs based on Tai Chi and Qigong to special populations in consultation with other Health and Fitness professionals where appropriate

6.50   CERTIFICATION AND ACCREDITATION

Successful completion of the course provides certification as a Tai Chi for Health Instructor by Tai Chi for Health & Community Fitness. The graduate is entitled to apply to be registered as an accredited Instructor member of Tai Chi for Health & Community Fitness (TCHCF) which also includes membership of Sakurakan-QUBBA. Accreditation and membership is not prescribed nor is it a necessary outcome for graduates of the course, it is a choice. Accreditation with TCHCF requires the TCH Instructor member to agree to abide by the "Code of Practice & Ethics" (see Unit 4.60) which includes the contractual obligation on the part of the accredited TCH Instructor member to be properly covered for liability insurance (see below for details).   TCHCF is a registered name for Elva's Fitness and Tai Chi for Health school. Elva is self-employed as a professional Fitness and Tai Chi Trainer and consultant. Both Elva and Denis are registered Instructor members of the non-profit organisation – Sakurakan-QUBBA, Queensland United Black Belt Association Incorporated.

TCHCF is also a registered school affiliated with Sakurakan-QUBBA. Sakurakan is the Japanese name for the "Academy of the Cherry Blossom" and QUBBA is the abbreviated name of the incorporated non-profit organisation - Queensland United Black Belt Association Inc. It is incorporated in accordance with the *Association Incorporations Act 1981 (Queensland),* and comes under the legal jurisdiction of the Queensland State Government Department, the Office of Fair Trading. Sakurakan-QUBBA was originally founded in 1959 by Geoff Geurts who introduced to Australia the Cherry Blossom or Sakura tradition of the martial arts, a tradition which emphasises the importance of the "ju" or "yielding" principle as the basis of a practical self defence (Seiryoko Zenyo) and the ethical standard of mutual benefit and respect (Jita Kyoei). He was 12th degree in Jujitsu and 5th dan in Judo trained within the traditions of the Japanese fighting arts introduced to Europe by Mikonosuke Kawaishi (see Kawaishi, 1955 and 1957). The Association is an official grading and accreditation authority being responsible for a comprehensive curriculum from beginner's levels through to advanced levels and over the years has been responsible for the grading of hundreds of Martial Arts Instructors, both women and men with a minimum age for grading to Black Belt and Instructor level of 18 years.

While the "core activities" of Sakurakan-QUBBA are the Japanese martial arts of Judo and Jujitsu, the constitution allows for the promotion and support of other martial, health and fitness activities. This is similar to the Budokwai, the non-profit British Martial Arts Association set up in London in 1918 by Gunji Koizumi, and includes a wide range of health and fitness activities including Yoga and Tai Chi. The Sakura tradition continues today as offering highly effective forms of self defence with Shihan William (Bill) Cadoo 9th Dan Jujitsu, 6th Dan Judo as the Chief Technical Adviser and has a number of individual Instructor members as well as Japanese and Chinese martial arts schools and Tai Chi for Health schools as affiliated members.

6.60   MEMBERSHIP & ACCREDITATION AS TAI CHI FOR HEALTH INSTRUCTOR

There are three categories of membership of Tai Chi for Health & Community Fitness (TCHCF) which is an affiliated school with Sakurakan-QUBBA. Students can apply for student membership of TCHCF after having completed the basic training at level 2.

1. **Student membership includes:**
    - Student Member of TCHCF school and associate membership of Sakurakan-QUBBA
    - Access to TCHCF community based classes & workshops
    - Eligible to attend advanced TCHCF classes and workshops
    - Mentoring for instructor training in Tai Chi for Health with TCHCF

2. **Individual Instructor Membership includes:**
    - Registered as accredited Tai Chi for Health Instructor (TCH) with TCHCF where Instructor provides evidence of appropriate liability insurance upon application
    - Instructor Member of TCHCF School and associate membership of Sakurakan-QUBBA
    - Support with application by provisional member for liability insurance for insurers who may require some form of accreditation or membership for obtaining liability insurance
    - Support with commencement and operating Tai Chi for Health Community based classes including appropriate use of TCHCF logo for publicity purposes and listing of Instructor on TCHCF website   A support network for Tai Chi for Health Instructor members
    - Forum for sharing ideas related to the promotion of Tai Chi for Health in the local community for Tai Chi for Health Instructors
    - Mutual support in development of Tai Chi for Health knowledge, expertise and training
    - Advice and support with accessing corporate and government sponsorship to fund community based projects and activities
    - Mutual encouragement and support for facilitating further research through the heath sciences and social sciences into Tai Chi for Health in the local community

3. **Individual Instructor & Affiliated School Membership includes:**
    - All the benefits listed under "Individual - Instructor membership"
    - Instructor Member School affiliated with TCHCF & Sakurakan-QUBBA
    - Support with promotion and publicity for affiliated school in developing and maintaining website on the World Wide Web for linking to TCHCF and Sakurakan-QUBBA websites
    - Membership of Sakurakan-QUBBA provides access to government and corporate funding where certain funding requirements necessitate membership of a non-profit organisation incorporated under the Association Incorporation's Act
    - Liability insurance for registered Instructors – professional indemnity, public liability
    - Personal accident insurance for registered student members
    - Insurance includes coverage for such Tai Chi activities as certification of students and two person physical contact such as sensitivity training and push hands

Appendix 1 – Open Letter re TCH Advanced Instructor Training Course

This "Open Letter" was included in Course Materials at the first Tai Chi for Health Advanced Instructor Training Workshop held on 21-22 July 2007. The intention of this letter was to explain the reasons for developing the Advanced Instructor Training course as being entirely consistent with a modern approach to "training the trainer" which includes graded levels not only of Tai Chi performance but also of teaching expertise. It also highlighted the need for these graded levels of competency as necessitating an alternative pathway different from that offered through the traditional martial arts approach and in Australia to the Level 1 Martial Arts Coaching course.

Open Letter re new Advanced Instructor Training for Tai Chi for Health - 20 July 2007

There has been a growing need in Australia for an advanced level of Instructor training in Tai Chi for Health, which offers a different and viable pathway from that of the traditional Tai Chi for Martial Arts Instructor training that exists at present. The need to develop this independent pathway of Tai Chi for Health Instructor training was something Elva and I both emphasised in the papers we wrote and presented at what was billed as the first International Tai Chi for Health Conference held in Korea in December 2006.

As the papers point out, Dr Lam's Tai Chi for Health programs do not offer levels of progression to become a Tai Chi for Health Instructor other than what is already available through the traditional Martial Arts approach, which specifies that you must complete the Level 1 Coaching course through the Martial Arts Industry Association (MAIA), which includes the Australian Kung Fu & Wushu Federation (AKWF), before you can be called a Tai Chi Instructor. This position is currently reflected on Tai Chi Productions website in advertising Dr Lam's TCA workshops offered in Australia through the global network of Master Trainers as follows:

> *This program (Tai Chi for Arthritis Instructor's Training) does not provide qualifications as a Tai Chi Instructor accredited with the Australian Sports Commission through the National Martial Arts Instructor Accreditation Scheme, which includes the Australian Kung-Fu (Wu-Shu) Federation (AKWF) but persons who successfully complete the TCA course will be accredited with Dr Paul Lam's Tai Chi for Health programs to teach the TCA program as a safe and effective form of exercise in the community... If you are currently qualified as an Instructor (Level 1 Coach) through the National Martial Arts Instructor Accreditation Scheme on behalf of the Australian Sports Commission (this includes the AKWF), you will be issued with a TCA Instructor certificate upon successful completion of the program. All other persons will be issued with a TCA Leader certificate. This requirement is for Australian Instructor/Leader's certificate ONLY.*

Originally, this was not to have been the case when Dr Lam first pioneered and introduced his Tai Chi for Arthritis Instructor training program in the late 1990s. For a number of years, there was no distinction between an "Instructor" and "Leader" as all graduates of the TCA Instructor Training program were accredited as Tai Chi for Arthritis Instructors. This changed in 2004, after Dr Lam had been lobbied by the traditional Kung Fu and Wushu community in Australia for him to recognise the AKWF as the only legitimate body for accreditation as a Tai Chi Instructor. Initially he agreed and made the change from "Tai Chi for Arthritis Instructor" to "Tai Chi for Arthritis Leader" for everyone who was not accredited with the AKWF. He was thus going to only recognise the AKWF as the accreditation body as acceptable for graduates of his Tai Chi for Arthritis program to be called "Instructor". It was only after it was drawn to his attention about the significance of the Martial Arts Industry Accreditation Scheme to the Level 1 Coaching qualification that he broadened the "Instructor" status to include Level 1 Coach accredited through the MAIA as the qualification to be a Tai Chi for Arthritis Instructor and not Leader.

This focus on "Leader" and "Instructor", however, really only served to highlight the more pertinent question about the need for further Instructor training specifically for Tai Chi for Health Leaders and others who did not wish to pursue the martial arts approach. In this regard, Elva approached Dr Lam shortly after in 2004 offering to facilitate and teach a new "Instructor Training" program linked to the Sun 73 course at his Sydney January workshop specifically at an advanced level, in particular, to extend the Tai Chi for Arthritis instructor training program and to increase the teaching expertise and confidence of the TCA Instructors now designated as Leaders. Dr Lam declined Elva's offer after he had consulted with his own Instructors at his own Sydney Tai Chi school - *Better Health Tai Chi Chuan Inc.* This now left Elva with the choice of either doing nothing, or doing something about it herself. Elva strongly believed then and now that there was and is a definite need to do something more, as the only option for so many new TCA "Leaders" was to continue their training through the local community with the traditional Kung Fu and Wushu trained Tai Chi for Martial Arts Instructor, which in Australia and the USA is invariably Yang Style and not Sun Style Tai Chi.

The papers, which Elva and I presented at last year's International Tai Chi for Health Conference, represent the culmination of this determination to do something concrete about the need for advanced level instructor training for Tai Chi for Health and TCA Leaders. The papers make a very strong case in a reasoned and practical way for a Tai Chi for Health Instructor training pathway independent from Tai Chi as a Martial Art. Elva is a qualified teacher of movement and dance with over forty five years teaching experience, she is an internationally recognised Sun Style Tai Chi for Health specialist, she is a Master Trainer with Dr Lam's Tai Chi for Health programs involved in "training the trainer" teaching in Australia, and she has taught Tai Chi for Health at overseas workshops in the USA, New Zealand and Korea. Elva has taken the initiative in developing the five levels of Tai Chi

Instructor Training and is now offering Advanced Levels of Tai Chi for Health Instructor Training. Sun Style Tai Chi features as the vehicle for "Advanced Instructor" training for those who do not wish to have to join some martial arts or kung fu organisation or learn the local Yang Style Tai Chi from the Kung-fu and Wushu Martial Arts Tai Chi Instructor in the local community as a necessary and only pathway to become a qualified Tai Chi for Health Instructor. Technically and legally, anyone can of course call themselves an "Instructor" without any training and some people do just that, unwittingly perhaps, leaving themselves, students and others exposed and vulnerable to Duty of Care issues, to the legal fine print of liability insurance and to other related legal and ethical matters.

After making the decision to proceed independently of Tai Chi Productions with the Advanced Level of Tai Chi for Health Instructor Training, Elva and I both spoke to Dr Lam in Sydney at the January 2007 Sydney workshop, not for the purpose of getting his approval, but as a matter of respect and courtesy to him. The outcome of that conversation was encouraging as he said that he had no objections and said that he supported the idea and wished us well. In short, Elva is now offering a valid alternative to the Tai Chi for Martial Arts pathway for those who may wish to progress and develop their teaching skills at an advanced level as part of becoming a Tai Chi for Health Instructor. We are not aware of any other similar course available within Australia or within the world. Elva will be teaching how to teach TAI CHI FOR HEALTH (NOT Kung Fu Tai Chi Chuan as a martial art) at an advanced level using the Sun Style and an In-Depth Study of the Sun 73 as the vehicle and as the form. This journey has already begun for those who have completed levels 1 and 2 of the Sun Style TCA course (Dr Lam's TCA Parts 1 and 2). Last year for the first time, Dr Lam offered the "Explore the Depth of TCA" workshop in Australia and also at the International Tai Chi for Health conference in Korea at which I assisted Dr Lam's Master Trainer Pat Webber in teaching in this program. This workshop offers an excellent opportunity for those who feel the need to develop a better performance of the Tai Chi for Arthritis (TCA) Sun 31 Form through an introduction to some new Tai Chi principles and martial applications, but it does not include any specific training on how to teach Tai Chi for Health, it does not include any knowledge on Tai Chi for Health and it does not have any Tai Chi for Health Instructor Training component at an intermediate or advanced level.

What is new with Elva's Advanced Instructor Training is the extension of an Instructor Training focus through intermediate to advanced Levels 3 and 4 through an In-depth Study of Sun 73 and then onto the final level 5 which represents a consolidation of a wide range of matters that is necessary as part of training in order to be an independent, responsible and proficient Tai Chi for Health Instructor. It is an exciting and pioneering development in the world of Tai Chi for Health. Elva's view is that Tai Chi for Health should be about making a difference and through this initiative we both feel we can make some small contribution to this end.

From a practical point of view, graduates of this program will be able to apply for accreditation as a Tai Chi for Health Instructor if they choose, which will include active membership of Tai Chi for Health & Community Fitness and the non-profit organisation, Queensland United Black Belt Association Inc (Sakurakan-QUBBA). Thus as an accredited Tai Chi for Health Instructor, one of the benefits will be to have access to various types of insurance relevant for a Tai Chi for Health Instructor either through Sakurakan-QUBBA or direct with a number of insurers who may require some form of accreditation. The two different types of accreditation, however, are strictly a matter of choice and are NOT necessary prerequisites for successful completion of any part of the Advanced Instructor Training program. The benefits of accreditation will also include registering your school with Tai Chi for Health & Community Fitness with the use of the logo and thus linking and listing your school in the community and on the World Wide Web for publicity purposes, as well having access to government and corporate funding where certain funding bodies require membership of a non-profit organisation incorporated under the Association Incorporation's Act.

Finally, it is important to know that after more than 25 years association with Queensland Keep Fit Association (QKFA), Elva resigned as an Instructor member in November 2006 and no longer has any association with QKFA, in particular, with any Fitness or Tai Chi activity or program that is offered or promoted by QKFA.

Dr Denis Arthy
Tai Chi for Health & Community Fitness
ABN: 73 482 976 952
260 Bloomfield St CLEVELAND Qld 4163
Phone: +61 7 3286 2779 **Email: ElvarMar@bigpond.net.au**

Appendix – 2 - Informed Consent about Health

TAI CHI FOR HEALTH & COMMUNITY FITNESS

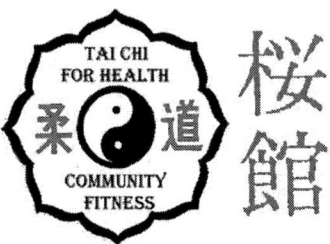

Personal Details

Name

....

Address

....

Email address

....

Dear Doctor/Physiotherapist/Health Professional

I am an accredited Tai Chi for Health Instructor with Tai Chi for Health & Community Fitness.

I teach ....classes in ....

(Please see over for information on these classes).

The following person

....

intends to make a commitment to participating in the **Tai Chi for Health class**

Could you please assess her/him for suitability to participate and make recommendations or suggestions, if necessary, which may assist in enhancing health benefits. Please feel free to contact me should you require further information.

Thank you for taking time to assist in the health management of my student.

Tai Chi for Health Instructor

Assessment/Recommendations/Suggestions:
....
....
Please print name: Dr ....   **Phone Nr** ....
....**Date** .... / .... / ....
Signed

Informed Consent about Health

Tai Chi for Health Classes Levels 1 to 2

All classes are Tai Chi for HEALTH classes and are NOT Tai Chi for Martial Arts classes as such do not involve physically pushing, throwing, grappling, break-falling, rolling, sparring and potentially dangerous or contra-indicated movements, some or all of which may be found in the traditional training of the Tai Chi as a Martial Arts class.

Beginners/Intermediate - levels 1 & 2

All classes at beginners' level include –

- Warm-up and cool down exercises
- Tai Chi for Arthritis program, Tai Chi for Diabetes program, Tai Chi for Back Pain program by Dr Paul Lam
- Tai Chi for Falls & Prevention Program by Alice Liping Yuan - Exercise Medicine Australia
- Relaxation and Qigong – breathing and relaxation techniques
- Importance of posture and balance training

Beginners start with the *Tai Chi for Arthritis (TCA)* program, which has the support of the Arthritis Foundation Australia and Osteoporosis Aust. The TCA program was developed in 1998 by the internationally recognized Tai Chi authority Dr Paul Lam assisted by a medical team including Professor John Edmonds (Professor of Rheumatology) and Rheumatologist, Dr Ian Portek at the St George Hospital, Sydney.

Tai Chi for Health & Relaxation Class – Levels 3 & 4

All classes are Tai Chi for HEALTH classes and are NOT Tai Chi for Martial Arts classes as such do not involve physically pushing, throwing, grappling, break-falling, rolling, sparring and potentially dangerous or contra-indicated movements, some or all of which may be found in the traditional training of the Tai Chi as a Martial Arts class.

Tai Chi for Health & Relaxation is a gentle form of exercise where the main focus is on learning and practising solo forms at an intermediate and advanced levels – such as Yang 24, Sun 73, Chen 36, Yang 42. Solo forms are a number of set movements flowing in a sequence with the emphasis on relaxation, mind-body co-ordination, and safety with modifications to suit the individual's age, health and general fitness levels.

The Tai Chi for Health & Relaxation class includes warm-up and cool-down routines appropriate to the type of activity, light stretching exercises for flexibility, co-ordinated breathing exercises, some gentle and controlled exercises with a partner (sensitivity training) to enhance the performance of the solo forms and movements. **Students are encouraged to work at their own levels, within their own comfort zone and at their own pace.**

Appendix 3 - Level 3 – Student Workshop Timetable

Day 1 8.30am - Registration

Session 1
9.00 am to 9.30 am - Introduction and
Workshop Plan - What is Tai Chi for
Health?
9.30 am to 10.30 am - Lecture/Discussion
AND Practical – Study of Sun 73
First demonstration by students of ALL Sun
73 Forms – First Reference Point (RP)
*Unit 300 Tai Ch Knowledge -Sub-Unit 3.30 Sun
Lutang's Eight Concepts*
*Unit 500 - In Depth Study Sun 73 - Refinement–
Sections I & II*

Morning Tea 10.30am to 11.00am

Session 2
*11.00 am to 1.00 pm – Lecture/Discussion AND
Practical – Warm-ups, Cool Downs, Training
Exercises*
*Unit 200 - Essential Knowledge of Human Body –
2.10 Anatomy & Posture*
*Unit 500 - In Depth Study Sun 73 Refinement–
Sections III*

Lunch 1.00pm to 2.00pm

Session 3
2.00 to 3.15pm — Lecture/Discussion &
Teaching Practice
*Unit 100 - Teaching Knowledge & Skills - Sub-
Units 1.10 Teaching Principles, and 1.40
Techniques of Teaching*

Afternoon tea 3.15pm to 3.30pm

Session 4
3.30pm to 4.30pm – Lecture/Discussion
AND Practical – Study of Sun 73 to focus
on specific principles
*Unit 500 - In Depth Study Sun 73 Refinement–
Sections IV & V*
*Unit 300 Tai Chi Knowledge -Sub-Unit 3.10
Modern Framework for Tai Chi for Health*

**4.30pm to 5.00pm – DAY 1 REVIEW -
Discussion** & Practical includes second
demonstration by students of ALL Sun 73
Forms - Second Reference Point (RP), Cool
Down and Australia Dreaming

Day 2 – 8.30am early practice

Session 5
9.00am to 9.15am – Overview for day &
Intro to *Unit 400 Legal & Other Responsibilities*
9.15am to 10.30am Lecture/Discussion
AND Practical – Study of Sun 73 practical
includes third demonstration by students of
ALL Sun 73 Forms
*Unit 500 - In Depth Study Sun 73 - Refinement–
Sections I to V*
*Unit 300 Tai Chi Knowledge -Sub-Unit 3.30 Tai
Chi Principles & Concepts*

Morning Tea 10.30am to 11.00am

Session 6
11.00am to 1.00pm – Lecture/Discussion &
Teaching Practice
*Unit 100 Teaching Knowledge & Skills, Sub-Unit
1.20 Communication, 1.30 Preparation. Discuss
preparation of ASSIGNMENT for next
workshop*

Lunch 1.00pm to 2.00pm

Session 7
2.00 to 3.15pm – Lecture/Discussion &
Teaching Practice
*Unit 100 Teaching Knowledge & Skills, Sub-Unit
1.20 Communication, 1.30 Preparation. – Review
of Teaching Performance*

Afternoon tea 3.15pm to 3.30pm

Session 8
3.30pm to 4.30pm – Lecture/Discussion
AND Practical – Study of Sun 73
Practical includes Assessment & Review
*Unit 500 In Depth Study Sun 73 - Performance
Review of Sections I – V*

**4.30pm to 5.00pm - WORKSHOP REVIEW –
Discussion & Feedback**
Demonstration of Sun 73 as final Reference
Point (RP) for workshop, Cool Down and
Australia Dreaming

Appendix 3 - Level 3 - Workshop Assignment

1. Review Dr Lam's DVDs Sun 73 Sections 1 to 4, and TCAI & II, analyse two forms or groups of forms – ONE from each list below. Task is to identify differences and similarities between – Dr Lam/Prof Men; TCA/Sun 73 (from List one only) and briefly and accurately as possible describe all movements in terms of the following – direction, shape, movement of hands, elbows, waist, knees, feet, toes, heel and ball of foot. (Main Focus is on choreography, physical posture, movement and relevant principles)

2. Prepare brief written Lesson Plan for teaching one form (or group) from each List as below. Identify your target student whether group with ages, levels, health conditions, beginners or advanced or mixture. Based on Lecture and Workshop Manual, include in lesson plan – need and how to modify, reason for modification, outcomes for lesson; Tai Chi principles /concepts involved; Qigong/ breathing factors.

List One	Form 10 – Brush Knee and Twist Step Left
	Form 11 – Playing the Lute
	Form 21 – Single Whip Left
	Form 26 – Leisurely Tying coat Left
	Form 30 – Waving Hands Like Clouds
List Two	Forms 6 & 7 – Lifting Hands and White Crane Flashes its Wings
	Forms 31 to 33 – Higher Horse, Toe Kicks Left & Right
	Form 34 – Step On Firmly to Punch Downwards
	Form 35 – Turn Body and Jump with both feet
	Form 36 – Subdue the Tiger
	Form 56 – Golden Cock Standing on One Leg
	Form 57- Fan Back

Assignment to be returned by mail on or before a fortnight prior to Level 4 Workshop

Level 3 - Workshop Assignment - Assignment Clarification

----- Original Message -----
From: Denis
Subject: Level 3 Assignment In-Depth Sun 73 Advanced Instructor Training
Date: Sat, 4 Aug 2007 13:42:41 +1000

Hello everyone

To put you in the picture, we had a question seeking clarification on the first assignment and prepared the following as a response to how to approach this exercise and get the best out of it, and thought I would pass it on to everyone.

In regard to the first assignment, there are two related tasks. The broad idea is to have a look at both performances of the Sun 73 all the way through. Then pick two forms you would like to focus on and analyse in detail. Rather than pick two forms you are already familiar with in regard to Level 1 and 2 (Sun 31 TCA), the idea is to ensure you pick a "new" form that is not one of the TCA 31, as well as selecting one that you are familiar with through the TCA 31. You should find this an interesting exercise as it will get you to examine the detail and initially see both similarities and differences, not between the forms but between the performances of Dr Lam and Prof Men.

However, the main task is analytical, to write down in a step by step manner what is happening in the particular movement in terms of the following which are offered as a guide only - direction, shape, movement of hands, elbows, waist, knees, feet, toes, heel and ball of foot. Also as part of your analysis you may also wish to include what you have observed about relevant or important principles which are outlined in Yang Cheng Fu's Ten Principles and Sun Lutantg's Eight Concepts. And as part of your detailed description of the choreography, you can note any significant differences between the performances of Dr Lam and Professor Men. And if you get inspired by this and feel you wish to do more, you could make a few notes on any differences as to how you might have interpreted and perform and or teach the particular form as there could well be some legitimate differences in regard to modification for the forms you choose.

Don't agonise over this, just be methodical and analytical, do not let it overwhelm, it is in principle a process that everyone goes through intuitively when trying to copy and modify according to a model or form, to gain as much precision as we can in accordance with what we might view as a good model or form to imitate until it becomes our own. Overall, what is important, I believe, are the principles behind the execution of the techniques and performance with the mind/body connections paramount. If you relate your analysis to this, you will or should find this very rewarding. I hope so anyway.

To summarise, the main task is to analyse and describe two different forms using Dr Lam and/or Prof Men as the model of the form and try and do so not only describing the choreography, but what you understand might be happening in regard to principles, such as - posture, transfer of weight, co-ordination of upper and lower body and so on.

Trust this assists, give it a go, and let us know if you need any further help or to check if you are on the right track.

Kind regards Denis

----- Original Message -----
From: M
Sent: Tuesday, August 21, 2007 6:38 PM
Subject: RE: Assignment In-Depth Sun 73 Advanced Instructor Training

Hi El, I just need another clarification. It is second question. Is it one lesson with a choice of one from the two lists or does that mean two lesson plans one from each list. Love M

----- Original Message -----
From: Elva
Sent: Thursday, August 23, 2007 1:22 PM
Subject: Level 3 Assignment In-Depth Sun 73 Advanced Instructor Training

The aim is to develop and fast track your ability to adapt your knowledge and training to any class, any setting and not feel unable to take on any project. By writing up a simpler lesson and then another taking more advanced students to show a different approach is what I would like to see.

 In saying that I really do not want pages and pages of every single thing you are going to do. I envisage about one to one and a half A4 pages - very brief notes in dot form, what you think is important to consider- everything in short form. I did this exercise straight as I would deliver it myself - just typing it onto the computer and it took me about half an hour not stressing for each class level.

I particularly do not want to cause you stress but hope you choose a form and students you would not normally teach - so that you can KNOW you can work it all out and plan it easily from your knowledge, from the matrix and from your own adaptability skills which you already have.

 The comparison study from the DVD is to compare a form from Paul and Professor Men (or Kam if you want) (or Robyn) and "spot the differences". This will confirm to yourselves that you can get a DVD and critically compare and note what it is you are seeing. Again this only has to be in dot form and I would be thrilled.

Luv El

Appendix 4 - Level 4 – Student Workshop Timetable

Day 1 - Warm-up and Early Practice

Session 1 (1hr 30mins)
9.00 am to 10.30 am - Lecture/Discussion
AND Practical – Study of Sun 73 –Unit 6
Lady at Shuttle in detail with Principles
including breathing
Unit 300 Tai Chi Knowledge
Sub-Unit 3.30 Tai Chi Principles & Concepts

Morning Tea 10.30am to 11.00am

Session 2 (1 hrs 30 min)
11.00 am to 12.30 pm – Practical - Teaching
Practice – Study of Sun 73
Unit 100 - Teaching Knowledge & Skills
Sub-unit – Teaching Practice – Assignment from
Level 3

Lunch 12.30 pm to 1.30 pm

Session 3 (1 hour 30 mins)
1.30pm to 3.00pm — Lecture/Discussion
AND Practical – Study of Sun 73
Unit 100 - Teaching Knowledge & Skills
Sub-Units 1.70 Modifications of Tai Chi for
Health

Afternoon tea 3.00pm to 3.30pm

Session 4 (1 hour 30 mins)
3.30pm to 4.30pm – Lecture/Discussion
AND Practical – Study of Sun 73
Unit 300 – Tai Chi Knowledge
Sub-Unit 3.60 –Martial Concept of Body and
Application

Day 2 – 8.30am early practice

Session 5 (1 hr 30 mins)

9.00am to 10.30am Lecture/Discussion
AND Practical – Study of Sun 73
Unit 200 Essential Knowledge of Human
Body
Sub-Unit 2.20 Stretching; Sub-Unit 2.30
Physiology & Breathing; Sub-Unit 2.40 Safety &
Health Management

Morning Tea 10.30am to 11.00am

Session 6 (1 hr 30 mins)
11.00am to 12.30pm – Lecture/Discussion
& Teaching Practice
Unit 100 Teaching Knowledge & Skills
Sub-Unit 1.50 & 1.60 Imagery, Concepts &
Music

Lunch 12.30pm to 1.30pm

Session 7 (1 hr 30 min)
1.30pm to 3.00pm – Discussion & Teaching
Practice
Unit 400 Legal Knowledge as related to
teaching
Unit 100 Teaching Knowledge & Skills –
Groups of Three with specific tasks

Afternoon tea 3.15pm to 3.30pm

Session 8 (1 hr 30 min)
3.30pm to 4.00pm – Practical – Study of Sun
73
Unit 500 In Depth Study Sun 73 - *Revision*
& Practice

4.00pm to 5.00pm - WORKSHOP REVIEW –
Discussion & Feedback
Demonstration of Sun 73, Cool Down and
Australia Dreaming & Presentation

Appendix 4 – Level 4 - Trainer Timetable

TIMETABLE – DAY 1

Day 1 - Registration from 8.30am

Session 1 – ELVA   **Unit 5.00 Sun 73 – (1 of 3)**

9.00am – 9.15am	WARM UPS- Basic Set – Elva
9.15am – 9.30am	Review of Manual Pt 1 & Overview for Workshop & Session – Elva
9.30am – 10.15am	First Reference Point of full performance of group alone
	Practical - Form 58 –61 - Revision/Teaching
	Break into two groups – 20 mins & rotate
10.15am - 10.30am	Two half groups – consolidate Forms 1 to 61 with Elva/Denis leading (one lead and other watch)
	Brief Comment by Group
	COOL DOWN

Session 2 – ELVA   **Unit 1.00 Teaching Practice (1 of 3)**

11.00am – 11.15am	Review of Assignment in General – Elva
	Overview of Practical session of teaching – Elva
11.15am – 12.15pm	Practical – Teaching/Review – Independent three groups of 4
	Rotation within each group – 10 mins each to teach prepared segment from 73 Form
	Elva & Denis to watch and assist each group
	COOL DOWN
12.15pm – 12.30pm	Large group review & discussion

Session 3 - ELVA   **Unit 1.00 – Teaching Theory - Units 1.70 & 1.**
                                                Unit 5.00 – Sun 73 (2 of 3)

1.30pm – 2.00pm	Presentation on Modifications & Special People – Elva
2.00pm – 2.45.pm	Practical – Revision/Teaching – Forms 62-67
	Break into two groups – 20 mins & rotate
2.45pm – 3.00pm	Two half groups – consolidate Forms 1 to 67 with Elva/Denis leading (one lead and other watch)
	Brief Comment by Group
	COOL DOWN

Session 4 - DENIS   **Unit 3.00 – Tai Chi Theory/Practice - Unit 3.60**
                                                Unit 5.00 – Sun 73 Revision & Application

3.30pm – 3.40pm	Presentation on Martial (50 minutes) – Denis Facilitator
	Brief Introduction to martial side – complexity and controversial aspects – differences of interpretation of movements – exceptional physicality not prerequisite for martial skill – reverse abdominal breathing and Kiai - sensitivity training as safe alternative to push hands – insurance perspective.
3.40pm – 3.50pm	Martial explanation of technique and principle – debate on this issue – give examples using "brush knee push" (power in hip), "move forward and punch down" (structure of body), "follow-step" (agility and speed – body evasion) and "play the lute" (static - fighting stance – movement evasion and control) and – challenge literal approach to application demonstrating multiple applications where principle is key focus
3.50pm – 4.20pm	Demonstration of sensitivity training – drills starting with gentle pushing eight directions explain purpose and focus – one and two hand push explain purpose – break into groups of two to demonstrate – sticky hands, one, two reverse and eyes closed.
4.20pm – 4.30pm	Warm-Up - Advanced Denis
4.30pm – 5.00pm	Practice section of 73 form (30 minutes) – Elva/Denis
	Consolidating Forms 1 – 67 with martial imagery with mind-body focus using principles – Separate focus for each of following – Denis to observe – Students three times each time focus on -
	Co-ordination body structure, Movement & power in hip Agility of follow step

CLOSE DAY WITH COOL DOWNS & ADVANCED STRETCHES

Appendix 4 – Level 4 Trainer Timetable- Eight Sessions over two days

TIMETABLE – DAY 2

Session 5 - ELVA	**Unit 2.00 – Knowledge Human Body – Units 2.20 & 2.30**
	Unit 5.00 – Sun 73 (3 of 3)
9.00am – 9.15am	Warm-Ups – Modified - Denis
9.15am – 9.30am	Overview - Stretching & Breathing – Elva
9.30am – 10.15am	Practical - Revision/Teaching Form 68–73
	Break into two groups – 20 mins & rotate
10.15am - 10.30am	Two half groups – consolidate Forms 1 to 73 with Elva/Denis leading (one lead and other watch)
	Brief Comment by Group
	COOL DOWN

Session 6 – DENIS	**Unit 1.00 – Teaching Theory – Unit 1.50**
	Unit 1.00 – Teaching Practice (2 of 3)
11.00am- 11.10am	Exercise on Mind-Body Focus (30 minutes) - Denis as Facilitator
	discussing Assignment - similarities & differences – viewing DVD
11.10am – 11.30am	Break into smaller sub-groups of two or three:
	(i) Denis to demonstrate static posture for four seconds - each person to observe and make notes, and then one person in sub-group to describe in words so as to make other student take shape of form based on the words alone. Rotate - Form will be - double open hand block - upper and lower (Yang form)
	(ii) Without comment from Denis or Elva, continuation of above - again static Form demonstrated for another 4 seconds. Sub-group now to use two fingers to replicate the shape.
	(iii) Then report back to larger group - discussion on observations on mind-body process.
	(iv) Second exercise building on first - Body movement is side step and look and return side step reversing form and look. Same process and in (i) & (iii) above combined.
	Comment: two factors in teaching mind-body focus -
	• Teacher needs to be able to have well developed skills of mind-body focus as a Tai Chi practitioner/student
	• Teacher needs to develop skills in being able to teach mind-body focus to significantly facilitate learning process - self-management
11.30am – 12.15pm	Practical – Teaching – Independent two groups of five
	Rotation within each group – 15 mins each Follow-on Session 2
	Form 35 as Mind-Body focus – Body Analysis (includes Static and Dynamic analysis of body) – linked to Concept Imagery
	Elva & Denis to watch and assist each group
	COOL DOWN
12.15pm – 12.30pm	Large group review & brief discussion

Session 7 – DENIS	**Unit 4.00 - Legal Theory – Units 4.40 & 4.50**
	Unit 1.00 – Teaching Practice (3 of 3)
1.30pm – 1.50pm	Discussion and presentation (20 minutes) – Denis Facilitator
	(a) Risk Management
	(b) Code of Practice & Accreditation
1.50pm - 2.45pm	Practical Teaching (55 minutes) – Elva
	• Groups of Three with specific tasks to practice
	• One person to teach Form 58 – Lady at Shuttle
	• Focus on Teaching method – copy, segment, 1/2/3 step, clock, breathing, shoulders relaxed – teaching principles and choreography
	COOL DOWN
2.45pm – 3.00pm	Group Discussion & Review

Appendix 4 – Level 4 Trainer Timetable- Eight Sessions over two days

Session 8 - ELVA　　　　**Unit 5.00 Sun 73 - Consolidation**
　3.30pm – 4.00pm　　　　Last Revision & Practice of Sun 73

- Break into two groups
- Focus on continuity
- Practice in Sections
- Rotate in Groups – one observe/other perform

　4.00pm to 4.15pm　　　　**WORKSHOP REVIEW**
　　　　　　　　　　　　Feedback Form AND Discuss next assignment

　4.15pm – 4.40pm　　　　Students demonstration and assessment of Sun 73

- Australia Dreaming
- COOL DOWN

　4.40pm – 5.00pm　　　　Presentation of certificates & photos

Appendix 4 - Level 4- Workshop Assignment

1.　**MIND-BODY ANALYSIS**
Analyse ONE form or a small group of forms by reviewing Dr Lam's DVDs Sun 73 from the three separate performances of -

(e)　Dr Lam
(f)　Professor Men
(g)　Person(s) demonstrating for Dr Lam

Specific Tasks
(a)　In what specific ways are the performances different in regards to choreography, that is, static physical posture and movement? Brief dot points ONLY.
(b)　Identify RELEVANT common principles for all performances using "Ten principles of Tai Chi for Health (Unit 3.33) as your reference. Brief dot points ONLY.
(c)　Identify safety issues for different groups using the Matrix (unit 3.40)– Brief dot point.
(d)　Describe in DETAIL ONE of the movements of the performance of either Dr Lam or Professor Men (your choice) in terms of the following – direction (use clock for orientation for precision), shape, movement and orientation of hands, elbows, eyes, head, shoulders, waist, knees, feet, toes, heel and ball of foot as well as co-ordination of upper and lower body.

2.　**LESSON PLAN** - Prepare BRIEF written Lesson Plan (No more than TWO pages) for teaching ONE form (or group of forms) (different from exercise 1 above) from Sun 73 Form.

You are beginning a new term with three continuing students at levels 2 and 3 and three new students who wish to start in your class and never done Tai Chi before. All are identified on a version of the Matrix of Performance as attached (*See next page*). Complete the tasks below considering your Duty of Care for all students, in particular with the three new students, with a view to preparing a lesson plan. To keep it all fairly simple, gender and cultural backgrounds are not relevant to your considerations.

Specific Tasks - your lesson plan should address each of the following factors:

(a)　What are the duty-of care considerations for each person, including those who wish to join your group?
(b)　Briefly identify the new form you are teaching from the Sun 73, the objectives and how you will teach the new form to the mixed group.
(c)　What are the Tai Chi Principles/concepts involved in teaching the chosen form relevant for the group and for each person in the group? In other words, what are your priorities in teaching principles as part of your first lesson plan?
(d)　Design a simple Qigong (Qigong) exercise (see unit 3.15) based on either the chosen form or from any of the Sun 73 forms and suitable for all persons in your group (please do not choose open/close or wave-hands-in-clouds). Briefly describe your objectives and how you would teach this as a group activity.
Assignment to be returned by mail or email before a fortnight prior to Level 5 Workshop

Level 4 - Workshop Assignment - Assignment Clarification

----- Original Message -----
From: Denis
Sent: Wednesday, October 17, 2007 9:38 PM
Subject: Level 4 Assignment In-Depth Sun 73 Advanced Instructor Training

Hello Everyone

We had an email from someone who needed clarification on the question, in particular, about the levels and the matrix. We thought that this might be helpful for everyone so here it is. Please remember to shout if you need any assistance, any clarification, only too pleased to assist.

Kind regards to you all Denis

Thanks for your Email, and glad to assist.
Rough rule of thumb for levels for the so-called average student is - one year per level. In other words, level 2 the person has been learning for two years and level 3 for three years. But the challenge is not to have an average class or average students ....whatever that might mean anyway. The matrix is a way of representing the variables that come into play for people in any Tai Chi for Health class to press the point that there should never be such a thing as an "average class" of one size fits all, your Duty of Care as a Tai Chi for Health Instructor cannot allow that to happen. Another way of representing the matrix below would be as follows:

There are six people in your class with different ages, levels of health and abilities. You have three people about to start brand new, never been to your class before, and the other three have been students for a couple of years and are ready to move to level 3 (or rule of thumb) or possibly into their third or even fourth year. Elva has sometimes up to 30 students in her class ranging from beginners to other students having been students for eight years. You have met two of those students who have stuck like glue to focussing on learning and progressing and not being intimidated by the challenges of learning the 73 Sun - Ann and Leon.

The hypothetical class below has six students and is mixed according to age, health conditions, physical ability and so on as described in the matrix. It is NOT an "average or traditional class" where everyone is considered the same with the teacher simply turning the back and getting everyone to follow. The assignment is set to challenge the teacher to be able to teach according to the safety principles that are central to Tai Chi for Health Advanced Instructor Training program to ensure a competent Tai Chi for Health Instructor to teach at all levels of competency, as distinct from a Tai Chi Leader with only two hours training in teaching and very basic understanding of a Duty of Care. The Tai Chi for martial arts world has challenged Paul Lam into recognising that Tai Chi Leaders are not properly trained to be instructors in their own right. This program is designed to address that very concern.

The main idea is for you to be able to structure your teaching to ensure that you run a safe and optimally, fun class ensuring that everyone is engaged in learning, not overloaded, and is able to progress at their levels of competency - taking account of the variable factors of age, health, ability etc - through focussed practice over time and effort ...... which is the true meaning of the word "KUNG FU"..... a great deal of practice through time and energy.

The hypothetical class is yours to structure, but the Sun Style is the style being used in this assignment with the Sun 73 as the framework within which your curriculum has been structured. This is a major part of your challenge and the challenge of any teacher teaching a mixed class. It is much ,much easier of course to only certain categories of people in your class as is the case for the TCA and TCD program. The advanced instructor training is aimed at encouraging the Tai Chi Leader to be able to teach beyond these two programs to teach what is essentially, not only a longer form, but bringing all the important Duty of Care principles into play moving beyond the mind-set of people being treated as "average" and embracing the diversity of people using the matrix from Level 3 as the conceptual tool to assist you in this regard.

As a Tai Chi for Health Instructor, as a specialist in Sun Style Tai Chi, you are challenged to teach Sun Style Tai Chi using.....and here is the key word........ using the Sun 73 as the framework of your Tai Chi expertise and structuring your class to suit the range of people who may wish to improve their health and fitness levels through your Tai Chi for Health program. You are a Tai Chi for HEALTH instructor and not Tai Chi as martial art, you are teaching a sophisticated type of exercise and movement using the brilliance, simplicity and depth of Sun Style Tai Chi as the vehicle. You have six students in your class, you need to ensure prior to beginning the new term that they are able to participate safely in your program .... what do you need to do to ensure that?..and the rest is up to you. Remember, be brief and dot point type responses, focussing on DUTY OF CARE considerations throughout, which of course includes modification and safety. Trust this assists, please get back to me if you need any further clarification.
Kind regards Denis

Level 4 - Workshop Assignment — Matrix of Performance

Matrix of Performance Levels for	Duty of Care					
		Students - Continuing & New				
Major Variables	Duty of Care Factors	1	2	3	4	5	6
Age	*Children*						
	Younger Adults			35		25	30
	Older Adults	55	45				
	Frail Aged				80		
Health	*Excellent - A*						
	Average-B		B		B	B	B
	Health – C			C			C
	- Chronic	Diabetes		Rh Arth	OsteoPor	OsteoAr	Paraplegia
	- Physical	Obese					Paraplegia
	- Psychological			Depression			Depression
Fitness - Aerobic	*Excellent -A*					B	
	Average-B			B	B		B/
	Poor -C	C	C				C
Fitness - Strength	*Excellent -A*					B	
	Average - B			B			B/
	Poor - C	C	C		C		C
Fitness - Flexibility	*Excellent - A*					B	
	Average - B			B	B		B/
	Poor - C	C	C				C
Skills - Capacity	*Level of Performance*	1	1	3	3	3	1
	Mobility (A, B, C)	B	B	B	C	B	Wheel Chair
	Sightedness (A, B, C)	B	A	A	B	A	A
	Hearing (A, B, C)	B	A	A	B	A	A
	Cognitive (A, B, C)	A	A	A	B	A	A

Appendix 5 - Level 5 - Workshop Timetable

Saturday 8.45am Registration

Session 1
9.00 am to 9.30am- Warm-ups and Review to date
9.30 am – 10.30am - Practical – Review of Choreography – Study of Sun 73
Focus: Structure & Co-ordination of Body – Whole Body moving together

Morning Tea 10.30am to 11.00am

Session 2
11.00 am to 12.30 pm – Practical – Mind & Intention – Study of Sun 73
Focus: Strategic Force – Relaxation and "Sung"

Lunch 12.30 pm to 1.30 pm

Session 3
1.30pm to 2.00pm - Review of Code of Practice
2.00pm to 3.00pm – Teaching Practice – Study of Sun 73

Afternoon tea 3.00pm to 3.30pm

Session 4
3.30pm to 4.30pm - Practical – Study of Sun 73
Focus: Sun Lutang's Concept - Diligent Practice with
            Yang Cheng Fu's Principle – Mind Enhancing Energy
4.30pm to 5.00pm - Cool-down, Australia Dreaming, Close

Appendix 5 - Level 5 - Assessment

You will have up to six months for completion of all assessment items, which can be posted on or before 31 May 2008 to:

Elva Arthy
Tai Chi for Health & Community Fitness
260 Bloomfield St
Cleveland QLD 4163

Please ensure you retain copies of your completed workbook, your DVD/video presentations of your solo performance and your teaching performance.

(a)   **Workbook** – The workbook is available in hard copy or electronically. It comprises 73 questions, which need to be completed within six months of the Level 5 workshop. If sent electronically this can be sent by email to Elvamar@bigpond.net.au

(b)   **Solo Performance of Sun 73 Competition Form** – a video or DVD presentation should demonstrate to a competent standard the complete form sequentially and without editing.

(c)   **Teaching performance** – a video or DVD presentation of no more than fifteen minutes of a segment of a Tai Chi for Health class, which demonstrates competent teaching to a student or group of students containing some specific aspect of the Sun Style Tai Chi form. A brief written outline of the Teaching Plan for this performance should accompany the DVD/Video.

Upon receipt of the above, you will be advised that the item has been received and every endeavour will be made to communicate to you the outcome of each assessment item within a reasonable time. You will be advised if you have or have not achieved a competent standard for each assessment item with constructive comments intended to assist you in your further development. If you are not considered competent in any area of the assessment, you can apply for an extension to undertake further work within the six-month period. If for whatever reason you do not complete the competency requirements for Level 5 by the end of the six month period, you will receive an attendance certificate for the Level 5 workshop.

When you have completed the competency requirements for assessment, you will be sent a "Certificate of Completion of Advanced Instructor Training for Tai Chi for Health – Level 5".

Also upon successful completion of the assessment, you will be eligible to apply for accreditation with Tai Chi for Health & Community Fitness. When applying for accreditation, the applicant agrees to abide by the "Code of Practice & Ethics".

If you decide not to apply for accreditation, you are advised that it is your personal responsibility to obtain appropriate liability insurance in regard to any Tai Chi for Health activity that you may conduct either in your professional capacity or in any other capacity including community based classes whether remunerated or otherwise.

WORKBOOK LEVEL 5

Surname

_____

First Name

_____

Address

_____

_____ Zip/Postcode: _____

Email Address

_____

Phone Home _____ **Phone Mobile** _____

1. List six of the most common barriers to participation in a Tai Chi for Health (TCH) class.

2. What attributes in a TCH Instructor would participants find discouraging?

3. List teaching habits and design practices which would make students feel and uncared for and uncomfortable.

4. Students often mirror the habits and behaviour of their teachers. Which teaching qualities are important for "leading by example" in the role of the teacher?

5. What are the four most important duties and responsibilities of the TCH Instructor?

6. How does your role as a teacher impact on the social needs of your students?

7. As the TCH instructor, how can you assist your students to be better informed about services and resources on health and exercise that are available in their community?

8. List three ways of networking with health professionals in your local area for optimal teaching outcomes for your students.

9. List four personal goals you hope to achieve teaching TCH.

10. . Which non-physical components of a class impact on lifting mood and satisfaction/comfort for your students (something to look forward to)?

11. Many physical factors limit the level of participation in a TCH class. List at least eight factors which impact physical activity.

12. Identify at least three techniques in a modern approach to teaching TCH which will minimise learning difficulties experienced by some students?

13. How can the TCH instructor find creative ways to assist learning? List three ways.

14. What is the most important consideration you have as a responsible teacher in a modern approach to teaching TCH for all students and in all classes and activities?

15. Students who have not received regular exercise prior to starting TCH may show the physical effects of a de-conditioned lifestyle. Which conditions decrease in a sedentary lifestyle?

16. Which personal attributes of the TCH Instructor will motivate students most?

17. How can the TCH Instructor communicate the students' progress or improvement within the class setting?

18. What education/information topics should the TCH Instructor introduce during the class?

19. Which three qualities of your teaching program will create a motivating learning environment for your students?

20. What are the functions of the warm-up phase?

21. After completing the stretches of the warm-ups, how could you extend this phase to further prepare your students for the conditioning phase?

22. In a TCH class of mainly older students, what percentage of class time should be spent on preparation (warm-up and drills)?

23. How can you explain to students about working at their "comfort level"?

24. Describe briefly the benefits of a modern approach to teaching Qigong breathing techniques within a TCH class.

25. What is the importance of the cool-down phase?

26. List six everyday "functional" activities which could be improved with TCH practice.

27. Students learn in different ways. Explain briefly the difference between "aural" learners and "visual" learners and why it is important for the TCH Instructor to be aware of this.

28. In a TCH class, how could you assist a person who responds to tactile cues?

29. How can frustration experienced by some students be minimised when learning new work?

30. List the main advantages of learning in small segments, for example, as appears in Dr Lam's "123 step progression method".

31. What are the potential risks in teaching TCH using the "copy-follow" method where the teacher turns the back to students?

32. What is the safety advantage of mirror teaching?

33. How is communication enhanced by teaching mirror image?

34. Why is "show me" important when learning new forms?

35. Is cueing necessary in the "show me" phase?

36. List six cue words useful in teaching practise?

37. What concept words could you use to enhance the efficiency of learning TCH?

38. With regard to student safety, what sorts of cues should the TCH Instructor look for to determine how students are feeling during the class?

39. Why is it important for the TCH Instructor to focus considerable attention to posture particularly for the beginning student?

40. How does improving posture impact on health?

41. Is it ever appropriate to try to physically re-align a student's posture? Explain.

42. How can posture enhancement be developed?

43. Which main muscle group is compromised by a posterior tilt of the pelvis?

44. Which is the main muscle responsible for "toe clearance"?

45. If you notice a significant postural condition with one of your students, what is your Duty of Care in this regard?

46. What are some of the features of skeletal muscle?

47. A person with moderately severe Kyphosis wants to join your TCH class? What is your Duty of Care to this student?

48. What is your understanding of Double Weighting?

49. How can you convey the concept of "Sung" to intermediate students?

50. What are the variables of the Matrix of Performance and what is the value of Matrix of Performance?

51. What is the feature of Chinese music which is ideal for the performance of Tai Chi?

52. Is there a place for other sorts of music in teaching Tai Chi in a modern setting? Give two examples and in what circumstances would you use them?

53. Why do we modify movement in a TCH class?

54. List at least two ways to teach side stepping to enhance performance and balance.

55. Why do we need to stretch? List four reasons.

56. List four main limitations to flexibility.

57. What is static stretching and what is dynamic stretching?

58. If one of your students has chronic pain, how should he/she participate in your class? What can you advise for safety and enjoyment and best results?

59. TCH is considered as an aerobic physical activity. How can the level of aerobic activity be increased or decreased?

60. When we are practising TCH, what are the Duty of Care considerations in relation to breathing?

61. Why should you not make exceptions with regard to medical screening policy in accordance with the Code of Practice for all students?

62. What are three benefits of the Badge system for identification and Duty of Care for your students?

63. Which two most important principles (from Yang Chen Fu and Sun Lu Tang) of Tai Chi for teaching falls prevention?

64. What is your Duty of Care if a student tells you they are on a course of antibiotics for an infection but wish to participate in your class?

65. At one of your Tai Chi for Health classes, you may be presented with the following scenarios:

(a)   After the class has started, one of your students tells you that he has a severe headache, he had taken some painkillers before the class and wants to do the class.

(b)   During a class, you observe that one of your students is being subjected to racial insults by another student.

(c)   During a class, one of your new students is being disruptive in the class by telling someone else that they are doing their Tai Chi wrong and attempting to correct them.

Describe briefly what you would do, or would not do, and what are the reasons, issues or considerations for your actions? Would your actions be different if the events happened before or after the class, and if so why?

66.   You are informed from a reliable source that the hall you have been hiring and teaching in for over ten years has asbestos somewhere in the building. How would you deal with this issue and what are the considerations?

67.   During a class you are teaching, you become aware that you can smell alcohol on a particular participant. How do you deal with this situation and what are the considerations for your actions?

68.   As an accredited Tai Chi for Health Instructor, the Code of Practice provides a legal and ethical framework .
Consider the following scenarios and briefly identify breaches (if any) of the Code of Practice and/or identify legal or ethical considerations, and give your reasons.

(a)   You advertise to the public that your "Tai Chi classes are guaranteed to improve the fitness and health of all participants".

(b)   You are unable to take a regular class and get your senior student (who is not accredited) to take the class in your absence.

(c)   One of your students has paid the full term fee for attendance at your Tai Chi for Health classes, but decides that she does not want to continue after the second class. She asks for a full refund.

69.   Identify the Acts and government agencies (both State and/or Commonwealth) that involve the following matters related to running a Tai Chi for Health activities:

(a)   Workplace Health and Safety

(b)   Discrimination and Sexual Harassment

(c)   Copyright material for music and DVDs, and general copyrighted publications

(d)   Advertising your classes

70.   Define the following terms and give an example of the associated behaviour relevant to teaching Tai Chi for Health classes in the community

(a)   Harassment

(b)   Discrimination

71.   One of your students has just moved into a retirement village and has asked you for advice on starting teaching Tai Chi to other residents. How would you advise her and what are the issues involved in relation to giving advice?

72.   Within a few minutes of starting a class, one of your students collapses and is not conscious. Briefly address the following:

(a)   In relation to this type of emergency, what have you previously considered and included in your Risk Management Plan for dealing with such an event?

(b)   Describe the specific steps as to you how you would deal with your unconscious student who was initially bleeding from having hit her head in the fall but has stopped breathing.

(c)   What are the follow-up issues in regard to this incident that you need to address?

73.   One of your students asks to borrow some music you are using in your class so as she can copy this for her own private use. What is your response and give reasons.

Appendix 6

REGISTRATION

Tai Chi for Health Advanced Instructor Training Workshop

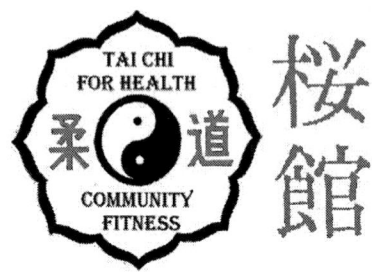

1. **Last Name**_____ **Given Names** _____

    Home Address _____ Post Code _____

    Private Email _____ Home Phone _____ Private Mobile _____

    Employer/ Work Address

    _____

    Employment Work Email _____ Work Phone _____

2. **Acknowledgment of Personal Responsibility /Consent /Waiver**

    (a) I understand that Tai Chi for Health is a gentle exercise, which may enhance my physical fitness and relieve discomfort. I also understand that Tai Chi for Health involves some degree of risk of personal injury.

    (b) During this workshop, I understand that some of the activities may be focused on two-person sensitivity training, which does not include any physical throwing, grappling or sparring with other participants of the workshop. I also understand that the practical focus of two-person sensitivity training as part of Tai Chi for Health is to learn to relax the body and mind and to understand the marital intention and the ebb and flow of energy within the performance of the Tai Chi form.

    (c) At all times during the workshop, I agree to take full personal responsibility for involvement in any activity, including two-person sensitivity training, and understand that I will work at my own level and be mindful of safety factors for myself and others.   This includes taking personal responsibility for taking the option in not participating in any activity, where I believe health and/or safety may be at risk.

    (d) I confirm that my physical condition is fit to safely participate in this two-day workshop and that at any time during the workshop I agree that I will advise the Instructors if my physical condition changes.

    (e) In consideration for admission to this workshop (i) I hereby accept full personal responsibility for and assume the risk of any injuries sustained because of my participation in this two day workshop involving Tai Chi for Health and (ii) I hereby release and hold harmless Tai Chi for Health & Community Fitness, the instructors Elva Arthy and Denis Arthy, and all persons in association with the Tai Chi two-day Workshop for any liabilities, injuries and expenses which may arise as a result of participation in this two day workshop involving the Tai Chi for Health Advanced Instructor program.

    (f) I agree to wear upon my person during the two day workshop a name badge which contains on the reverse side personal information about a contact person and phone number in the event of illness and information about my health conditions and medications. In the event of my illness, I consent to allow this information to be provided to the Instructors, to paramedics and medical doctors.

    (g) I consent to the use of any photographs or videos taken of me, as well as any feedback or written comments by me in connection with the Tai Chi Workshop, for publicity, promotion, demonstration or other business purposes, in any medium, including the internet, and I waive any right to compensation in connection with such use.

    Signature of Workshop Participant _____ Date ...... / .... /

POSTURE AND MOVEMENT

1. **Posture Head – Golden Thread**

2. **Posture Shoulders – Chest and Back**

3. **Posture Waist - Loosen the Waist and Hips**

4. **Body Movement – Weight Shifting**

5. **Posture Arms - Sink Shoulders, Drop Elbows**

MIND AND FOCUS

6. **Mind Directing the Body - Use Will, Not Strength**

7. **Whole Body Moving Together – Co-ordination Between Top and Bottom**

8. **Training the Mind - Internal and External Unity**

9. **Continuous Body Movement – Regulated by Controlled Breathing**

10. **Mind Enhancing Energy – Relaxed Continuous Movements through Breathing**

Bibliography

ACCC, (2009), Australian Competition and Consumer Commission, see website - www.accc.gov.au

AON, (2009), Allied Health Insurance Policy, on AON website - www.aon.com.au/pdf/proposal_forms/allied_health_practitioners_insurance_policy.pdf

Arthy, D (1996), "Shaping the Good Citizen", Chapter 2 in *The Vocational Personality: Guidance and Counselling Practices in Queensland Education*, unpublished PhD thesis, Faculty of Humanities, Griffith University, Brisbane

Arthy, D (1996a), "Vocational Guidance and Government Reconstruction of the Good Citizen", paper presented at Australian and New Zealand History of Education Society – 26th Annual Conference – Childhood, Citizenship, Culture, published by ANZHEZ in *Proceedings of the ANZHES 26th Annual Conference* – Volume 1, Brisbane

Arthy, D (1997), "Governance of the Vocational Personality in the Origins of Vocational Guidance", in *Journal of Career Development*, Vol 24, Nr 2 Winter, Human Sciences Press Inc, New York

Arthy, Dr Denis (2005), *Legal and Ethical Responsibilities of Tai Chi for Health (TCH) Instructor Training*

Arthy, Dr Denis (2006), *Genius of Sun Lutang: Origins and Concepts of Tai Chi for Health*, paper presented at "The First International Conference of Tai Chi for Health", 4-7 Dec, Seoul

Arthy, Elva and Arthy, Dr Denis (2006), The *"Text and Context" of How to Teach Tai Chi for Health Effectively*, joint paper presented by Elva Arthy at "The First International Tai Chi for Health Conference", 4-7 Dec, Seoul

Arthy, Elva and Arthy, Dr Denis (2008), *Australia Dreaming: Tribute to the Ancestors - Sun Style Tai Chi*, unpublished book containing the Australia Dreaming Chi Kung by Elva with colour prints of art work by Elva's sister, Gail Higgins and an article titled *Sun Style Tai Chi – Tai Chi for Health in a Modern World* by Denis

ATSIC, 1999, *Our Culture: Our Future -- Report on Australian Indigenous Cultural and Intellectual Property Rights*, by Aboriginal and Torres Straight Islander Commission (ATSIC), Canberra

Atwood, Brian and Markus, Andrew (2009), article The Myth of the 1967 Referendum" in website of Reconciliation Australia, http://www.reconciliation.org.au/home/reconciliation-resources/1967-referendum/perspectives-on-the-referendum/the-myth-of-the-1967-referendum

Australian Government (2009a), website for information on 1967 Referendum – National Archives of Australia, http://www.naa.gov.au/about-us/publications/fact-sheets/fs150.aspx

Australian Government (2009b), website - http://www.bom.gov.au/iwk/climate_culture/rainbow_serp.shtml

Australian Government (2009c), website for information on liability insurance - www.business.gov.au

Australian Privacy Foundation, (2009), *Privacy Laws States and Territories of Australia*, website providing access to laws relevant to privacy, and to other related matters - http://www.privacy.org.au/Resources/PLawsST.html -

Australian Sports Commission, (2007a) website for information on "Ethics in Sport – Harassment Frees Sport" - http://www.ausport.gov.au/ethics/hfs.asp

Banner, S (2005), "Why *Terra Nullius*? Anthropology and Property Law in Early Australia", in *Law and History Review*, Vol 23 Nr 1 Spring, see website - www.historycooperative.org

Barrett, R (2006), "Understanding Xu and Shi", article in *T'ai Chi -The International Magazine of T'ai Chi Ch'uan*, Vol. 30, No 2 April, pp47-49

Barthes, Roland (2001), *Mythologies*, Granada, London

Baumgartner, R.N., Koehler, K.M., Gallagher, D., Romero, L., Heymsfield, S.B., Ross, R.R., *et al*, (1998), "Epidemiology of sarcopenia among the elderly in New Mexico", *American Journal of Epidemiology*, Vol 147 No 8, pp 755-63

Binder, Dr Brad (1999), *Psychosocial Benefits of the Martial Arts: Myth or Reality? A Literature Review, Articles and Guidelines from Waboku Jujitsu group*, website http://userpages.itis.com/wrassoc

Borg, G. (1982), *Medical Science Sports Exercise*, 14:377-87

Bibliography

Brianmac Sports Coach (2007) "Energy Pathways", website - http://www.brianmac.co.uk/energy.htm

Brown, D, Wang, Y, Ebbeling, C, Fortlage, L, Puleo, E., Benson, H, Rippe, J. (1995), "Chronic Psychological Effects of Exercise and Exercise plus Cognitive Strategies", *Med-Sci-Sports-Exerc,* May: 27 (5), pp 765-75

Brudnak, M; Dendero, D; and van Hecke, F (2002), Fall preventing effects of the Korean Martial art, TaeKwon-Do, in senior citizens, April, Medical Hypotheses, Vol 59 Issue 4, October, pp485-91

Cartmell, Tim (1992), *Internal vs External What Sets Them Apart,* July, Inside Kung-fu Magazine

Cartmell, Tim (2003), Foreword to Sun (1921)

Cartmell, Tim (2006), Spine Curling, see Shen Wu website www.shenwu.com

Chang, Han-liang (2003), *The Rise of Chinese Literary Theory: Intertextuality and System Mutations in Classical Texts,* Paper by Professor of Semiotics at National Taiwan University, available from world wide web - http://homepage.ntu.edu.tw/~changhl/changhl/Am%20semiotics%20mss.pdf

Chen, William (2006), "William C.C. Chen on Breathing", article in *T'ai Chi - The International Magazine of T'ai Chi Ch'uan,* Vol 30, No 6, December, pp6-11

Cheryl (2001), *Tai Chi for Arthritis–Amazon.com Customer Review,* www.amazon.com reviews of TCA Video

Cisar, C. & Kravitz, (1989), M, "Turning Back Time: Exercises and Ageing." *American Academy of Physical Education Papers,* No 22

Chu, Vincent (2006), "Relaxation and Tension in Tai Chi Chuan", article in *T'ai Chi - The International Magazine of T'ai Chi Ch'uan,* Vol 30, No 2, pp24-29

Chu, Vincent (2006a), *Yin and Yang,* from website http://www.gstaichi.org/english/yinYang.php

Cisar, C. & Kravitz, (1989), M, "Turning Back Time: Exercises and Ageing", *American Academy of Physical Education Papers,* No 22

CLR (1992), *Mabo v.Queensland,* 175 CLR 1

Cobb, Thomas and Grannis, Phyllis (2006), *How to Find a T'ai Chi Teacher,* Life Matters Champions for Living Well, web site address - http://lifematters.com/taiteach.asp

Colbert, B., Ankney, J. and Lee, K. (2007) *Anatomy and Physiology for Health Professions,* Prentice Hall Health, New Jersey

Cross, I, (2001), "Music, Cognition, Culture and Evolution", *Annals of the New York Academy of Sciences,* 930-25-42

Crouch, J (1975), *Functional Human Anatomy,* Lea & Febiger, Philadelphia

Dalai Lama, (2000),*The Little Book of Wisdom,* Rider

Daley, M.J. & Spinks, W.L. (2009), "Exercise, mobility and aging", *Sports Medicine,* 29:1-12

Davies, A D (2006)*, Dan Docherty: Tai Chi Gladiator,* interview with Dan Docherty on website - http://www.taichichuan.co.uk/information/articles/tai_chi_gladiator.html

Douris, P; Chinan, A; Gomez, M; Aw, A; Steffens, D; and Weiss, S (2004), *Fitness levels of middle aged martial arts practitioners,* in British Journal of Sports Medicine, 33: 142-147

Dunn, T (1990), *T'ai Chi Ruler – Chines Yoga for Health and Longevity,* North Atlantic Books, Berkeley

Eco, Umberto (1976), *A Theory of Semiotics,* Indiana University Press, Bloomington

Ehrlich, Prof Fred; Zheng, Henry; and Yuan, Alice L (2006), *Tai Chi for Health & Falls Injury Prevention Program,* Exercise Medicine Australia, on web site, http://www.fallsprevention.org.au/thaichi.htm

Emory University, (2009), *The Vertebral Column and Spinal Cord,* Emory University, Atlanta, USA , see website http://www.emory.edu/ANATOMY/AnatomyManual/back.html

Bibliography

Evenson, Brad (2004), *Benefits for Adults*, National Post, Canada – reported on website - http://www.kikara.ca

Exercise Medicine Australia (2009), Alice Liping Yuan's website for Tai Chi for Health programs including DVDs/Videos: Tai Chi for Health & Falls Injury Prevention, Tai Chi for Health Heart, Keep Active and Healthy with the Ring, 18 Form Tai Chi Fan for Wellness, 8 Form Mulan Qi Gong, 24 Form Mulan Bare Hands – see website - www.exercisemedicine.com.au

Foster, B (2006), "Knee Problems and the Tai Chi Player", article in *T'ai Chi - The International Magazine of T'ai Chi Ch'uan*, Vol 30, No 4, pp44-46

Foucault, Michel (1977), *The Order of Things – An Archaeology of the Human Sciences*, London, Tavistock.

Fransen, M., Nairn, L., Winstanley, J., Lam., P & Edmonds, J. (2007), "Physical activity for osteoarthritis management: a randomized controlled clinical trial evaluating hydrotherapy or tai chi classes", *Arthritis Rheumatism (Arthritis Care & Research)*, 57:3 pp407-14

Fried, R. (1993), *The Psychology and Physiology of Breathing*, New York, Plenum

Gilman, Michael (1998), *108 Insights Tai Chi Chuan – A String of Pearls*, YMAA Publication Center, Jamaica Plain

Golden Glow, (2008), "The Art of Tai Chi, Poetry in Motion", article in hard copy magazine – *The Best of Golden Glow Health Products*, May, pp 28-9, see website http://www.goldenglow.com.au

Gregson, Brian (2004), *More on the debate – Tai Chi for Health, Tai Chi for Self-Defence,* Article on website of Tai Chi Association of Australia, http://www.taichiaustralia.com

Grigg, Pastor Fred (1990), *The Deception of Martial Arts and Yoga*, Palm Beach, Mandate Ministries

Hammersley, M and Atkinson, P (1980), *Ethnography, Principles and Practice*, London, Routledge

Hirst, P and Woolley, P (1984), *Social Relations and Human Attributes*, London, Tavistock

Ho, Anthony (2008), "The Meaning of Doubleweight in Taiji", in *T'ai Chi – The International Magazine of Tai Chi Chuan*, Vol 32, No 1

Human Biodyssey (2008), *Human Biodyssey – Exploring Anatomy and Physiology*, see website http://www.gwc.maricopa.edu/class/bio201/skeleton.htm

Hwa-Yu T'ai Chi Health and Wellbeing (2006), *Eight Methods of Hwa-Yu T'ai Chi*, from website - http://www.gmaf.org/methods.html

Hyon, Yong-Ha Dr and Park, Sae-Woon Dr (1988), *A New Two-Dimensional Double-Entry Bookkeeping System and Three-Dimensional Accounting, paper* presented at the Second Asian Pacific Interdisciplinary Research in Accounting (APIRA98) Conference held on August 4th-6th, 1998 in Osaka, Japan, from School of Economics and Management, Chang-Won National University, Chang-Won, Korea

Iannuzzi-Sucich, M., Prestwood, K.M. & Kenny A.M., (2002), "Prevalence of Sarcopenia and Predictors of Skeletal Muscle Mass in Healthy, Older Men and Women, *Journals of Gerontology Series A: Biological Sciences and Medical Sciences*, 57:M772-7

Jacobson, B, Chen H, Cashel, C, Guerrero,L, (1997), "The Effect of Tai Chi Chuan Training on Balance, Kinesthetic Sense and Strength", *Percept-Motor-Skills*, Feb: 84 (1), pp 27-33

Jiang, LW Chang (2006), On Skeletal Posture and Muscle Function, article in *T'ai Chi - The International Magazine of T'ai Chi Ch'uan*, Vol 30, No 3, pp6-8

Jin,P. (1989), "Changes in Heart Rate, Noradrenaline, Cortisol and Mood During Tai Chi", *J-Psychosom-Res*, 33(2), pp 197-206

Jin,P. (1992), "Efficacy of Tai Chi, Brisk Walking, Meditation and Reading in Reducing Mental and Emotional Stress", *J-Psychosom-Res*, May: 36(4), pp 361-70

Jou, Tsung Hwa (1984), *The Tao of I Ching – Way to Divination*, Tai Chi Foundation, Taiwan

Kano, Prof Jigoro (1994), *Kodokan Judo*, Tokyo, Kodansha International

Kano, Prof Jigoro (2005), *Mind over Muscle, Writings from the Founder of Judo*, Kodansha International, Tokyo

Kawaishi, Mikonosuke Shihan (1955), *My Method of Judo*, C. Timling & Co Ltd, London translated and edited by EJ Harrison

Kawaishi, Mikonosuke Shihan (1957), *The Complete 7 Katas of Judo*, W. Foulsham & Co Ltd, London, 1957 translated and edited by EJ Harrison

Kelly, Dr M (2007), The Science Behind Dim Mak, see website http://www.dimmak.net/

Kirschner, P A; Sweller, J; and Clark, R E (2006). "Why minimal guidance during instruction does not work: an analysis of the failure of constructivist, discovery, problem-based, experiential, and inquiry-based teaching". Educational Psychologist 41 (2): 75-86

Knott, M., Voss, D. (1968), *PNF Patterns and Techniques*, New York, Harper & Row

Kuhn, Thomas (1970), *The Structure of Scientific Revolutions*, Chigago, Chigago University Press

Kurz, T. (1994), *Stretching Scientifically A Guide to Flexibility Training*, (3rd edition), Island Pond, Stadion Publishing

Kutner, N., Barnhart, H., Wolf, S., McNeely, E., Xu, T. (1997), "Self-Report Benefits of Tai Chi Practice by Older Adults", *AU:Jour-Gerontol-B-Psychol-Sci-Soc-Sci*, Sept: 52(5), pp.242-6

La-Forge, R (1997), "Mind-Body Fitness: Encouraging Prospects for Primary and Secondary Prevention", *Journal CardV Nurs*, April, 11(3), pp 53-65

Lakatos, I Worral, J and Currie, G (1980), *The Methodology of Scientific Research Programmes, Philosophical Papers Volume I*, Cambridge, Cambridge University Press

Lai,Y, (1999), "Effect of Music Listening on Depressed Women in Taiwan", *Issues in Mental Health Nursing*, May 20:3, pp229-46

Lam Dr Paul, Horstman, Judith (2002), *Overcoming Arthritis, A holistic plan including a unique tai chi programme to relieve pain and restore mobility*, Melbourne, Dorling Kindersley Book

Lam, Dr Paul (2005), *Tai Chi Breathing*, Tai Chi Productions, Sydney, http://www.taichiproductions.com/articles/individual_article.php?id=19

Lam, Dr Paul (2006), *Acceptance Through Science*, Tai Chi Productions, Sydney, www.taichiproductions.com/articles/individual_article.php?id=58

Lam, Dr Paul (2006a), *Teaching Tai Chi Effectively*, Tai Chi Productions, Sydney

Lam, Kam Chuen, (1994), *Step-by Step Tai Chi*, Sydney, Random House Pty Ltd

Laronge, Joseph (1999), The 7 Levels To Mastery Of Tai Chi, – http://www.willamette.edu/~jlaronge/seven.html

Laughlin, K. (1999), *Stretching & Flexibility*, Simon & Schuster, Sydney

Lee, James S. (2009), "Scientific Explanation of Chi Kung No. 8 – Have Chi, Will Have Strength", see website – www.self growth.com

Levi-Strauss, Claude (1977), *Structural Anthropology*, London, Penguin

Lexell, J., (1997), "Evidence for nervous system degeneration with advancing age", *The Journal of Nutrition*, 127:1011-3

Li, J., Hong, Y. and Chan, K. (2001), "Tai Chi: physiological characteristics and beneficial effects on health", *British Journal of Sports Medicine,* June, 35 (3):145-56

Liu, Yao-ting, (2006), "The Development of T'ai Chi Ch'uan", article in *T'ai Chi - The International Magazine of T'ai Chi Ch'uan*, Vol 30, No 4, p47

Lorig, K & Fries, JF (1998), *The Arthritis Helpbook – A tested self-management program for coping with arthritis and fibromyalgia*, 4th Edition, Reading Mass, Addiston-Wesley Publishing Co

Bibliography

Luskin-FM; Newell-KA; Griffith-M; Holmes-M; Telles-S; Marvasti-FF; Pelletier-KR; Haskell-WL: (1998), "A review of mind-body therapies in the treatment of cardiovascular disease. Part 1: Implications for the elderly", *Altern-Ther-Health-Med.*, May; 4(3): 46-61

MacHose, M and Peper, E. (1991), "The effect of clothing on inhalation volume", *Biofeedback and Self-Regulation*, 16, (3), 261-265

Mahoney, J.E, (1998), Immobility and falls", *Clinical Geriatric Medicine*, 14:699-726

Marieb, Elaine (2006), *Essentials of Human Anatomy & Physiology*, Pearson Benjamin Cummings, San Franscisco

McCarthy, Patrick (1995), *The Bible of Karate: Bubishi*, translated with commentary by Patrick McCarthy, Tuttle Publishing, Boston

McCraty, R, Barrios-Choplin, B, Atkinson, M, Tomasino, D, 1998,"The Effects of different types of music on mood, tension and mental clarity", *Alternative Therapies in Health and Medicine*, Volume 4, Issue 1, January, pp75-84

Medicine on Line (2004), "Martial Arts Defend Against Aging, Sports like karate boost strength and balance, study finds", summary medical article in March 25, 2004, *British Journal of Sports Medicine*, Peter Douris, Ed.D., physical therapist, New York Institute of Technology, Old Westbury, N.Y.; Douglas McKeag, M.D., M.F., director, Indiana University Center for Sports Medicine, Indianapolis

Miller, Dan (2000), in Sun (1915)

Mills, John (2004), *Tai Chi for Health or Tai Chi for Self Defence?* Article on website of Tai Chi Association of Australia, http://www.taichiaustralia.com

Montaigue, E (2004), *The Deadly and Deceptive Hands of T'ai Chi Ch'uan*, article on Tai Chi Association of Australia website - http://www.taichiaustralia.com

Montaigue, E. (2007) – Video - *Tai Chi: The 3 Energy Systems of the Human Body*: Montaigue, Website http://www.youtube.com/watch?v=yIjhEXMVevY

Mulhauser, Dr Greg (2009), *Welcome to Counselling Rescources.Com* – see website – www.counsellingresource.com

Myers, A & Gonda, G. (1986), "Research on Physical Activity in the Elderly: Practical Implications for Program Planning", *Canadian Journal on Aging*, pp 175-85

Noakes, T.D., (2000), "Physiological models to understand exercise fatigue and the adaptations that predict or enhance athletic performance", *Scandinavian Journal of Medicine and Science in Sports*, 10, 123-145

Obama, Barack (2006), *The Audacity of Hope – Thoughts on Reclaiming the American Dream*, The Text Publishing Company, Melbourne

Oliver, Rose (2007), "Working with the Taiji Energy Circle", *T'ai Chi -The International Magazine of T'ai Chi Ch'uan*, Vol. 31, No 2 April, pp22-31

Pan, Da'An (1996), *Tracing the traceless antelope: Toward an interartistic semiotics of the Chinese sister arts*, College Literature, February, from world wide web - http://findarticles.com

Peper, E. & Tibbetts, V. (1994), *Effortless diaphramatic breathing*. Physical Therapy Products. 6(2), 67-71

Popper, Karl (1974), *The Poverty of Historicism*, London, Routledge & Kegan Paul

Preston, Diana (2002), *A Brief History of the Boxer Rebellion China's War on Foreigners 1900*, London, Robinson

Queensland Government, (2008), *Civil Liability Act 2003* , Reprinted on 25 November Reprint No. 2B, see website - http://www.legislation.qld.gov.au/LEGISLTN/CURRENT/C/CivilLiabA03.pdf
Queensland Government, (2009a), *Workplace Health and Safety Act 1995*, Reprint no 8C reprinted on 23 February, see website http://www.legislation.qld.gov.au/LEGISLTN/CURRENT/W/WorkplHSaA95.pdf
Queensland Government, (2009b), Workplace Health & Safety section of website as follows – http://www.deir.qld.gov.au/workplace/law/legislation/act

Bibliography

Queensland Government, (2009c), for Queensland State government responsibility for consumer affairs - see website - http://www.consumer.qld.gov.au/

Rantanen, T., Era, P. & Heikkinen, E., (1997), "Physical activity and the changes in maximal isometric strength in men and women from the age of 75 to 80 years", *Journal of American Geriatrics Society*, 45:1439-45

Reinman, William (2009), Rainbow Serpent, 12 C Panama, see website - www.williamreimann.com

Reptilian Agenda, (2009), see website - www.reptilianagenda.com

Reynolds, Henry (2000), *Why weren't we told?* Penguin, Melbourne

Reynolds, Henry (2005), *Nowhere People - How international race thinking shaped Australia's identity*, Penguin, Melbourne

Riso, D. and Hudson, R. (1996) *Personality Types,* Houghton, Mifflin Company

Robertson, Geoffrey (2005), *The Tyrannicide Brief – The Story of the Man sho sent Charles I to the Scaffold*, Chatto & Windus, London

Rolf, F., (1998), "Effect of training on muscle strength and motor function in the elderly", *Reproduction Nutrition Development*, 38:167-74

Romel El-Sheik v Australian Capital Territory Schools Authority (1999) ACTSC 90, 27 August 1999

Rosenberg, I.H., (1989), "Summary comments", *The American Journal of Clinical Nutrition*, 0:1231-3

Rosenberg, I.H, (1997), "Sarcopenia: origins and clinical relevance", *The Journal of Nutrition*, 127:990S-1S

Rose, Hilary and Rose, Steven (1977), *Science and Society*, London, Penguin Books

Rudd, Kevin (2008), Speech by Prime Minister of Australia – *Apology to Australia's Indigenous Peoples, House of Representatives, Parliament House, Canberra,* see Australian Government website - http://www.pm.gov.au/media/speech/2008/speech_0073.cfm

Ryan, Alan (Ed), (1973), *The Philosophy of Social Explanation*, London, Oxford University Press

Shaffer, F., Sponsel, M., Knight, D. & Peper, E. (1994), *Tight shoulders and designer jeans prevent diaphragmatic breathing*, quoted in Peper & Tibbets

Song, R., Lee, E., Lam, P. & Sang-Cheol, B., (2003), *Effects of Exercise on Pain, Balance, Muscle Strength, and Perceived Difficulties in Physical Functioning in Older Women with Osteoarthritis: A Randomized Clinical Trial.* , The Journal of Rheumatology Publishing Company Limited, Volume 30: No. 9 September

Sports Fitness Advisor (2007)– "Energy Systems in Sport and Exercise ", website - http://www.sport-fitness-advisor.com/energysystems.html

Stookey, Lorena (2004), *Thematic Guide to World Mythology*, Greenwood Press, Abingdon

Sun, Master Jian Yun (2006), *A Brief Introduction to Sun Style Taijiquan*, by Beijing, China, translated and compiled by Ted W. Knecht – see website - http://www.geocities.com/yongnian

Sun, Lutang (1915), *The Study of Form-Mind Boxing*, by Sun Lutang, Burbank, Unique Publications, 2000, translated by Albert Liu, compiled and edited by Dan Miller, originally published in 1915

Sun, Lutang (1921), *A Study of Taijiquan,* Berkeley, North Atlantic Books 2003, translated by Tim Cartmell, originally published in 1921

Swiercz, A (2005), *The Physical and Psychological Benefits of Martial Arts Training,* article on the DCTaekwondo, Training, Education and Excellence website - http://www.dctkd.org

Tabrett, Mike (2005), *T'ai Chi and the Martial Arts, Grey Heron Internal Arts,* linked to an extensive bibliography of articles on the martial arts including 51 articles on Tai Chi reviewed on website – DCTaekwondo, training, education, excellence, George Washington Taekwondo Club, Washington DC – http://www.dctkd.org/index.cfm

Bibliography

Tai Chi Society of University of Nottingham, (2009), see website –
http://www.su-eb.nottingham.ac.uk/~taichi/index.php

Tai Chi Productions (2009), Dr Paul Lam's website for Tai Chi for Health programs including DVD/Videos: *Tai Chi for Arthritis, Tai Chi for Diabetes, Tai Chi Anywhere, Tai Chi for Health, Qigong for Health, Tai Chi for Older Adults, Tai Chi for Beginners, Tai Chi for Work* - Tai Chi Productions - see websites www.taichiproductions.com and www.taichiforarthritis.com

Toguchi, S (1987), *Okinawan Goju –Ryu The Fundamentals of Shorei-kan Karate*, Ohara Publications, Burbank

Tuovinen, J. E. and Sweller, J. (1999), "A comparison of cognitive load associated with discovery learning and worked examples", *Journal of Educational Psychology,* 91(2), 334-341

Tunneshende, Merrilyn (2001), Don Juan and the Art of Sexual Energy: The Rainbow Serpent of the Toltecs, Inner Traditions International Ltd, see website - www.innertraditions.com

Turner, Roy (Ed), (1975), *Ethnomethodology*, London, Penguin Education

Tzu, Lao (2005) *The Tao Te Ching*, a new translation, commentary and introduction by Ralph Alan Dale, Watkins, London

UFC (2006), *Ultimate Fighting Championship* – website - http://www.ufc.com/

Voukelatos, A., Cumming, R., Lord, S., & Rissel, C., (2007), "A Randomized, Controlled Trial of tai chi for the Prevention of Falls: The Central Sydney tai chi Trial", *The American Geriatrics Society,* 55:1185–1191

Weiser, M; Kutz, I; Kutz, S; and Weiser, D (1995), "Psychotherapeautic aspects of the martial arts", *American Journal of Psychotherapy*, 49: 118-127

Wientjes, CJE. (1993), *Psychological Influences Upon Breathing: Situational and Dispositional Aspects,* Soeserberg: TNO Institute for Perception.

Wikipedia (2007a), on world wide web for "Qigong" at   http://en.wikipedia.org/wiki/Qigong

Wikipedia, (2007b), on world wide web for "Universal dialectic"
http://en.wikipedia.org/wiki/Universal_dialectic

Wikipedia, (2007c), on world wide web for "Kiai", http://en.wikipedia.org/wiki/Kiai

Wikipedia, (2007d), on world wide web for "Jin and Jing" http://en.wikipedia.org/wiki/Nei_jin

Wikpedia, (2009), article on Kano Jigoro - http://en.wikipedia.org/wiki/Kano_Jigoro

Wile, Prof D (1993), *T'ai Chi Touchstones: Yang Family Secret Transmissions*, New York, Sweet Ch'i Press

Wile, D (2006), "The Confucian Influence on Tai Chi Chuan", article in *T'ai Chi - The International Magazine of T'ai Chi Ch'uan*, Vol 30, No 4, August, pp50-51

Wolf, S.L., Barnhart, H.X., Ellison, G.L., Coogler, C.E., (1997), "The effect of Tai Chi Quan and computerized balance training on postural stability in older subjects, Atlanta FICSIT Group. Frailty and Injuries: Cooperative Studies on Intervention Techniques", *Physical Therapy*, 77:371-81; discussion 82-4

Wolfson, L., Whipple, R., Derby, C., Judge, J., King, M., Amerman, P., *et al,* (1996), "Balance and strength training in older adults: intervention gains and Tai Chi maintenance", *Journal of American Geriatrics Society*, 44:498-506

Wong, Kiew Kit (1996), *The Complete Book of Tai Chi Chuan – A Comprehensive Guide to the Principles and Practice*, Element, Melbourne

Wong, Kiew Kit (2006a), *Sifu's Comments,* in Zhang, Wuji (2006a)

Wong, Kiew Kit (2006b), in Zhang, Wuji (2006b)

Wong, K Y (2001), *First Steps to Chi Kung,* Axiom, South Australia

Xu, G. (2007), "Harnessing Taiji's Wave-Like Energy", article in *T'ai Chi - The International Magazine of T'ai Chi Ch'uan*, Vol 31, No 2, April, pp6-11

Yang, Dr Jwing Ming (1991), *Qigong for Arthritis,* Jamaica Plain, YMAA Publication Center

Yang, Dr Jwing Ming (1996), *The Essence of Shaolin White Crane Martial Power and Qigong – the foundation of White Crane kung fu and the root of Okinawan karate*, YMAA, Jamaica Plain

Yang, Dr Jwing Ming (1997), *The Root of Chinese Qigong – Secrets for Health, Longevity, & Enlightenment*, Rosindale, YMAA Publication Center

Yang, Dr Jwing Ming (1999), *Taijiquan, Classical Yang Style - the complete form and qigong*, YMAA Publicatin Center, Boston

Yeo, Alex (2008), "Chan See Meng on: Martial Arts Training Methods", in *T'ai Chi The International Magazine of T'ai Chi Ch'uan*, Vol 32 No 1, pp 14-22

Yun, Kun-Ho (1984), *A Study on the Accounting History* in Korea. Korean Studies Series, Volume 51, The Korean Research Center, Seoul, Korea, 1984

Zhang, Wuji (2006a), *Questions on Taoist Philosophy and Concept of Open and Close,* from Sifu Wong Kiew Kit's Homepage http://www.wongkk.com/general/comparison-12.html

Zhang, Wuji (2006b), *Yin Yang God and Health,,* from Sifu Wong Kiew Kit's Homepage http://wongkk.com/general/comparison-08.html#Yin-Yang

Zhou, Lishang (2006), *Jiang Yukun's Notes on Taijiquan - Part 2*, in T'ai Chi The International Magazine of T'ai Chi Ch'uan, Vol 30 No 4, pp 22-29

Zorya, Joanna (2006), Top Quality Instruction in Chinese Martial Arts, Reeling Silk Kung Fu School, references on website - http://www.reelingsilk.co.uk

Index

172

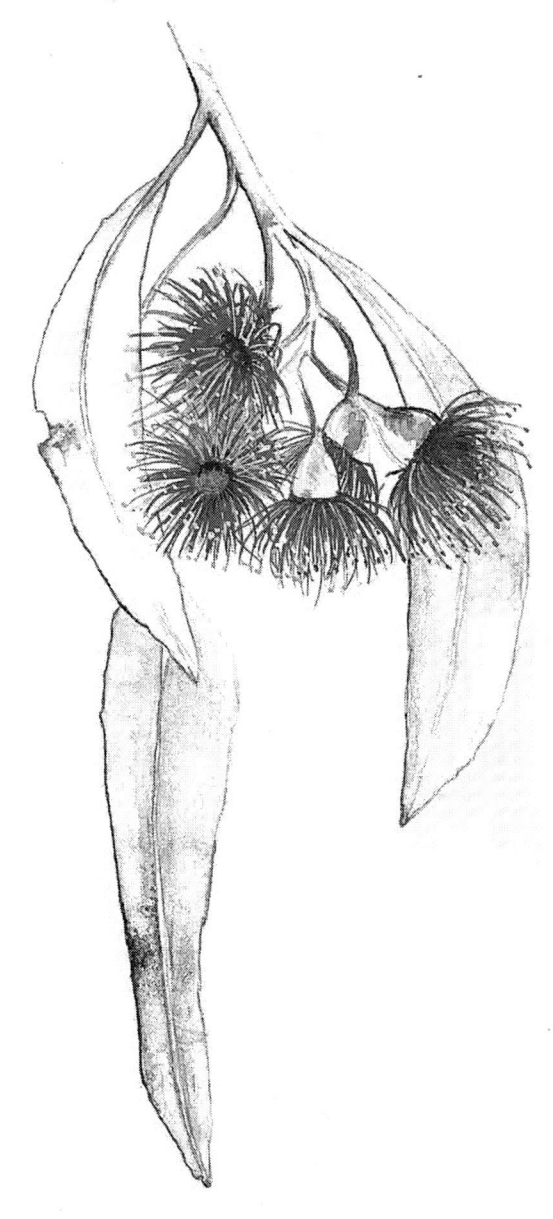